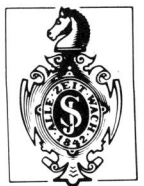

B. M. Wroblewski

Revision Surgery in Total Hip Arthroplasty

With 179 figures

Springer-Verlag
London Berlin Heidelberg New York
Paris Tokyo Hong Kong

B. M. Wroblewski, MB, ChB, FRCS
Consultant Orthopaedic Surgeon, The Centre for Hip Surgery,
Wrightington Hospital, near Wigan, Lancs WN6 9EP, UK.

ISBN 3–540–19618–8 Springer-Verlag Berlin Heidelberg New York
ISBN 0–387–19618–8 Springer-Verlag New York Berlin Heidelberg

Cover
Fig 18.4b. A sinogram showing extensive sinus. The line drawing is adapted from the graph illustrated in Fig. 10.4.

British Library Cataloguing in Publication Data
Wroblewski, B. M. (Boguslaw Michael) *1934–*
Revision surgery in total hip arthroplasty.
1. Man. Hips. Arthroplasty
I. Title
617.581059
ISBN 3–540–19618–8

Library of Congress Cataloging-in-Publication Data
Wroblewski, B. M., 1934–
Revision surgery in total hip arthroplasty/B.M. Wroblewski.
p. cm. Includes bibliographical references.
ISBN 0–387–19618–8 (U.S.: alk. paper)
1. Total hip replacement—Reoperation. I. Title. [DNLM: 1. Arthroplasty. 2. Hip Joint—surgery.
3. Hip Prosthesis. 4. Surgery, Operative. WE 860 W957r] RD549.W76 1990 617.5'810592—dc20
DNLM/DLC   90-9747
for Library of Congress   CIP

Typeset by Wilmaset, Birkenhead, Wirral
Printed by Henry Ling Ltd, The Dorset Press, Dorchester
2128/3916–543210 Printed on acid-free paper .

For Peggy, Michael, Paul, Ania and John
in appreciation of their patience, understanding and support

Mike/Tatus

Preface

Revision surgery defines secondary operative intervention in cases of total hip arthroplasty for whatever reason this has to be undertaken. Thus it includes a broad spectrum of operative procedures from minor ones to a full-scale exchange. The very rapid development of this field brings with it new demands and necessitates the continuous availability of the operative and design skills of the surgeon who remains under obligation to provide indefinite follow-up and revision facilities for the patient.

The increase in the number of revisions is in some measure the result of longer follow-up and improved identification of problems and provision of solutions for individual patients. It is the success of revision surgery for the individual patient that has made this type of work worthwhile. Success cannot be readily quantified and is often a very personal aspect of clinical practice.

The use of total hip arthroplasty as a method of choice for the treatment of the arthritic hip is so extensive that certain suggestions must be given serious consideration. The complexity of this type of treatment is such that revision surgery must be concentrated in the hands of surgeons devoted to this type of work. This must be recognized at the professional and administrative level as being of long-term benefit to the patient, the surgeon and the system which provides such care.

The purpose of this book is to present to the surgeons involved in total hip arthroplasty ideas and methods for the management of problems in revision surgery. It is based on 20 years of practical experience with the Charnley low-friction arthroplasty and over 5000 operations including over 1200 revisions performed personally. It is not intended to be a collection of all the references on the subject; the reader must study these personally. Nor is it a *vade mecum* for a "do-it-yourself" enthusiast containing the latest diagnostic procedures and practical solutions in this rapidly developing and changing field. It is primarily a practical approach to revision surgery, evolved over a number of years. The lessons learned from revisions are used for the benefit of patients undergoing primary operations. It is for this reason that the two types of operation must continue to evolve simultaneously and not be separated for administrative or other reasons.

The author offers no apology for expressing personal views which at times may be in disagreement with the views of others. As with so many studies of this nature it is bound to be changed and modified with time. A certain degree of repetition in the text is inevitable and even deliberate. Some of it is to avoid the nuisance of repeated interruption by frequent referral to other parts of the book, some to maintain the continuity of argument, or line of evolution, but most of it is to stress the importance of the topic under discussion.

Having accepted the benefits of the operation, the patient and the surgeon must realize and accept that there are certain responsibilities inherent to the procedure. The operation marks the beginning and not the end of the treatment. No patient can be formally discharged from follow-up. Regular follow-up by serial radiographs is essential, the time interval depending on the age and life style of the patient and on radiographic appearances. Revision surgery may have to be undertaken on the basis of radiographic changes alone, each operation bringing with it the risks associated with major surgery and an ever diminishing bone stock. This responsibility must be understood and shared by the patient and surgeon alike, *before* the primary operation.

Defining clinical success of the operation for an individual patient is of very personal or anecdotal value only and yet is the essence of clinical practice. The aim of total hip arthroplasty for most, if not all, patients is the long-term success of the method. Failing that, the least that should be offered is the predictability of the outcome of the operation for an individual patient, accepting that statistical probabilities derived from large numbers do not apply to the individual patient.

The Centre for Hip Surgery,   B. M. Wroblewski
Wrightington Hospital
Near Wigan, Lancs
June 1989

Acknowledgements

Any study involving clinical, experimental and research aspects cannot be satisfactorily carried out by an individual working alone. In this the author has been very fortunate to be associated with a number of helpful and co-operative people. It is not possible to mention them all individually for fear of omitting some.

However, I would like to acknowledge the late Professor Sir John Charnley, who was the prime mover in encouraging the study and management of revision surgery, and a number of anaesthetists – Drs. George Brittain, Dec Ryan, John Crook, Maurice Girgis and the late Rasheed Sobhy – who have made surgery safe for the patient and enjoyable for the surgeon.

I would also like to thank Theatre and Anaesthetic Department staff, including Staff Nurse, now Sister Maureen Abraham and Sister Cathy Platt, who patiently put up with long operating sessions; Geoff Halliwell, the late Mr. David Jones, Brian Blundell, Brian Spencer and Andrew Burrows ("the leg holders") who could "winkle out" any hip without trouble; the residents and the nursing staff caring for the patients on the wards and for out-patients; physiotherapists, radiographers and all hospital staff; and Biomechanical Research Laboratory staff including the late Mr. Ken Marsh, Mr. Frank Brown and, more recently, Drs. Phillip Shelley and Graham Isaac, who were ready to put new ideas into workable form but who always tempered the enthusiasm with constructive criticism and the knowledge of practical possibilities. Dr. Shelley's role as Research Fellow and his extensive knowledge of mechanics and computers as well as their practical application to clinical practice has been invaluable.

I thank Dr. Randolph White who by his encouragement and critical analysis often added statistical respectability to the finished product, and Chas. F. Thackray Ltd. of Leeds who were always ready with practical help and patiently awaited the completion of this study. Lack of commercialism and pressure was greatly appreciated.

My thanks also go to Mr. Peter Kilshaw and the Department of Medical Illustration for their help with photography and graphics; to my secretary Mrs. Brenda Lowerson who so sympathetically dealt with patients, retyped numerous manuscripts and acquired the new skills of dealing with computers and authors' hieroglyphics; and to the publishers, Springer-Verlag, who patiently waited during the long gestation (and transverse arrest) of this work.

Thanks must be given to my colleagues who showed their confidence by referring their patients for revision surgery, who offered constructive comments when visiting the Unit and who gave the author the privilege of addresssing them at various meetings both nationally and internationally.

My special thanks go to the patients themselves who were prepared to undergo surgery and who kept in touch and attended follow-up clinics, often travelling long distances. It is true to say that without their involvement all this would not have been possible.

Acknowledgements for Illustrations

The author wishes to thank the following journals and publishers for permission to reproduce previously published illustrations:

Acta Orthopaedica Scandinavica: Figs. 16.4, 16.5
Clinical Orthopaedics and Related Research (J.B. Lippincott): Table 9.1
Engineering in Medicine (by permission of the Council of the Institution of Mechanical Engineers): Fig. 9.6b
Journal of Bone and Joint Surgery: Figs. 3.5, 5.5, 5.6a and b, 10.5b and c, 10.6, 10.13b and c, 12.1b and c, 13.6a, 13.12, 13.13a
Orthopedic Clinics of North America (W.B. Saunders): Figs. 10.1a–d, 11.1a
Springer-Verlag: 1.1, 3.1c and d, 3.6, 5.13, 8.2, 8.3, 9.5, 10.4, 14.7, 14.9a, b and c, 14.10a and b, 14.12a, 14.13a and b, 19.10
Wear (Elsevier Sequoia S.A.): Figs. 10.8a, c and d, 10.9a and b, 10.10a and b, 11.1a–e

Contents

Preface vii

Acknowledgements ix

1 **Introduction** 1

SECTION I: COMPLICATIONS LEADING TO REVISION SURGERY 5

2 **Haematoma** 7

    Introduction 7
    The Role of Anaesthesia 8
    Classification of Haematoma 9
        Superficial Haematoma 9
        Deep Haematoma 10
        Infected Haematoma 10

3 **Problems Arising from an Inadequate Exposure** 11

    What is Required at the Time of the Exposure? 11
        Exposure of the Acetabulum 14
        Exposure of the Medullary Canal 16
        Preservation of the Integrity of the Abductors 18

4 **Trochanteric Osteotomy and Problems Resulting from It** 19

    Introduction 19
    Trochanteric Osteotomy 22
    Problems Related to Trochanteric Osteotomy 24
        Increased Blood Loss and Operating Time 24
        Trochanteric Bursitis (or Trochanteric Pain) 26
        Trochanteric Non-union 27
        Pain 27
        Limp 27
        Dislocation 28

5 Dislocation 29

Introduction 29
The Mechanism of Dislocation 30
   Impingement 30
   Distraction 31
Dislocation Following Primary Surgery 31
   Loss of the Abductor Mechanism 32
   Shortening of the Limb 32
   Malorientation of the Components 35
Practical Approach to Dislocation: Non-operative Methods 41
Operative Procedures 42
   Recent Advances 43

6 Infection 47

Introduction 47
Incidence of Deep Infection 48
   The Size of the Sample Studied 48
   The Length of the Follow-up 48
Deep Sepsis in Osteoarthritis 48
Deep Sepsis in Rheumatoid Arthritis 48
Deep Sepsis Following Previous Hip Surgery 48
Patients at Risk for Deep Sepsis 49
   Males with Post-operative Urinary Retention, Catheterization and
      Prostatectomy 49
   Diabetics 49
   Patients with Psoriasis 49
Prevention of Deep Infection 49
Review of the Use of ALAC in Total Hip Arthroplasty 50
   Leaching out from Acrylic Bone Cement 50
   Revisions for Deep Sepsis Using Plain Acrylic Cement 50
   Revisions for Deep Sepsis Using ALAC (Palacos plus 0.5 g Gentamicin) 50
   Release of Gentamicin from Acrylic Cement: Ex Vivo Study 50
   Comparison of Plain CMW Acrylic Cement and ALAC (Palacos plus 0.5 g
      Gentamicin) 51
Diagnosis of Deep Infection 51
Classification of Infection 53
   Late Infection 53
Management of Deep Infection 55
   Conservative 55
   Operative – One- or Two-Stage Revision? 56
   The Principles of One-Stage Revision for Deep Infection 56
   Results of Revisions for Deep Infection 58
The Use of Antibiotic-Loaded Acrylic Beads 61
   The Concept 61
   Clinical Use 61

7 Loosening of the Components 63

Introduction 63
What is Required for Component Fixation? 65
Containment and Pressurization of Cement 65
Socket Fixation 66
The Femur 67

8 The Socket: Changes at the Bone–Cement Interface 71

Demarcation of the Socket 71
Socket Migration 72
Correlation Between Radiographic Appearances and the Clinical Results 73
Correlation Between Radiographic Appearances and the Operative Findings .. 73
Correlation Between the Depth of Socket Wear and the Incidence of Socket
     Migration 74
Correlation Between Radiographic Appearances and Long-Term Clinical
     Results 74
Socket Demarcation and Loosening 75
     Surgical Technique 75
     Socket Wear 76
     Natural History of the Hip Condition 77

9 Loosening of the Socket 81

Introduction 81
The Time Lag Between Primary and Revision Surgery 82
The Correlation Between the Clinical, the Radiological and the Operative
     Findings 83
     Wear of the Socket: The Mechanical and Histological Changes Resulting
          from It 86

10 Wear of the Socket 87

Introduction 87
Radiographic Measurement of Socket Wear 89
Wear Measurement of Explanted Sockets 91
     Correlation Between Real and Radiographic Wear Measurements 91
     Direction of Wear 92
     Impingement 92
     The Effect of Cement Ingress into the Socket 96
Reduced Diameter Neck Stem 96
     Mechanical Testing of the Reduced Neck Stem 97
Summary 97

11 Tissue Reaction to High-Density Polyethylene Wear Particles 99

Introduction 99
Teflon 99
High-Density Polyethylene 101

12 Metal Backing of the Socket 105

13 Loosening of the Stem 109

Introduction 109
Intramedullary Bone Block 112
The Pacheco Study 112
     Unchanged Radiographic Appearances 112
     Demarcation of Distal Femoral Cement 113
     Separation of the Stem from Cement 113
     Fracture of the Femoral Cement at the Tip of the Stem 113
     Endosteal Cavitation of the Femoral Cortex 113

Position of the Stem Within the Medullary Canal 115
Previous Hip Surgery 115
Primary to Revision Surgery 116
Radiological Appearances of Failure of Stem Fixation 117
Patterns of Failure of Stem Fixation 117
Slip of the Stem Within the Cement Mantle 119
Slip of the Stem–Cement Complex Within the Medullary Canal 119
Tilt of the Stem 120
Tilt of the Stem–Cement Complex 120
Pivoting of the Implant Within the Cement 120
Pivoting of the Implant Within the Bone 120
Pivoting of the Stem–Cement Complex 121
The Sequelae of Failure of Stem Fixation 123
Lack or Loss of Proximal Support in the Presence of Good Distal Fixation ... 123
Endosteal Cavitation 123

14 Fracture of the Stem 125

Introduction 125
Patients' Function 128
Patients' Weight and Time to Fracture 128
Surgical Technique 129
Radiographic Appearances 129
Fracture of the Femoral Cement 129
Endosteal Cavitation of the Femur 129
Early Radiographic Signs of Failure of Stem Fixation 129
Position of the Stem Within the Medullary Canal 130
Comparison of Cases from Two Sources 131
The Mechanism of Fracture of the Stem in Total Hip Arthroplasty 131
Obliquity of the Fracture 131
Bending of the Proximal Fragment 133
Fracture Wave 134
Fracture Lip 134
The Level of Fracture of the Stem 135
Fracture of the Stem Following Revision Surgery 135
The Pattern 136
The Specimens 136
Radiographs 136
Mechanism of Stem Fracture 137
Experimental Confirmation 137
Clinical Implications 137
Recent Developments 138
Fracture of the Stem in the Uncemented Metal-to-Metal Arthroplasty 138

15 Fracture of the Shaft of the Femur 139

Introduction 139

16 Heterotopic Ossification 145

Introduction 145
Proposed Definition 145
The Incidence 146
The Site 147
The Extent 147
Inclusion of Cancellous Bone in the Operative Site 147
Periosteal Stripping 148
Excision 148

Contents

SECTION II: PRACTICAL APPROACH TO REVISION SURGERY 153

17 Timing of Revision Surgery 155

Introduction 155
Problems to be Anticipated at Follow-up 155
    Deep Infection 155
    Dislocation 156
    Fracture of the Stem 156
    Loosening of the Stem 158
    Loosening of the Socket 159
Correlation Between Radiological Appearances and Clinical Function 160

18 Assessment of the Patient 163

Introduction 163
Assessment of the Arthritic Hip 163
Assessment of a Patient with Failed Total Hip Arthroplasty 164
    Clinical History 164
    Pain in Failed Total Hip Arthroplasty 164
    Function 165
    Straight Leg Raising 165
    Local Examination 165
    Special Investigations 165
Discussion with the Patient 167
Anaesthetic Assessment 168

19 Instrumentation for Revision Surgery 169

Introduction 169
The Diagnosis 169
The Availability of the Instruments and the Components 169
Removal of Trochanteric Wires 172
Trochanteric Osteotomy 172
Mobilization of the Proximal Femur and Dislocation 172
Extraction of the Femoral Stem 172
Socket Exposure, Testing and Extraction 173
Removal of the Femoral Cement 173
Removal of the Distal Cement Plug 173
Extraction of the Complete Cement Mantle from the Medullary Canal 174
Extraction of the Distal Fragment of Fractured Stem 174

20 Selection of Components 175

Introduction 175
The Acetabulum 175
The Femur 176

21 Revision Surgery: The Technique 179

Introduction 179
Positioning the Patient 179
The Incision 180
    Incision in the Deep Fascia 181
The Landmarks 181
Removal of the Trochanteric Wires 182
    The Claw Hammer Method 183
    The Sardine-Can Method 183

Exposure of the Hip Joint 183
    Trochanteric Osteotomy 183
    Examination of the Components 186
    Exposure and Examination of the Acetabular Cavity 189
    Preparation of the Acetabulum and Fixation of the Socket 189

**22 Revision with Trochanteric Non-union: Reattachment of the Un-united
Trochanter** 191

    Introduction 191
    The Series 191

23 The Femur 193

    Introduction 193
    Extraction of the Femoral Component 193
    Removal of the Acrylic Cement 193
        The Proximal Part 194
        The Middle Part 194
        The Distal Part 195
        Femoral Cement Restrictors 195
    Removal of Fibrous or Pyogenic Granulation Tissue from the Bone–Cement
        Junction 196
    Removal of a Thin Layer of Condensed Cancellous Bone 196
    Excavation of the Lesser Trochanter 196
    Selection of a Femoral Stem and Trial Reduction 197
        Trial Reduction 198
    Distal Closure of the Medullary Canal and Stem Insertion 198
        Reattachment of the Greater Trochanter 198
        Reattachment of the Greater Trochanter when the Stem has not Been Changed 199

24 Loss of Bone Stock 201

    Introduction 201
    Acetabular Defects 201
        Central Acetabular Deficiencies 202
        Superior Acetabular Defects 203
        Disruption of the Acetabular Rim 203
        Support and Reinforcement Rings 204
        Future Developments 204
    Femoral Defects 205
        Minor Femoral Deficiencies 205
        Major Deficiencies of the Proximal Femur 205
        Practical Approach: The Modular Stem System 206
        Future Developments 206

25 Wound Closure 209

    Introduction 209
    The Acetabulum, Femur and Total Hip Components 209
    The Capsule, the Abductors, the Greater Trochanter and the Vastus Group of
        Muscles 209
    The Deep Fascia 209
    Subcutaneous Fat 210
    The Skin 210
    The Use of Drains 210

26 Post-operative Management 213

SECTION III: THE ULTIMATE CHALLENGE OF SURGERY 215

27 Girdlestone Pseudarthrosis for a Failed Total Hip Arthroplasty 217

    Introduction 217
    Indications for Pseudarthrosis 217
    The Operative Procedure 219
    Post-operative Management 219
    Clinical Results 219
    Conclusion 219

28 Pulmonary Embolism 221

    Introduction 221
    Prediction 221
    Prevention 221
    Treatment 222
    Reviews of Pulmonary Emboli Trends 222
        Yearly Variations in Incidence 223
        Seasonal Variations in Incidence 223
        Variations in the Incidence Between Different Patient Groups 223
        The Incidence of Fatal Pulmonary Emboli During the Post-operative Period . 224
    Mortality Due to Causes Other than Pulmonary Embolism 224

SECTION IV: CONCLUSIONS 225

29 Conclusions 227

References 229

Subject Index 233

1 Introduction

Acrylic cement has been available for component fixation for many years. When high-density polyethylene was introduced by Charnley in 1962 as the material of choice for the socket, the operation of total hip arthroplasty became widely practised. Since then, numerous component designs have become commercially available, each one advocating or extolling some newly discovered "principle".

There are three important aspects to this type of surgery: the components (material and design), the surgical technique and the bone stock.

When considering the components, due respect must be paid to the underlying engineering principles, the materials, the methods of manufacture and testing as well as the examination of the components after years of normal function in the body. This involves many basic sciences, most of them unfortunately outside the scope of an ordinary clinician.

Surgical technique includes the methods of exposure and of component fixation and orientation, as well as instrumentation. Like any technical skill it cannot be improved indefinitely. Herein lies the dilemma. The manufacturer cannot and dare not attempt to sell "surgical technique". Surgical technique is not a commodity that can be sold at a profit except through the medium of a design. Detailed instructions must be provided and even then repeated use is required if the operative skills involved are to be improved. Thus repeated instruction from the manufacturer on the technique would alienate the surgeon.

An alternative route may be taken; attempts may be made to equate design with the surgical technique thus implying that design takes priority over the surgical technique, the former now becoming a saleable commodity.

Acrylic cement is another such saleable commodity. Although implanted at the time of surgery it really is a part, and a reflection, of the surgical technique. It readily makes up for the defects of bone preparation, component fixation and, at times, even of component design.

The long-term results of surgery readily point to the defects of the design or technique. The time interval between primary and revision surgery should be a minimum of 6 years but preferably at least 8–10 years. Furthermore the number of cases included in a study must be substantial – somewhere in the region of 2500. What is really being examined in a long-term study is a certain number of total hip arthroplasties subjected to normal daily activities over a period of time, i.e. the fatigue and wear of the components in clinical practice.

Clinical impressions over a short period of time contribute little. Radiographic appearances give better information. However, there is no substitute for a large series and long-term, well-documented follow-up.

In recent years there has been an explosion in the number of designs being used for various reasons, some less obvious than others. More than ever attempts are being made to equate design with component fixation when cement is used. However, some surgeons advocate "cement-free, bony ingrowth" designs, probably to avoid the difficulties of the surgical technique by suggesting that, given time, nature will provide the solution to any problems of component fixation. There is probably nothing more attractive to a surgeon than a procedure that is technically undemanding and always effective, or to a physician than a drug that is always effective and has no side-effects.

In a specialty as vast as that of orthopaedics, surgeons yearn for an easy hip operation, or if a good operation is difficult they hope that having mastered its performance through trial and tribulation it should be universally applicable. The only type of operation that could ever be universal would be an arthroplasty. This would eliminate the intellectual task of choosing the best operation for the individual problem, but until that happy day arrives it is obvious that the surgery of the hip is the beginning of a large subject. It demands training in mechanical techniques; liaison with departments of engineering and technology would be most rewarding. (Charnley 1960)

And yet one further aspect must be seriously considered – that of the bone's or the patient's response to the implant; although reasons are often hinted at it has never been satisfactorily explained. Why should an identical set of components and an apparently standard (and yet unsophisticated) technique produce widely varying results? Are we looking at minutiae of technique that escape standard scrutiny or should we be hoping for "the bones to give up their secrets". The natural history of the arthritic hip is something that has yet to be studied in detail.

Innovations and changes are inevitable sequelae of a mechanical procedure such as total hip arthroplasty and follow from study of long-term results and of complications or findings at revision surgery. One must reflect on the need to depart radically from a method which is backed by 26 years of clinical experience but there can be two basic reasons for change.

First, dissatisfaction with the principles of the method because of poor results and the need for frequent surgical interventions because of failures may indicate a change.

A second indication for change is a genuine belief, backed by scientific evidence, that introduction of fundamentally new principles will offer better or longer lasting results.

If there is dissatisfaction with the long-term results of the Charnley low-friction arthroplasty then this is not reflected in the statistics from the Hip Centre. Detailed analysis of some aspects have already been published; other aspects will be analysed in the pages of this volume.

It must be pointed out at this stage that in the 24 years from the inception of the Charnley low-friction arthroplasty (November 1962–December 1986), 20 588 Charnley low-friction arthroplasties have been performed. During this time 607 revisions are known to have been carried out, 37 for dislocation, 351 for loosening of the components and 219 for fracture of the stem, a revision rate of 3% over a 24-year period. (No particular meaning is attached to percentages and the numbers are presented only to give some indication of the patterns of revisions.) With improvements in the design and the surgical technique brought about as a result of long-term studies and revision surgery, the rate of revision will almost certainly be reduced further. These operations have been carried out by some 180 surgeons either in training at or on the Staff of, the Unit of Wrightington Hospital. No attempt must be made by any individual to monopolise that success!

If a new principle or design genuinely appears to offer better or longer lasting results then long-term follow-up to confirm this is essential. The statistics from the Hip Centre show quite clearly that a follow-up for 6 years of a series of 2500 cases without change in design or technique and without a revision (Fig. 1.1) is required. Neither short-term follow-up of small series nor frequent changes in design inspire confidence.

How often is it that surgeons are ready to put into practice new and unproved ideas because they have failed to study well-tried methods already in existence?

The most essential aspect of cemented total hip arthroplasty is that of soundness of fixation of components when under load, both in primary and in revision surgery. Poor fixation of components is a feature easily recognized in cases of failure. However, sound fixation is more difficult to define in terms which reflect the component design, operative technique, postoperative radiological appearances and long-term follow-up results. Components can be said to be soundly fixed when the most recent radiograph of a patient with normal function looks indistinguishable from the one taken shortly after surgery, for it is on this soundness of fixation of the components when under load that the ultimate success of the operation depends. The principle is not usually appreciated by the young surgeon, and is often forgotten by the old hand. Not until this sound fixation of components under load is achieved consistently should we even consider other modes of failure such as "cement being the weak link", "failure of acceptance of the cement by the body", "histiocytic reaction", "metal sensitivity" or

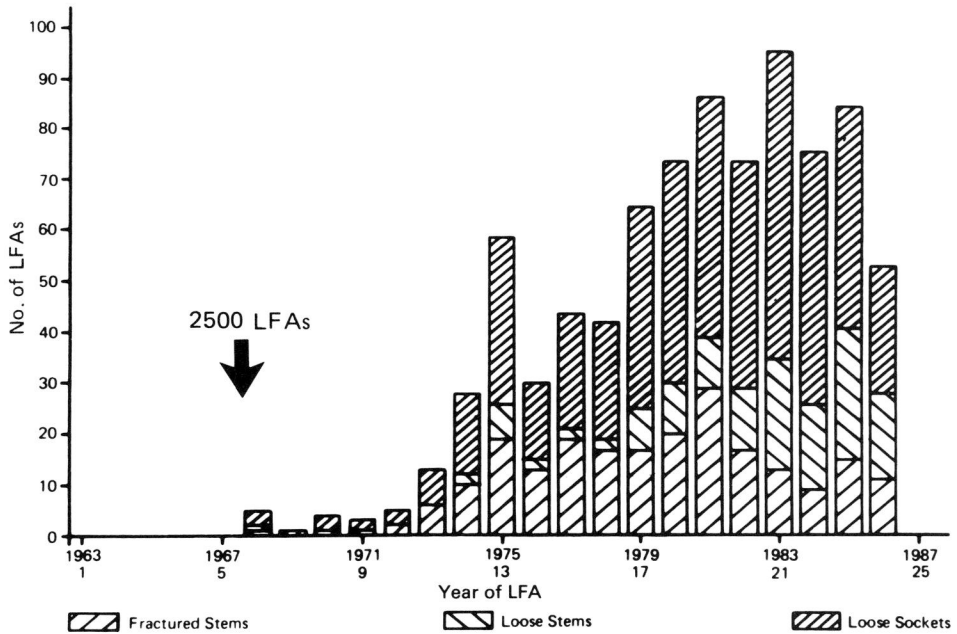

Fig. 1.1. The Charnley Standard. (2500 cases with a 6-year follow-up. There were no revisions for loose or fractured stems and no revisions for loose sockets.)

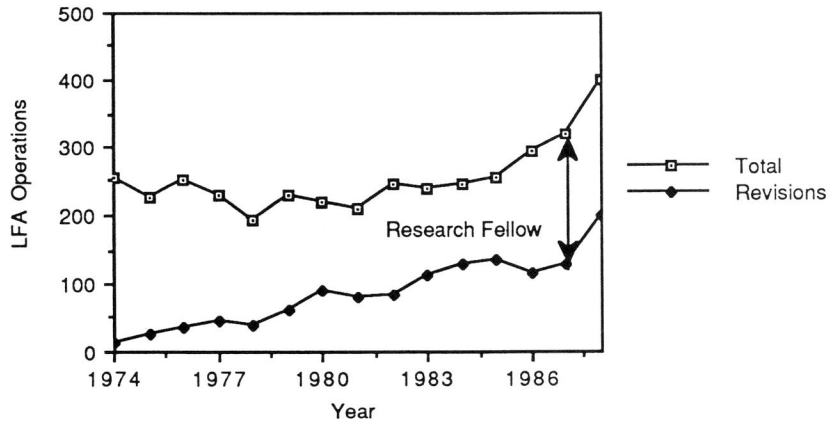

Fig. 1.2. Graph showing the increasing number of revisions, from all sources, over a 15-year period. In 1987 a Fellowship in Research and Revision Surgery was established.

even "aseptic loosening". Only when the materials, the design, the surgical technique and the terminology have been standardized can we meaningfully discuss long-term results. Even then the elusive "quality of the bone stock" must be considered. The problem of wear is a separate issue.

The author's own involvement in revision surgery includes a 15-year period as a Consultant at the Centre for Hip Surgery, Wrightington Hospital. While the number of operations carried out each year has remained more-or-less constant, the number of revisions has steadily increased to over 50% of the total (Fig. 1.2). This dramatic increase in the workload reflects the demand for this type of surgery and the excellent support offered by the staff of the hospital. The level reached is probably the maximum possible for an individual and it is with gratitude that the author acknowledges help in establishing the post of Research Fellow in Revision Surgery. It is visualized that this will offer an in-depth involvement for surgeons interested in this expanding subspecialty.

Revision surgery gave a unique opportunity, hitherto not available, to examine several aspects of total hip arthroplasty: clinical and radiological studies were made of cases which had failed and which had fully documented histories; the correlation between the clinical performance, radiological appearances and the operative findings was studied; and at surgery there was the opportunity to examine the components in their "natural environment" and then to examine them in detail *ex vivo*. The effects of the various complications on the bone stock has always been a revelation. Studying cases of revision it was often possible to work out predictable patterns of failure which could then be applied not only to prospective studies but also could be used as a base line when applying new techniques in primary surgery. This particular aspect of the work allowed simultaneous studies of revision and prospective studies of primary surgery to be carried out. New techniques and instrumentation had to be developed. Lessons learned from revision surgery have their application in primary interventions, for this is the real meaning of experience.

Complications Leading to Revision Surgery

2 Haematoma

Introduction

The management of haematoma is always more obvious retrospectively. To suggest that haemostasis should be a routine part of any surgical procedure is to state the obvious; to seek out known bleeding points routinely is to avoid problems.

When performing total hip arthroplasty using a lateral transtrochanteric approach the following constant bleeding areas can be easily identified:

1. Several veins running transversely in the fat layer.
2. When separating the fascia and the muscle fibres of the tensor fascia lata above the greater trochanter brisk bleeding can be seen from the posterior flap. This must be attended to. With the initial incision retractor in place bleeding may cease only to reappear at the time of closure.
3. Two and sometimes three bleeding points are seen on the anterior capsule between the vastus lateralis ridge and the anterior margin of the acetabulum (Fig. 2.1).
4. A collection of vessels, often a plexus, in the piriform fossa.
5. Small individual points in the posterior capsule.
6. The acetabular branch of the obturator artery at the exposure of the inferior margin of the acetabulum, the pulvinar and the tear drop.
7. Branches of the profunda femoris artery when the capsule is stripped extensively off the medial femoral neck or when the proximal femur is to be resected.
8. Intrapelvic sources of bleeding are fortunately rare provided care is taken during exposure and preparation of the acetabulum.

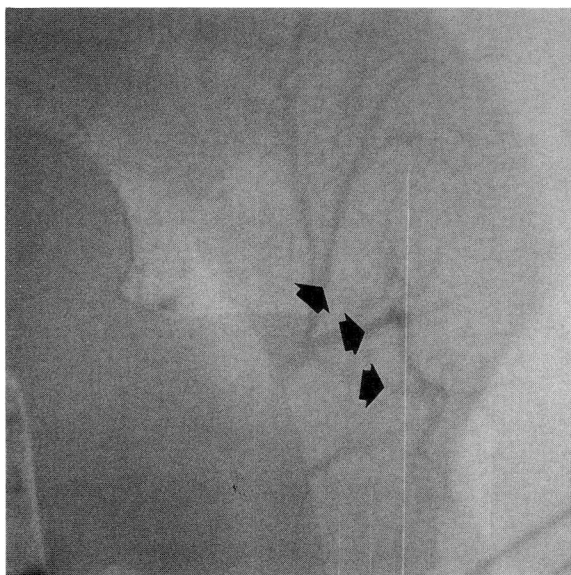

Fig. 2.1. Bleeding points encountered at trochanteric osteotomy.

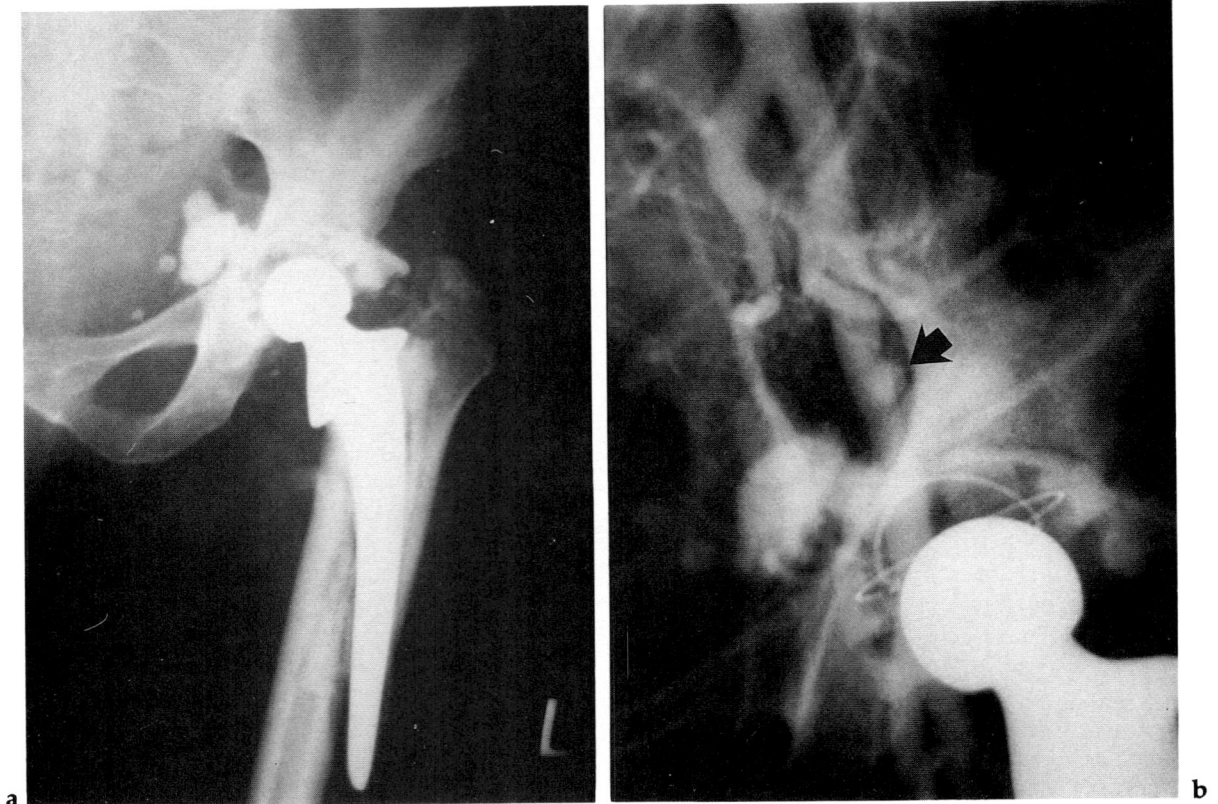

Fig. 2.2. Intrapelvic source of bleeding. **a** A problem for solution. The arthroplasty has been infected with two episodes of fresh bleeding from a wound sinus. **b** Arteriogram outlining a small aneurysm of the external iliac artery in relation to the extruded acrylic cement.

(Use of the Hohman retractor for the anterior acetabular exposure is best avoided. Its sharp end may damage femoral or even iliac vessels.) In cases of prolapsed socket, especially when this has occurred early in the post-operative period, which usually implies deep sepsis, arteriography may be indicated (Fig. 2.2).

9. Other sources of bleeding may be present and are created by the need to dissect various tissue planes, as occurs during the mobilization of the proximal femur and its separation from the pelvis prior to and after dislocation.

10. The bleeding in the piriform fossa may be started again during manipulation of the femur or insertion of the femoral retractor or the trochanteric wires. This may become obvious as the hip is being reduced and should be checked for before final reduction.

Despite knowledge of all the above and the details outlined in Chap. 25, haematomas do occur.

The Role of Anaesthesia

Far be it for a surgeon to venture into making comments on anaesthesia in relation to bleeding or post-operative haematoma; however, some observations, thought to be relevant, may be worthwhile recording. Adequate sedation, gentle induction and intubation and an anaesthetic without "peaks and troughs" is almost guaranteed to give a bloodless field, especially if combined with judicious use of hypotensive agents. An anxious patient and a difficult intubation associated with coughing spasm will lead

Haematoma

9

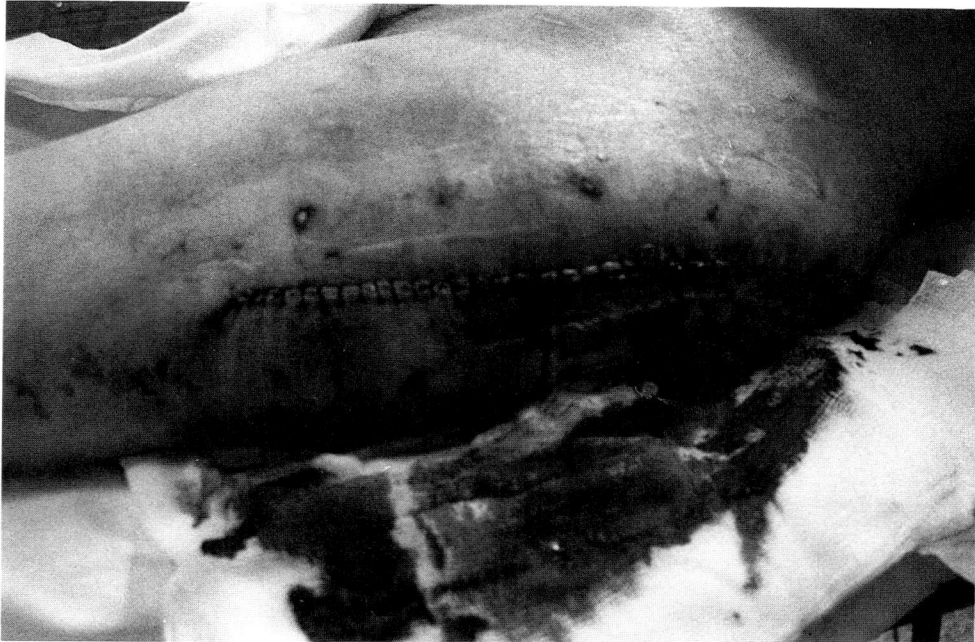

Fig. 2.3. Superficial haematoma. Note the oedema and oozing blood.

to a congested operative field. The worst situation is probably the patient who is beginning "to come out of the anaesthetic" as the operation is coming to an end. A sudden increase in muscle tone sets off bleeding points which were hitherto quiescent and which at this stage may well be out of reach as the various tissue layers will have been closed. The state manifests as an immediately post-operative restlessness or even a struggle; the patient takes time to settle and invariably requires extra sedation. The result is excessive drainage, bruising or haematoma. It is even more serious if during this period the drains become dislodged. The problem becomes obvious days later when the drop in haemoglobin level is greater than anticipated from the measured blood loss.

It is almost certain that in an adequately sedated patient bleeding is less likely to occur than in a patient with venous engorgement and raised arterial pressure resulting from an untimely recovery or inadequate sedation. In this context the role of epidural anaesthesia is worthwhile investigating.

Classification of Haematoma

Haematoma can be classified as superficial, deep or infected. The diagnosis is not difficult but the treatment may be.

Superficial Haematoma

There is oedema localized to the area immediately adjacent to the incision. It does not reach the femoral triangle, but may extend along the tensor fascia lata as far as the knee or even more distally. The skin has a "peau d'orange" appearance and after a day or two it will look blue due to the collection of blood deep to it (Fig. 2.3). The skin stitches look to be too tight and the incision itself may appear as a thin blue membrane ready to burst open. The patient may be pyrexial. Bruising is obvious. Skin under strapping or fat sutures may blister from tension.

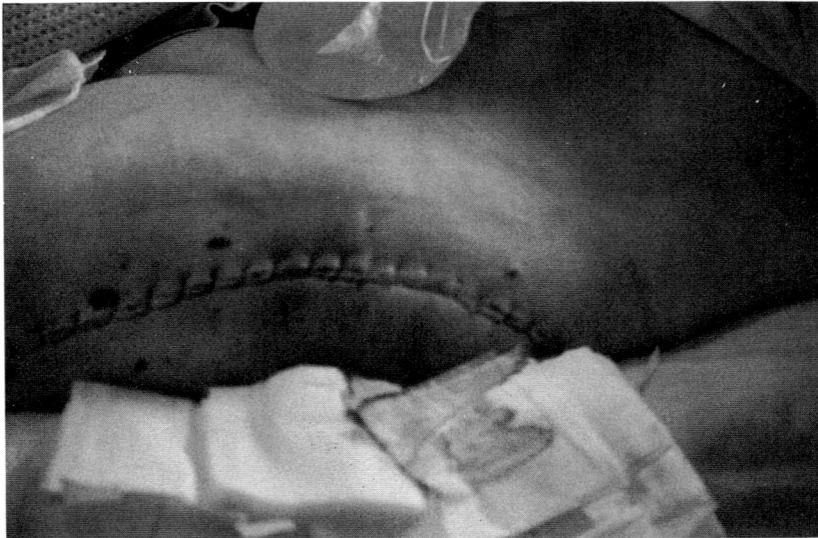

Fig. 2.4. Infected haematoma. Note the sutures now under tension due to oedema, bruising, blistering and thin serous discharge. (Note also the proximity of the stoma bag.)

Management

Under general anaesthetic and in an operating theatre some or all of the skin sutures should be removed and the haematoma evacuated. Bacteriological specimens should be taken. The cavity should contain clotted blood only. A careful check should be made for any defects in the deep fascia, but probing is to be avoided. After removal of all the clot any obvious bleeding points should be coagulated with diathermy and the cavity *gently* packed with *dry* sterile gauze. Forceful packing leads to ischaemia of the tissues while wet packs do not allow any exudate to be soaked up and leave a mess in the bed. The pack should be changed every 24–48 hours until the wound is clean enough for either secondary suturing or gentle taping of the skin edges. Prophylactic antibiotics should be given. The benefits of this method of management are often more obvious in retrospect.

Deep Haematoma

The wound itself looks fine, there being no oedema. There is swelling however of the anterior and medial aspects of the thigh and these areas may be somewhat tender. The patient is pyrexial.

Unless there is an indication that bleeding may be continuing, an expectant approach is indicated; several days' bed rest and antibiotics are all that is usually needed. As the haematoma is lysed the swelling settles very rapidly.

Infected Haematoma

This type of haematoma may follow superficial or deep haematoma but more often than not it is really deep sepsis that is presenting itself. The diagnosis is made obvious by oozing from either the incision, the sutures or the drain sites (Fig. 2.4). Such haematomas should always be evacuated and the cavity packed until clean and then either sutured or taped. Antibiotics should obviously be given. Serous oozing from the wound must be viewed with suspicion; the problem is most likely to be deep sepsis, the bacteria producing lysis of the haematoma. Exploration here does not give the satisfactory result obtained with a superficial sterile haematoma. The oozing often persists and may even result in a sinus. Deep sepsis will become obvious with time, will affect the outcome of the operation and will have to be dealt with as a separate issue at some future date.

3 Problems Arising from an Inadequate Exposure

The socket should be fully covered and supported within the acetabulum; the intramedullary portion of the stem, not the femoral neck, decides the exposure of the femur.

There is little doubt that total hip arthroplasty can be performed successfully utilizing any of the common exposures. What is less obvious is that only some of them allow consistently good access, more so in difficult primary or revision cases.

Some of the problems probably arise from the fact that the surgeon performing the operation often "graduates" from management of fractures of the femoral neck where the exposure needs to be limited, some from the spectacular early clinical results of total hip arthroplasty which may give the surgeon and the patient a false sense of security and some may arise from the failure to appreciate that the long-term success of the operation largely depends on the quality of component fixation and that this can be severely tested by the grateful patient over years of normal function. In fact there is no other orthopaedic operation where so much depends on the mechanical aspects of the procedure.

Problems resulting from an inadequate exposure, although often easy to recognize in individual cases, are yet to be quantified. They may at times be put down to the joint being "stiff" or the "osteophytes being extensive", the "deformity being rather severe", the patient being "obese" or "muscular" or the medullary canal being "narrow". The net effect is a collection of problems which span the whole spectrum seen in this type of surgery. Immediately obvious is the fracture of the shaft of the femur at various stages; this can be at the moment of attempted dislocation, during forceful reduction while applying torsion to the femur or during the penetration of femoral cortex by the stem. Malposition or malorientation of components may lead to early dislocation.

In the long term it is the loosening of the components which is the penalty that may have to be paid. But then, after a spell of normal function, the term "aseptic loosening" may become the diagnostic label which unfortunately fails to identify the root of the problem. It is also probable that physical difficulties encountered by the surgeon may result in tissue damage and a higher incidence of deep sepsis. That there may be some correlation between the two has been previously hinted at (Wroblewski 1984b): in some 10% of cases of known deep sepsis an element of "difficulty" was noted at primary surgery. Examples of problems resulting from inadequate exposure are given in Fig. 3.1.

What is Required at the Time of the Exposure?

Three main things are required at the time of exposure:

1. A circumferential view of the acetabulum.
2. Unimpeded access to the medullary canal.
3. Preservation of the integrity of the abductor muscles.

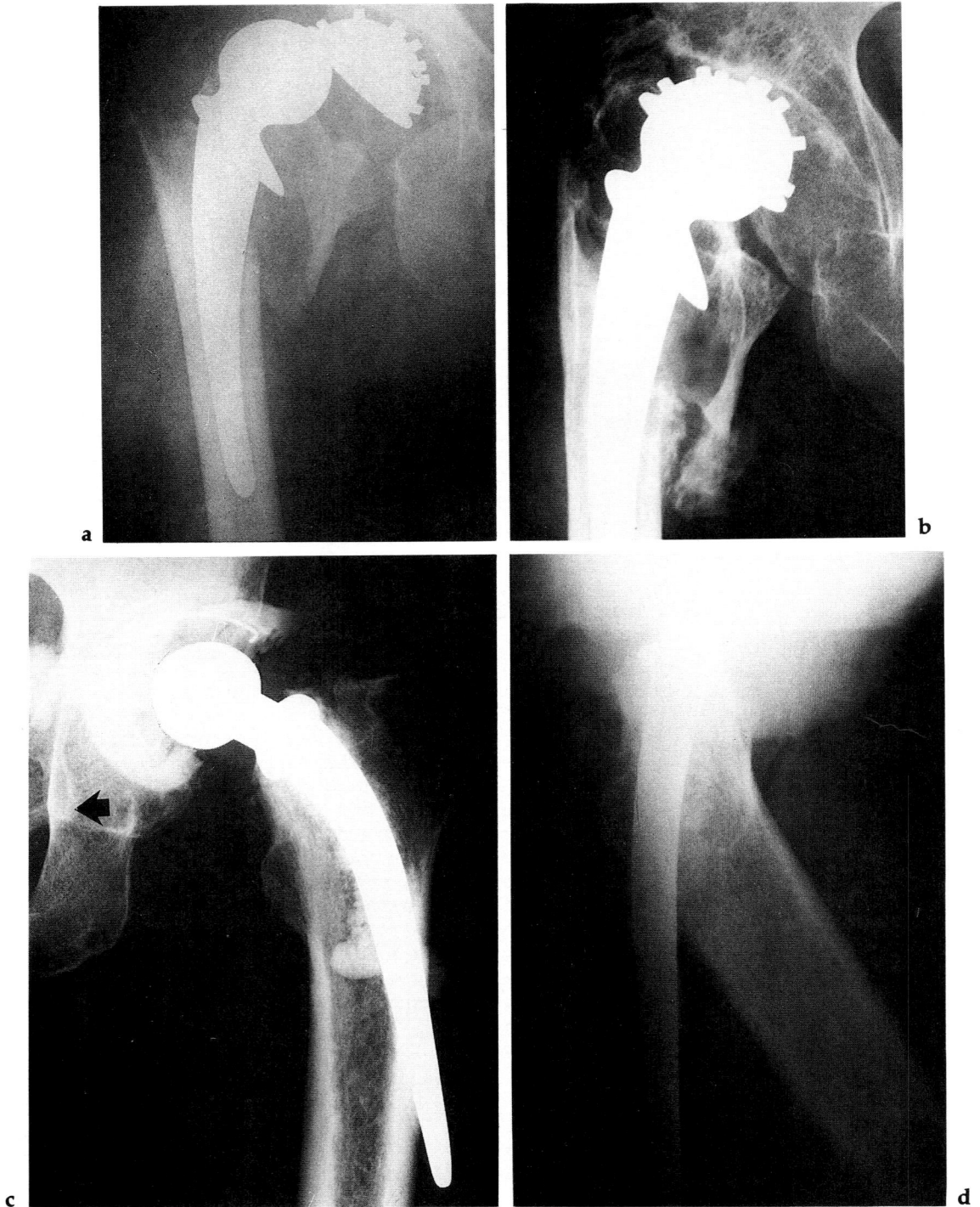

Fig. 3.1. Some of the problems resulting from an inadequate exposure of the acetabulum and the medullary canal. **a** McKee–Farrar arthroplasty, 1969 post-operative appearance with immediate post-operative dislocation. Note the medial proximal femoral cortex and the greater trochanter. **b** 1988 appearance. Almost 20 years of clinically successful result now symptomatic and presenting a challenge for revision. **c** Limited exposure of the acetabulum and the medullary canal. The result is high placement of the socket and subcutaneous stem. **d** Lateral view.

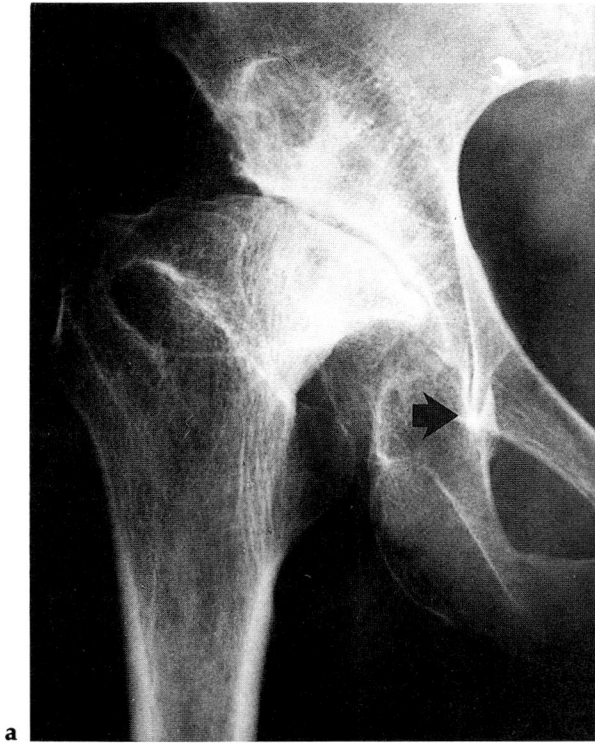

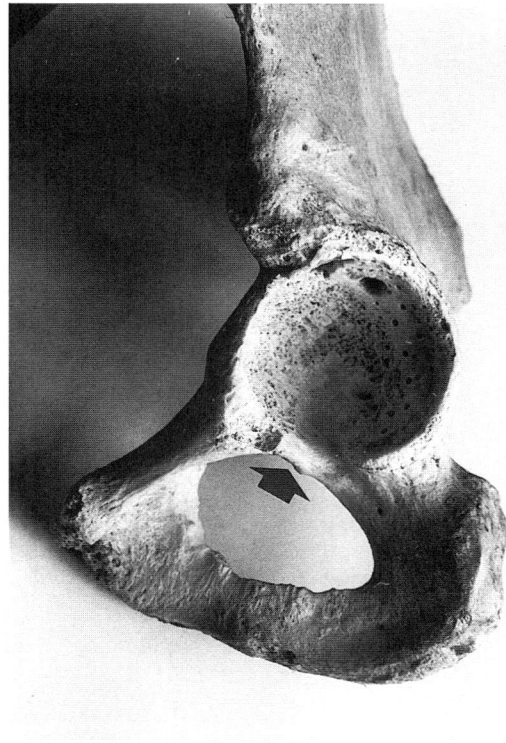

Fig. 3.2. The "tear drop". **a** The rolled edge of the lower margin of the acetabulum at its junction with the obturator foramen. **b** Circumferential view of the acetabulum. **c** Coronal section of hemi-pelvis through the "tear drop".

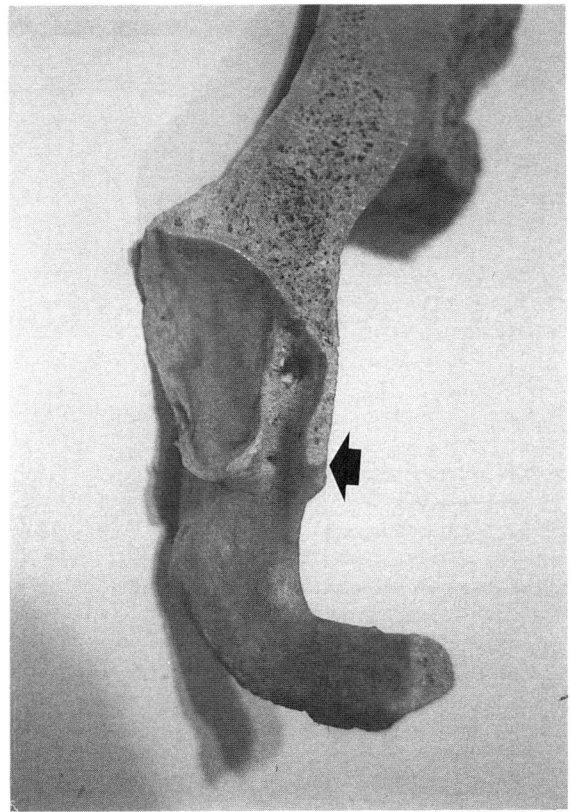

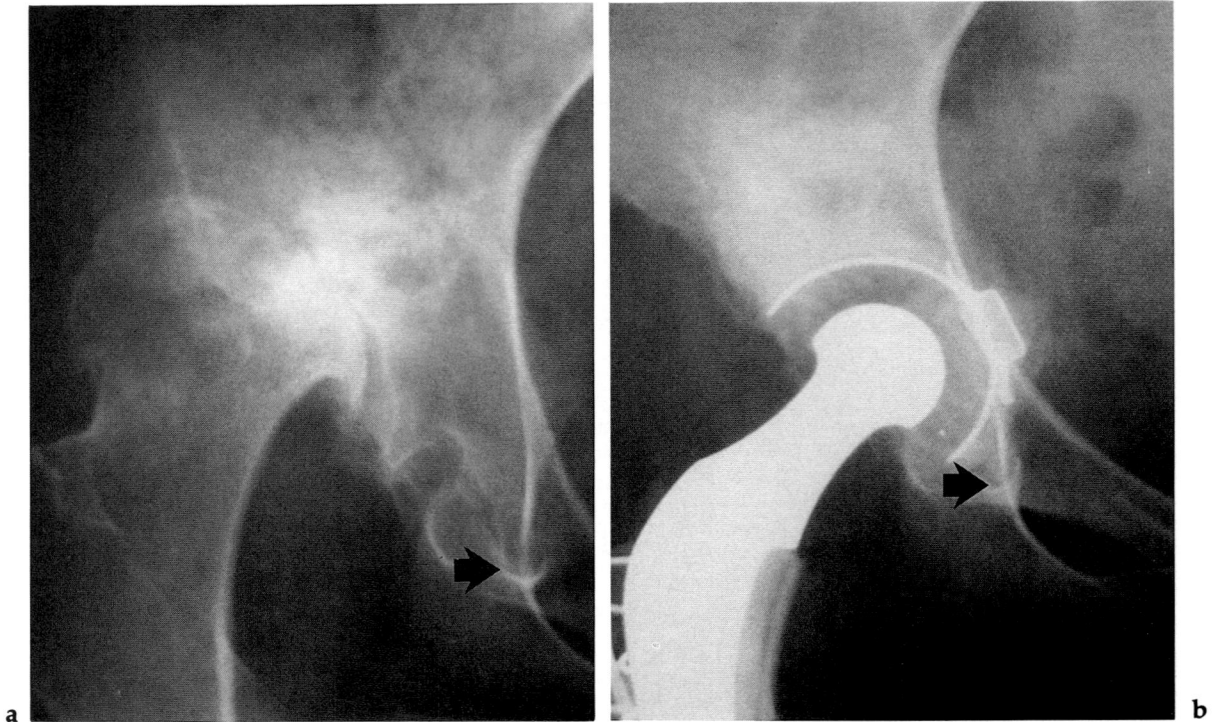

Fig. 3.3. Primary surgery. **a** Congenital dislocation of the right hip with secondary degenerative changes. **b** Post-operative radiograph. Socket fixed at the anatomical level with respect to the "tear drop".

Exposure of the Acetabulum

An unimpeded circumferential view of the acetabulum is required, from the "tear drop" distally to the superior margin proximally, with clear exposure of the anterior and posterior acetabular margins. The tear drop serves as an indispensable landmark of the inferior margin of the acetabulum (Fig. 3.2). Its exposure in primary surgery allows careful preparation of the acetabulum. Its importance may not be appreciated in straightforward primary surgery, but becomes obvious when dealing with dysplastic hips and in revision surgery (Figs. 3.3 and 3.4). A retractor designed for the purpose (Fig. 3.5) inserted at the lower margin of the acetabulum will expose the shining cortical bone of the tear drop, retract the soft tissue at the inferior acetabular margin and serve as a guide for the correct placement of the socket. In some cases the postero-inferior acetabular osteophyte may have to be removed and the transverse ligament excised before this area can be fully exposed.

The superior margin of the acetabulum is exposed using the Charnley pin retractor which is introduced transversely above the superior acetabular margin. The east–west retractor is then placed with one jaw on the pin retractor (thus protecting the abductor muscles and facilitating the exposure by retracting the femur distally) and the second on the femoral neck just above the lesser trochanter. (Full proximal to distal exposure may not be achieved immediately; it may be necessary to apply more pressure to this retractor as the operation progresses.)

The antero-posterior exposure is achieved by using the Charnley north–south retractor. The posterior blade is placed postero-inferiorly on the thick capsule which is usually present in this area, thus protecting the sciatic nerve. In cases of revision or when the capsule may be non-existent it is advisable to place a folded swab so that the teeth of the retractor will not press on the sciatic nerve. The sharp spike of the Hohman retractor is best avoided, especially anteriorly, for fear of damaging the contents of the femoral triangle. The acetabular retractor, placed below the tear drop, completes the exposure.

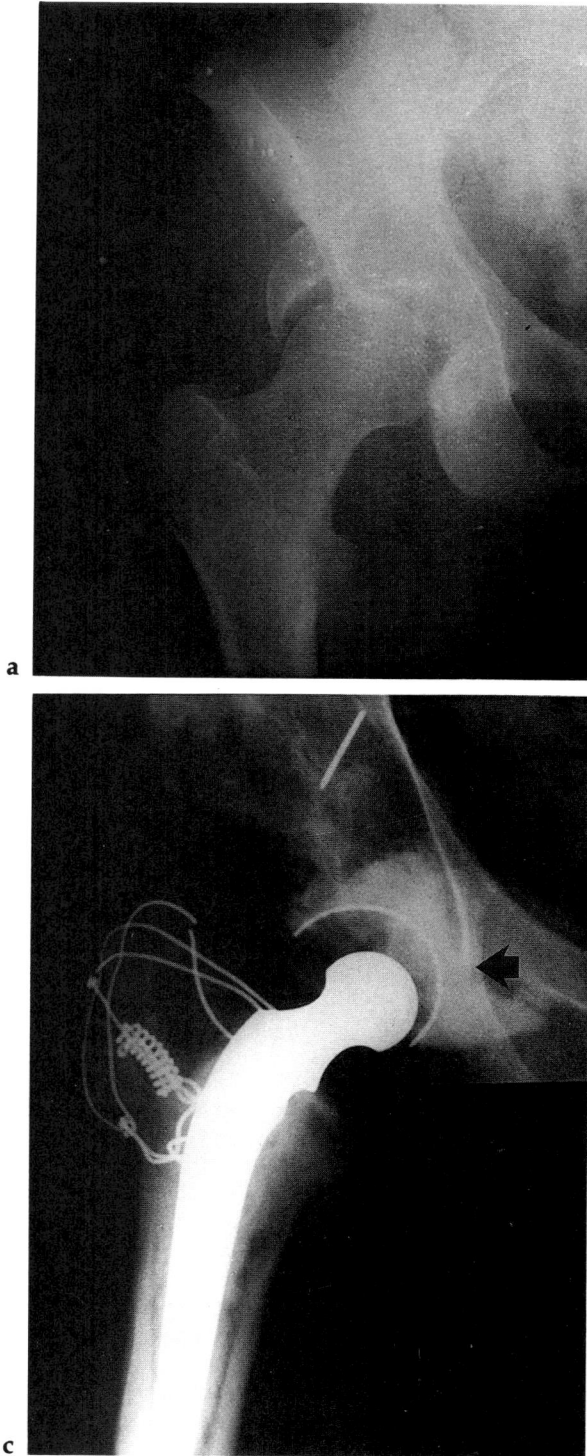

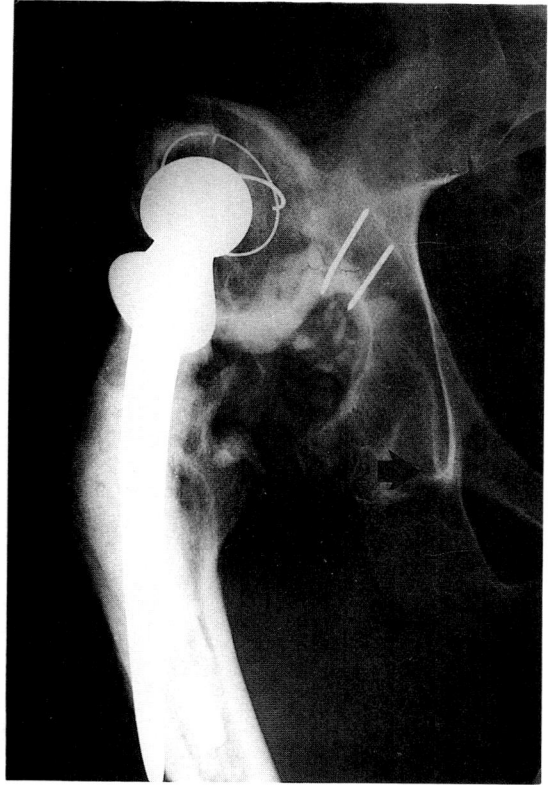

Fig. 3.4. Revision surgery. **a** Fracture dislocation of the right hip treated initially by open reduction and pin fixation of the fracture. Early failure demanding further treatment (total hip arthroplasty). **b** Total hip arthroplasty with good initial clinical result. Socket high and migrating. Stem as seen. **c** Six years after revision. Note the offset-bore socket fixed in the only reasonable quality bone available at the level of the "tear drop".

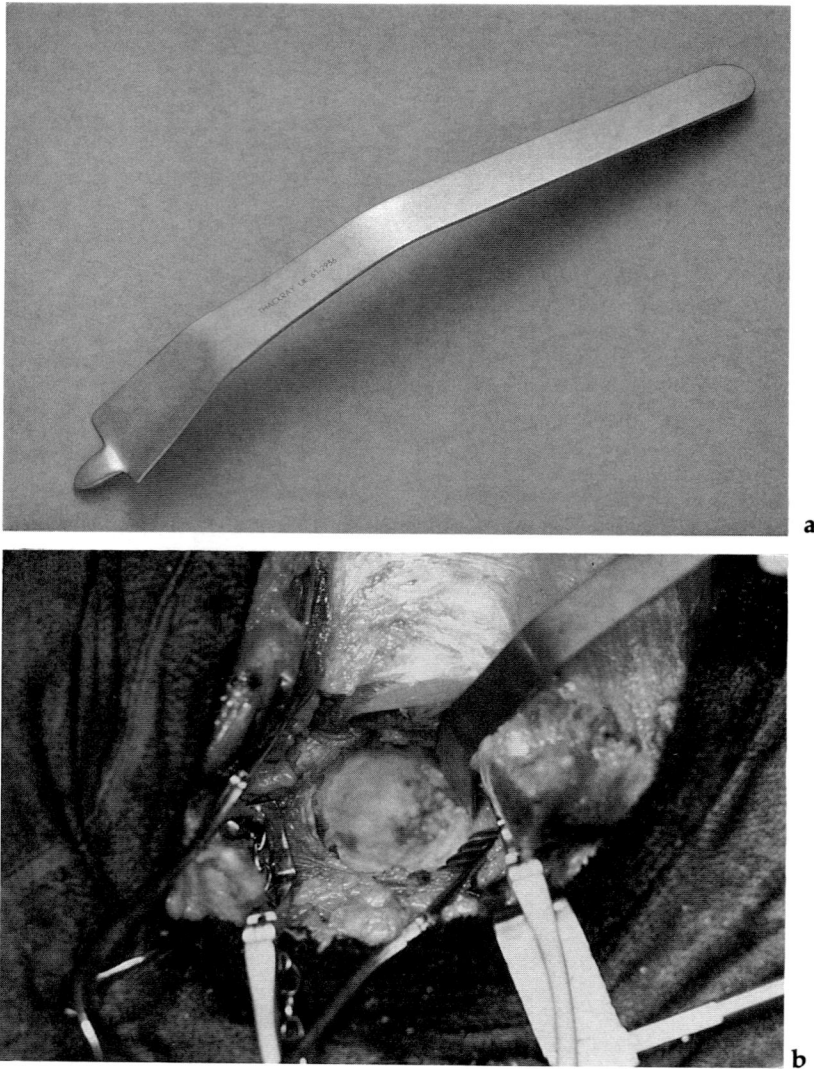

Fig. 3.5. a Acetabulum retractor. (Note the blunt end to avoid damage to the obturator structures.) **b** Acetabulum retractor in place defines the most inferior part of the acetabulum, the "tear drop".

Exposure of the Medullary Canal

On the femoral side, a full view and direct access to the medullary canal (and not just the sectioned femoral neck) is essential. It is probably not readily appreciated, or more likely it is forgotten, that the neck and the shaft of the femur lie in different planes and at an angle to each other. Access to the femoral neck does not guarantee access to the medullary canal. A number of problems arise in this context of which penetration of the back of the femoral cortex (the femoral neck being anteverted) is probably only secondary to inadequate positioning and fixation of the stem.

Irrespective of the exposure used, the access to the medullary canal required is that which can be compared to the retrograde placement of a Kuntscher nail – the nail comes out through the postero-lateral part of the greater trochanter (Fig. 3.6). That is the direction along which the stem should enter the medullary canal. In the

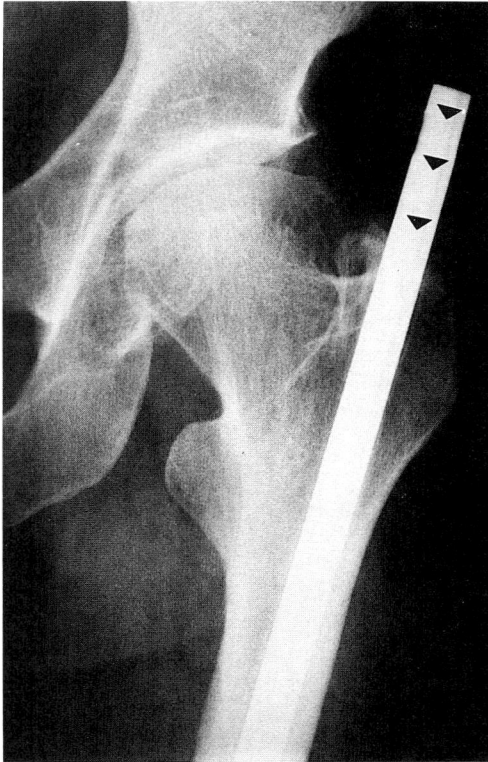

Fig. 3.6. Access to the medullary canal. Kuntscher nail in place: its exit is at the junction of the piriform fossa and the posterior aspect of the greater trochanter. That is the port of entry for the intra-medullary portion of the stem, not the femoral neck.

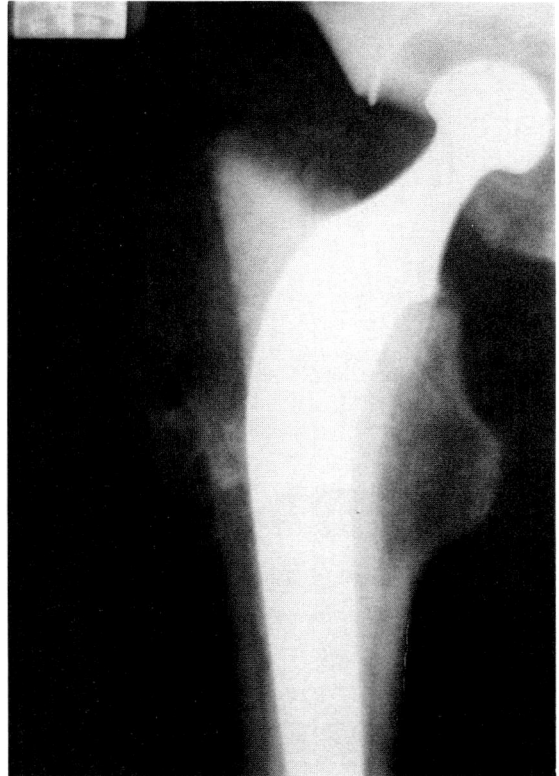

hands of the surgeon skilled in the method, it doesn't matter whether this direct access to the medullary canal is offered by trochanteric osteotomy or by excavation of the greater trochanter and the posterior aspect of the femoral neck. What does matter is the careful preparation of the medullary canal, proper cement injection and correct placement of the stem. It must be appreciated that even with a trochanteric osteotomy the final position of the stem may depend on the "attitude" of the stem in relation to the

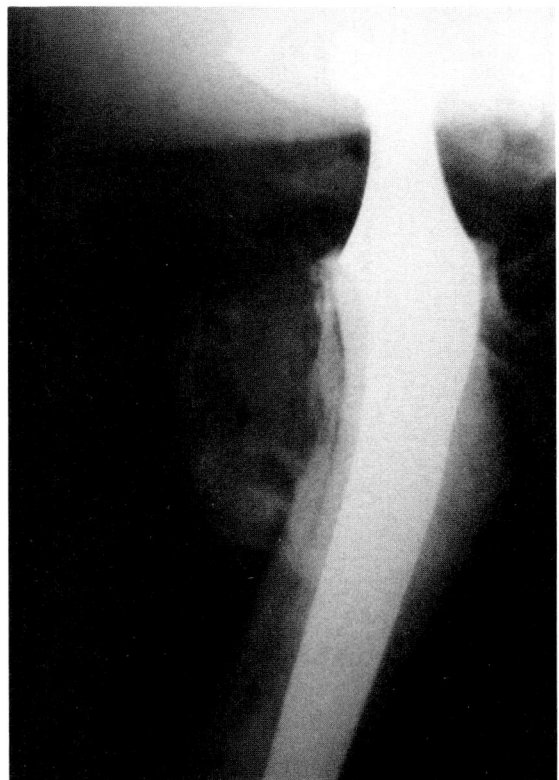

Fig. 3.7. "Direct" exposure of the hip with partial elevation of the abductors. The complaint is of restricted painful flexion and a palpable mass anterior to the greater trochanter. **a** AP radiograph offers no clues. Stem position and cement distribution appear adequate. **b** Lateral radiograph reveals the problem, i.e. heterotopic ossification resulting from elevation of the anterior abductor mass off the bone.

femoral shaft at the moment of stem insertion. Unless the thigh is held parallel to the ground the tendency will be for the stem to be directed towards the posterior femoral cortex. In order to avoid this, the leg holder must be instructed to roll the patient gently away from the surgeon until the tibia is vertical and the thigh on the operation side is parallel to the ground.

Preservation of the Integrity of the Abductors

Exposure and operation should be carried out with the minimum of soft tissue trauma, muscle damage or periosteal stripping, for it is pointless to undertake complex hip replacement surgery if the muscles needed for its normal function have been damaged or denervated by careless or forceful exposure. That the integrity of the abductors must be preserved is no doubt obvious. Yet none of the exposures in common use, except for the transtrochanteric, address that problem by enumerating complications. Could this be something to do with "what the eye does not see . . . "? The recent upsurge of alternative exposures is in some measure responsible for increased abductor damage (Fig. 3.7).

It cannot be stressed strongly enough that adequate exposure, proper bone preparation and cement injection and correct placement of the components are the most essential aspects of the procedure, and the only aspects within the surgeon's control. It is from these aspects that the long-term results will be judged.

Review of the author's revisions (from various sources), which are by no means a representative cross-section, have shown that some 10% of the problems arise from inadequate exposure at primary operation.

4 Trochanteric Osteotomy and Problems Resulting from It

If it could be guaranteed that the greater trochanter would unite within three weeks when reattached, and without imposing restrictions which would impede rehabilitation, few surgeons would fail to avail themselves of the easy and beautiful access to the hip joint provided by the lateral approach. (Charnley 1979a)

Three weeks for trochanteric union may be an unrealistically short time and some restrictions on the speed of rehabilitation must be imposed, especially in the young and following revision surgery. The statement, however, remains basically correct.

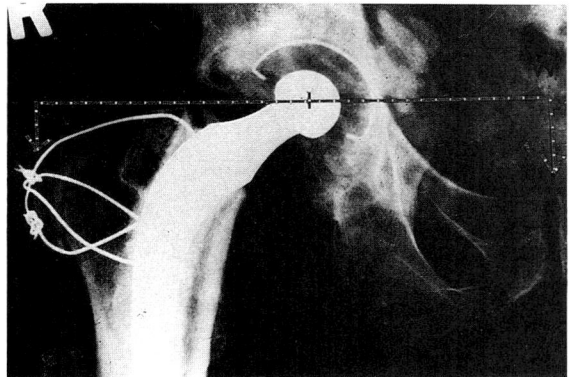

Fig. 4.1. Diagrammatic presentation of improvement in the lever ratios following low-friction arthroplasty. (A copy of a framed photograph from Sir John Charnley's office.)

Introduction

In order to understand the reasoning behind this method of exposure of the hip it is essential to know something about the evolution of the trochanteric osteotomy as practised by the late Professor Sir John Charnley.

According to Sir John himself this was the method to which he was introduced by Sir Harry Platt and it would probably be correct to say, on Sir John's own admission, that this was the only method he had ever used routinely for the purpose of total hip arthroplasty.

In the design, evolution and practice of the low-frictional torque arthroplasty, the perfection of the mechanical aspects of the procedure, took priority. In carrying out the operation, the teachings of Pauwels were followed. Directed to that aim was the reduction of the medial lever by deep placement of the socket, and an increase of the lateral lever by the lateral and distal placement of the greater trochanter (Fig. 4.1). It was at this stage that the positions of reattachment of the trochanter were designated by the number 1, 2 or 3 (Fig. 4.2), each one indicating the most advantageous mechanical improvement in the lateral lever (Charnley and Ferreira 1964). (It may be of interest to point out that the surgeons who do not perform trochanteric osteotomy have never entered into the discussion directed towards the restoration of the lever ratios as part of the operation of total hip arthroplasty.)

The concept of the low-frictional torque was of the utmost importance, for loosening of the

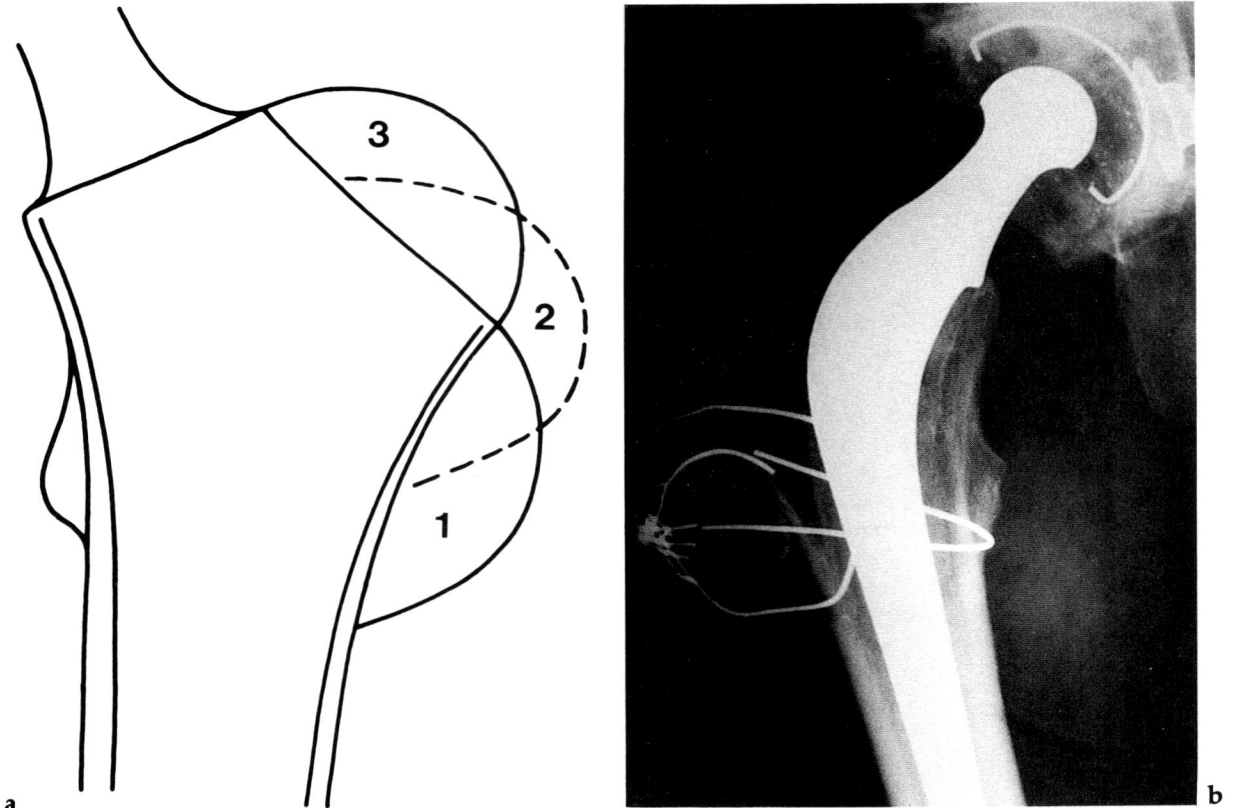

a   b

Fig. 4.2. Position of the greater trochanter in the Charnley low-friction arthroplasty. **a** "The first position denotes the site of the trochanter with the cut surface in contact with the lateral surface of the shaft of the femur. The third position denotes that the detached part of the greater trochanter returned to its original position in relation to the femur. The second position denotes a site intermediate between the first and third positions" (Charnley and Ferriera 1964). **b** The "first position" of the greater trochanter, probably somewhat over-enthusiastic.

components has always been considered to be the most likely long-term complication to be overcome. Also important was the consistently full exposure for the preparation of bone and placement and fixation of the components in a way that could easily be followed by other surgeons. The socket was invariably placed deep and high. The stem had a short neck. The trochanteric bed was not encroached upon, the stem being in a varus position. Simple trochanteric fixation was used with a consistently high incidence of bony union. With time, in order to avoid impingement of the femur on the acetabular rim, the length of the neck was increased.

In the early 1970s the concept of the anatomical placement of the socket in relation to the "tear drop" became established as part of the technique, as did the preservation of the strong,

load-bearing subchondral bone of the acetabulum. It was at this stage of the evolution of the low-friction arthroplasty that fracture of the stem presented as an important clinical entity (Fig. 4.3). With its management and prevention came the call for valgus placement of the stem. Actually the statement was " . . . too much concentration on teaching the valgus position had distracted attention from the *quality* of contact between cement and calcar femoris" (Charnley 1975 p.116).

It was not readily appreciated that at trial reduction the stem tilts into the varus position and may even subside down the medullary canal, thus resulting in shortening (the trochanteric fragment readily returning to its original position). With the stem cemented in the valgus position the overlengthening becomes obvious,

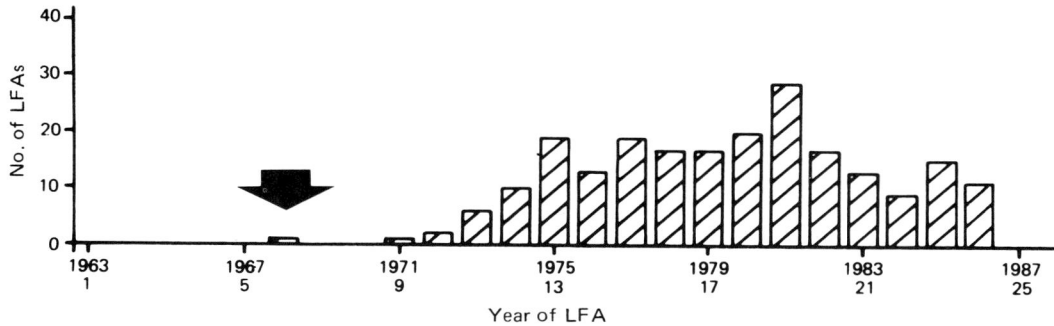

Fig. 4.3. Fracture of the first stem of the low-friction arthroplasty, 1968. Increasing numbers of fractured stems presented for revision surgery from 1971 to 1981.

and at a stage when it cannot be corrected. An omission to study the second part of the statement by some surgeons has probably resulted in over-emphasis of the valgus position of the stem at the expense of its fixation.

Thus, anatomical and less deep placement of the socket allowed some correction of the leg-length discrepancy before the level of the section of the femoral neck was determined. (The original concept was based on the deep placement of the socket by judging the thickness of the medial acetabular wall; later, full coverage of the socket and preservation of the subchondral plate was the standard.) Since the level of the femoral neck section has been more or less uniform and the length of the neck of the femoral stem unchanged (it has actually been increased compared with the earlier design), with the stem now in a valgus position a new set of problems has inadvertently crept in.

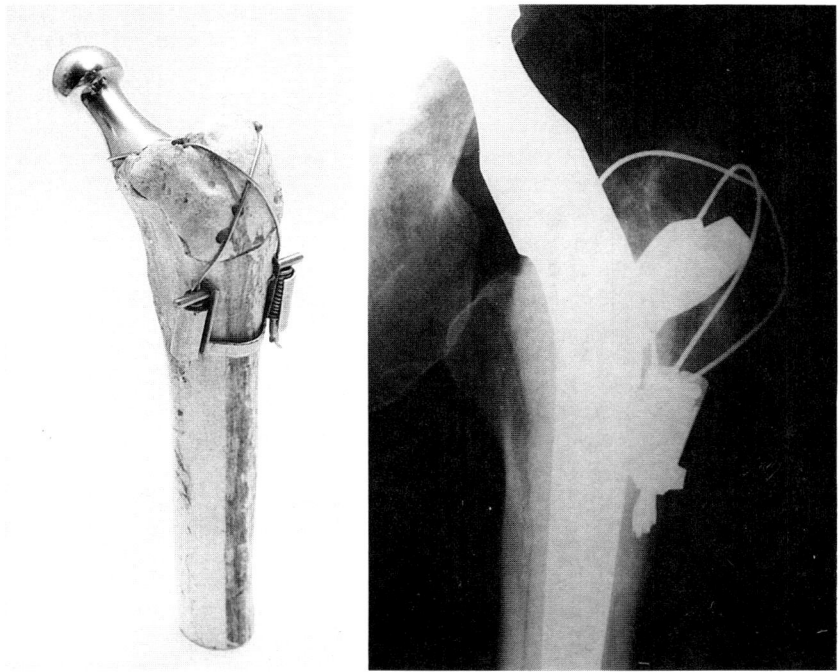

a   b

Fig. 4.4a,b. One of many attempts by the late Professor Sir John Charnley to improve and simplify the method of trochanteric reattachment. The long wire loops were prone to fatigue failure while the compression springs below the vastus lateralis ridge proved bulky.

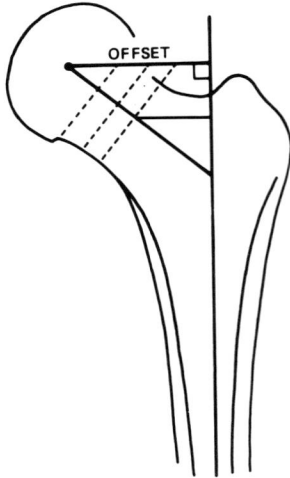

Fig. 4.5. Reducing the offset of the stem demands a lower level of section of the femoral neck in order to maintain the effective length of the limb constant.

The valgus position of the stem increased the leg length further, while the back of the stem now encroached on the previously intact trochanteric bed, reducing the area of contact of the cancellous bone for trochanteric fragment fixation. Overlengthening of the limb and trochanteric detachment followed. It was for these reasons that this period saw numerous attempts to improve the methods of trochanteric reattachment (Fig. 4.4). The offset of the stem was reduced from 45 to 40 mm (reduction of offset demands that the neck be sectioned at a lower level, see Fig.4.5) and a flange was added to the round back stem to improve proximal fixation of the stem; however, of necessity it encroached on the trochanteric bed posteriorly as all stems should do. Panic had by this stage set in. It is this sequence of developmentally essential changes following each other in rapid succession that has been responsible for increasing controversy and polarization of individual surgeons on the exposure of the hip joint.

In retrospect it becomes obvious how the anatomical placement of the socket, encroachment of the valgus stem into the trochanteric bed, the unchanged level of the femoral neck section, the increased length of the neck of the femoral stem and finally the reduced offset flanged stem all added up to the necessity for the trochanter to be reattached with the hip in an

abducted position, while at the same time reducing the area of the trochanteric bed. The result was trochanteric detachment. It was not until the Adjustable Trial Prosthesis (ATP) was introduced (unfortunately often erroneously regarded as "yet another gimmick") that the whole problem was corrected. The ATP prosthesis allowed correct (neutral) placement of the stem and the correct level of section of the femoral neck while the tension of the abductors and the capsule, as well as the position of the greater trochanter, could be checked at trial reduction. At that stage the cruciate wire system and the staple bolt became firmly established and gave uniformly successful results. By now it was too late to stop the tide and yet too early to have the benefit of the knowledge of the advantages as shown by long-term results. Unfortunately, human nature being what it is, an easy option is apparently preferable, and long-term results are a long way away.

The controversy surrounding trochanteric osteotomy need not exist and this "bone of contention" should be put to rest. Surgeons will each have their preferred methods which will be judged in the light of long-term results. One aspect of this type of surgery is obvious, that is, the need for revision. This, now a more complex procedure, will demand trochanteric osteotomy for most if not all cases. Primary surgery offers ample opportunity to perfect the method for any surgeon committed to this method of treatment. Beyond that each surgeon must make up his or her own mind, not only as to the method of exposure of the hip in general, but if need be, for individual cases in particular. If trochanteric osteotomy is to be used in a particular case then the operation must be planned accordingly; it is not a "cure all" when brought in as a panic measure (Fig. 4.6).

Trochanteric Osteotomy

When considering trochanteric osteotomy as a method of exposure in the context of total hip arthroplasty, certain clinical observations must be taken into account. An osteotomized trochanter, especially if some of the external rotators have been divided, has a tendency to rotate anteriorly in relation to its bed, thus tightening the posterior part of the capsule attached to the greater trochanter. Before its reattachment the

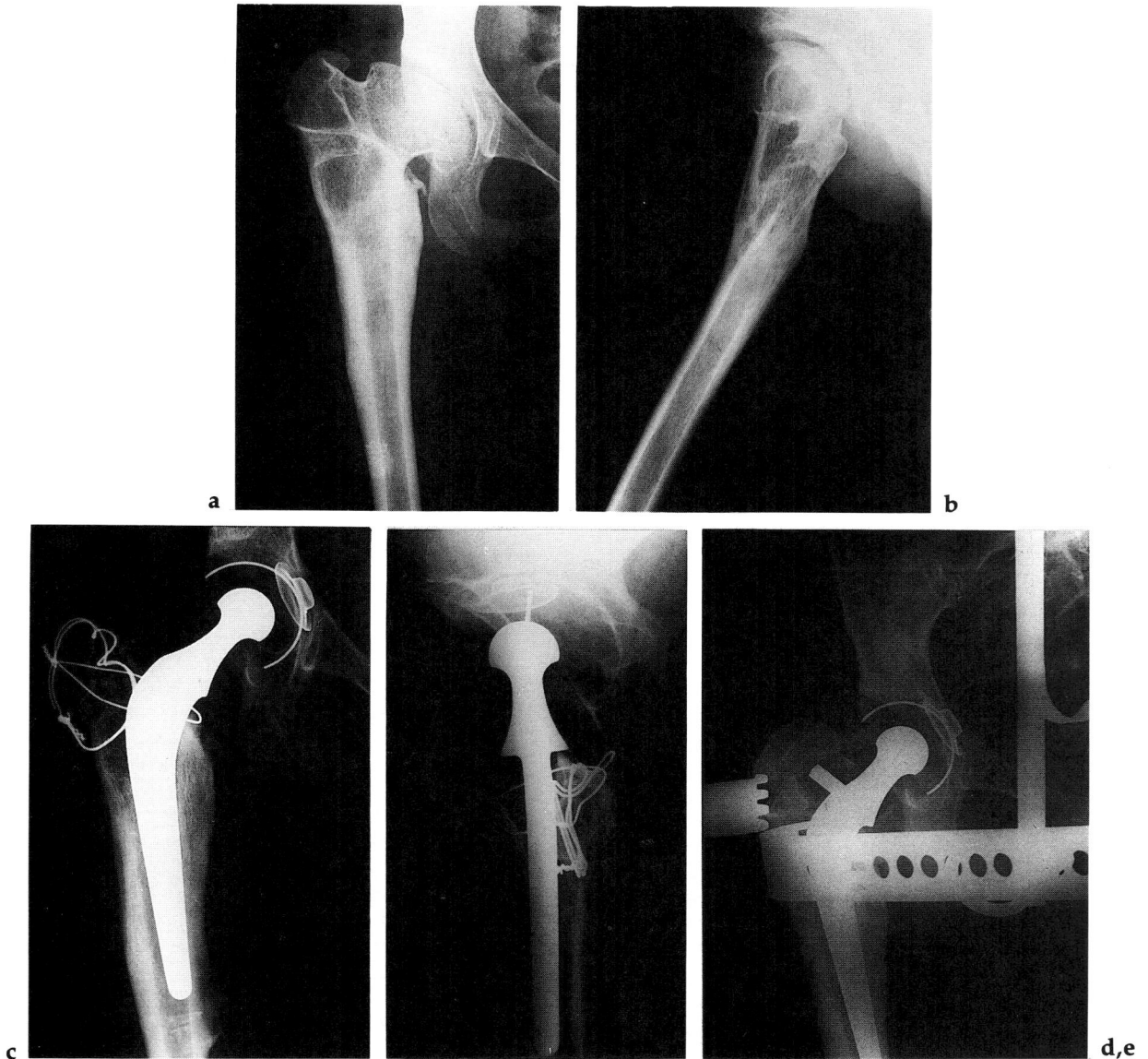

Fig. 4.6. Trochanteric osteotomy. Was the trochanteric osteotomy carried out only when difficulties with preparation of the medullary canal became apparent? **a,b** Pre-operative problems. **c** Post-operative radiograph. Operation clinically successful for several years, now becoming painful after a stumble. **d** The stem is positioned anteriorly to the shaft of the femur. **e** Radiograph taken at surgery. Note the trial stem and the Charnley initial incision retractor in place.

trochanter must be rotated posteriorly into its original position. Failure to do this leaves the posterior part of the capsule tight; this will become more obvious when the hip is in flexion. The tendency will be for the trochanter to separate from its bed by a shearing movement. With the trochanter rotated onto its anatomical bed, the hip can be fully flexed without the tendency for the trochanter to become displaced, even before its reattachment. However, when the hip is adducted, or adducted in flexion, the distal part of the greater trochanter will be seen to lift away from its bed, a position often observed radiologically before the trochanter becomes

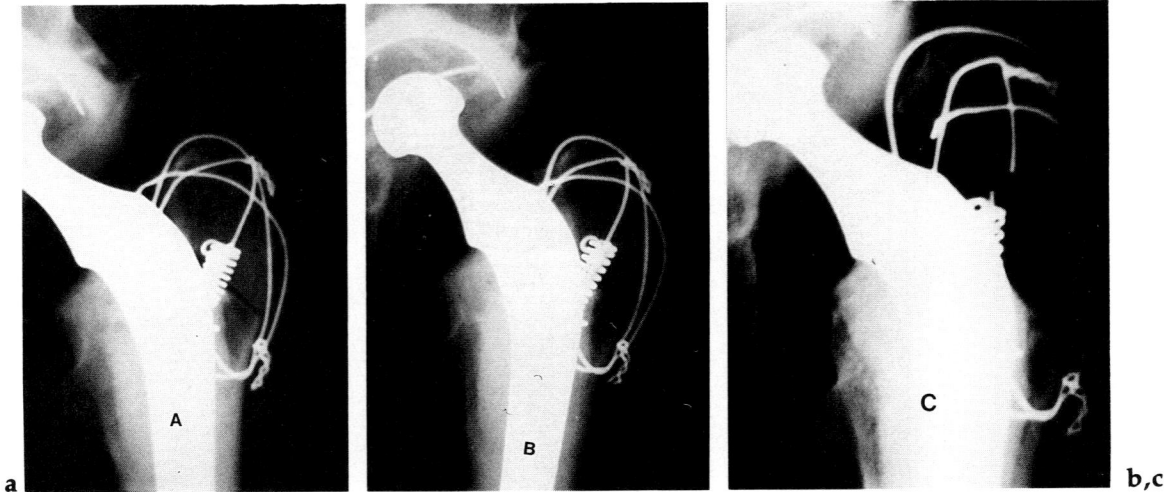

Fig. 4.7. Stages of post-operative trochanteric detachment. **a** Immediate post-operative radiograph. The stump of the neck of the femur is long and the hip is in an abducted position. **b** Radiograph at 2 weeks: distal part of the greater trochanter elevated from its bed. **c** Radiograph at 3 months showing trochanter detachment.

detached (Fig. 4.7). The elevation of the distal part of the trochanter from its bed was observed by Sir John Charnley in 1980 (Fig. 4.8). Its significance did not become clear until some time later.

At surgery, adduction of the hip by some 10 degrees must be possible without the distal part of the trochanter becoming elevated from its bed. If this is not possible then the femoral neck should be shortened, the greater trochanter released or a shorter neck stem used before the trochanter is reattached.

It must be pointed out here that at trial reduction the stem, unless firmly secured in its position by the ATP or some such method, will tend to tilt into the varus position and sink down the medullary canal. Both will give shortening and a false sense of security of the trochanteric stability. With the stem cemented, and if it is in a valgus position, the overlengthening will become obvious, and at a stage when it is too late to correct.

The evidence points to the fact that correct placement of the trochanter in relation to its bed, avoidance of overlengthening and attention to the details of the method of trochanteric reattachment should result in a high incidence of trochanteric union.

Reconstruction of the hip mechanics can thus be achieved by the anatomical placement of the socket, section of the femoral neck at the correct level and the use of the appropriate offset stem centred within the medullary canal.

Trochanteric osteotomy has now become the method of choice of exposure and is now as much a part of total hip arthroplasty as is incision in the skin or the deep fascia. It allows the operation to be carried out without any trauma to the abductors and gives full view for preparation of bone, component orientation and fixation, these now becoming the most important aspects of the operation.

Problems Related to Trochanteric Osteotomy

Problems of trochanteric osteotomy can be divided into three main categories as follows:

1. Increased blood loss and operating time.
2. Trochanteric bursitis.
3. Trochanteric non-union leading to pain, a limp and dislocation.

Increased Blood Loss and Operating Time

Suggestions that trochanteric osteotomy increases blood loss and operation time are

KING EDWARD VII HOSPITAL

President:
HER MAJESTY THE QUEEN

M. R. Geake, Esq., M.B., B.Chir., F.R.C.P.,
Senior Physician.,
Major General S. E. Large M.B.E., M.D., F.R.C.P.,
Director of Medical Services.

Vice-President and Chairman:
LAVINIA, DUCHESS OF NORFOLK, C.B.E.

Deputy Chairman:
BRIGADIER SIR GEOFFREY HARDY-ROBERTS
K.C.V.O., C.B., C.B.E., D.L., J.P.

MIDHURST
SUSSEX GU29 0BL

MIDHURST 2341/4
(07 3081 2341)

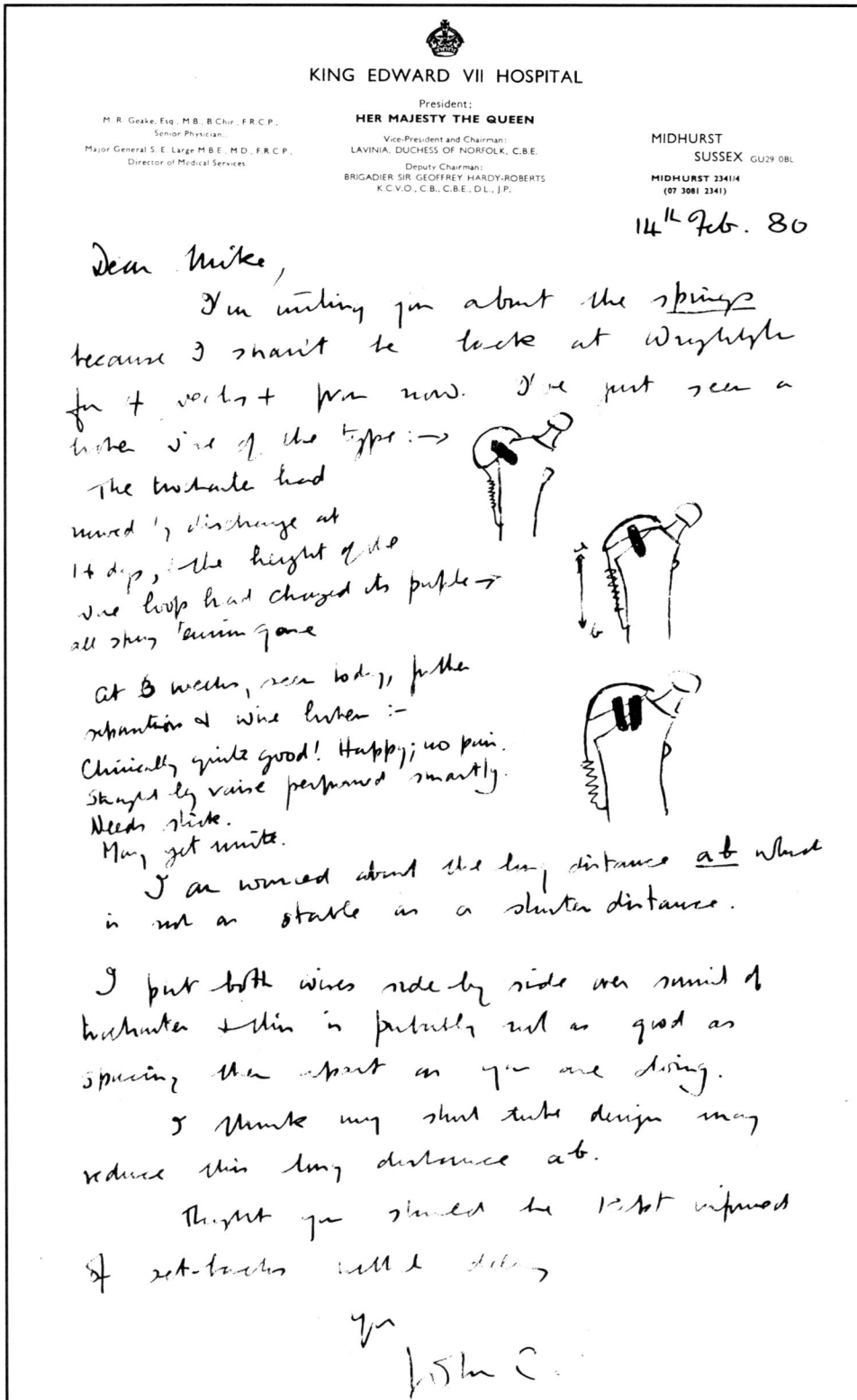

Fig. 4.8. A problem observed is quickly communicated. Copy of a letter from Sir John Charnley to the Author.

Table 4.1. Blood loss and operation time in cases with and without trochanteric osteotomy

| | Wiesman et al. (1978) | | del Sel et al. (1981) (all cases with trochanteric osteotomy) | | |
	Without trochanteric osteotomy	With trochanteric osteotomy	Primary surgery	Conversions	Revisions
No. of cases	12	12	149	26	19
Blood loss (ml)	1248	1820	180–1350	390–1680	520–2080
Operating time (min)	156	186	40–110	60–150	75–150

unfounded. The often-quoted paper of Wiesman et al. (1978), although scientifically excellent, is based on such a small sample that it must surely reflect only a certain level of surgical expertise. The answer to it has been published (del Sel et al. 1981) and is summarized with the Wiesman results in Table 4.1.

Trochanteric Bursitis (or Trochanteric Pain)

The trochanteric bursa, or the "abductor muscle-mass fascia", is a structure not described accurately in the standard textbooks of anatomy. It is a sheet of dense areolar tissue which extends from the anterior margin of the abductor mass and the tensor fascia femoris in the front, to the insertion of gluteus maximus posteriorly. Its free border lies just distal to the vastus lateralis ridge. Proximally it blends intimately with the intermuscular septa of the abductor mass. The greater trochanter can be seen to move deep to it when the hip is rotated.

In the exposure of the greater trochanter the bursa must be elevated proximally. This is best done with a pair of dissecting forceps inserted under the free edge; the bursa is then elevated, intact if possible, over the abductor mass. This manoeuvre allows direct access to the greater

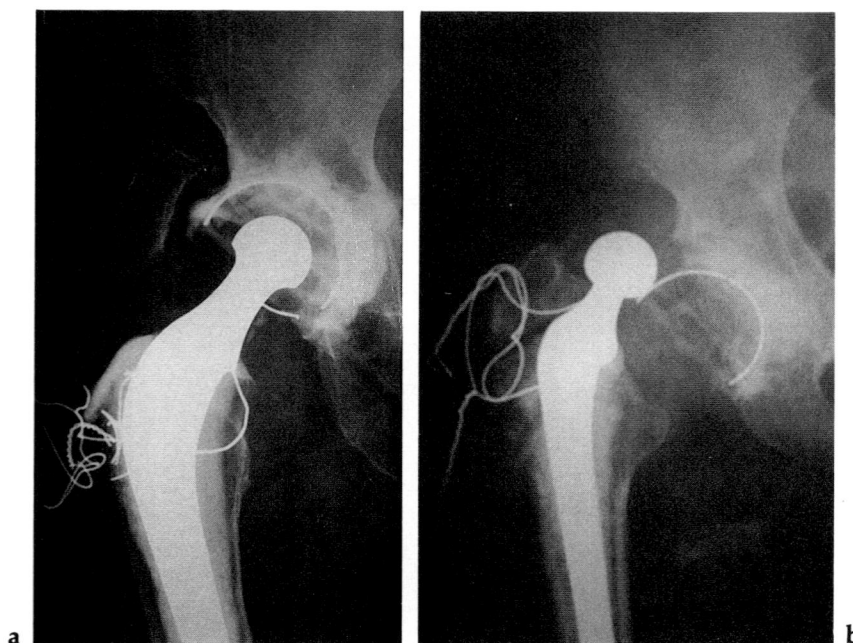

Fig. 4.9. Trochanteric reattachment – a problem? **a** The trochanter cannot be expected to unite to acrylic cement. **b** Long loops show lack of appreciation of the method of fixation.

Table 4.2. Identifiable causes of trochanteric pain

Cause	No.	% of whole group
Projecting trochanteric wires	34	6.9
Trochanteric non-union	22	4.5
Trochanteric union with displacement	19	3.9
Heterotopic ossification	21	4.3
Deep sepsis	12	2.4
Degenerative changes of lumbar spine (referred pain)	10	2.0
Loosening of components	5	1.0
Total	123	25.0

trochanter, an essential step before trochanteric osteotomy; to fail to do this is to run the risk of picking up the sciatic nerve.

Until the advent of total hip arthroplasty, trochanteric bursitis had not featured prominently in the orthopaedic literature. Since then it has commonly been used as an argument against trochanteric osteotomy. (It is cases such as those shown in Fig. 4.9 that give this method of exposure a bad reputation.) That trochanteric bursitis can follow total hip replacement even without osteotomy is a fact that is not well documented. Also that gross crepitus over the trochanteric area is often asymptomatic is not usually appreciated. What is beyond argument is that repeated surgery, using the same skin incision, often results in loss of the subcutaneous fat and some degree of tenderness over the scar though not necessarily over the most prominent trochanteric area. Whatever the label attached to this very definite clinical entity, any patient undergoing revision surgery must be made aware of and accept this nuisance aspect of the operation.

Trochanteric bursitis can be defined as pain or tenderness localized to the area of the greater trochanter severe enough to affect the result of the operation and necessitate the patient to seek advice and treatment. Hook reviewed the results (as yet unpublished) of 12 100 Charnley low-friction arthroplasties (LFAs) where trochanteric osteotomy had been performed. His findings can be summarized as follows: of the 12 100 cases, 491 had trochanteric pain – an incidence of 4%. The majority of those with pain were treated successfully by local infiltration of the tender area with a mixture of 1% lignocaine and a steroid. In the remaining 123 (25.0%), the causes were identified as shown in Table 4.2.

Trochanteric Non-union

Trochanteric non-union per se is seldom, if ever, an indication for surgical intervention. That a very careful assessment of the problem is essential is obvious from the review carried out by Hook. Exploration for trochanteric non-union must not be undertaken lightly for fear of being faced with a full-scale revision unprepared and without any guarantee of achieving success.

In Hook's series, exploration and attempted reattachment in 16 patients with trochanteric non-union failed to achieve either union or relief of symptoms. In a series reported by Fraser and Wroblewski (1981) bony union was achieved only in four out of ten such cases. In each one of them an element of compression was incorporated in the method of fixation of the greater trochanter.

Three problems can really be attributed to trochanteric non-union: pain, limp and dislocation.

Pain

Pain, or more often discomfort or tenderness, over the trochanteric area is not a constant finding in cases of non-union. It is surprising how often the patient is unaware of the radiological problem as judged by clinical methods of observation of the patient or hip function. What is interesting is that it may distract the surgeon's attention from other pathology, deep sepsis or loosening of the stem being the most serious of these. If need be, careful observation over a period of 6–9 months using serial radiographs will often reveal the true cause. During that time the symptoms from the non-union would be expected to have subsided. Non-steroidal analgesics/anti-inflammatory drugs and use of a stick in the opposite hand may be of help. Local steroid injections are best avoided unless the diagnosis of sepsis is excluded. Bacteriology of aspirate of the joint or the local area may be of value.

Limp

That limp should result from trochanteric non-union due to the defective function of the abductors is not unexpected. What is unexpected is that it is the degree of trochanteric displacement rather than the non-union per se that is responsible. This has been pointed out by Nutton and Checketts (1984). Presumably whether the abductors act through a bony or a fibrous union is of little consequence; what matters is the effective length of the muscles. It could be expected that with time some degree of adaptation will take place and during this period the use of support in the opposite hand is to be advocated. It is, however, aesthetically pleasing and clinically desirable to achieve bony union in all cases, if possible. Then at least the surgeon can be confident that the mechanics of the hip joint have been restored to normal and a possible cause of complication avoided.

Dislocation

That trochanteric non-union, and with it the loss of the stabilizing action of the abductor mechanism, may be a potent, albeit rare, cause of dislocation has been pointed out before (Fraser and Wroblewski 1981).

A single dislocation, although very alarming to the patient, need not be a source of worry.

Manipulation under general anaesthetic when reducing the hip will also give an opportunity to assess the position which allows the hip to dislocate. Until recently the routine practice following dislocation has been a 3-week period of bed rest with an abduction mattress. As the pressure on beds has increased it is now the author's practice to mobilize the patient as soon as the pain has settled, usually after several days. Coupled with well-directed exercises this is probably more logical than the inactivity of bed rest. There is however, a need to support this statement by results.

Recurrent dislocation, however, soon undermines a patient's confidence due to the inability to rely on the hip, especially in situations where quick action, with the hip in flexion and internal rotation, is required. The subject is discussed at length in Chap. 5. Suffice it to say here that treatment of such cases can be the most taxing of all revisions and requires careful assessment and, if need be, well-directed surgery which may turn out to be a full-scale revision.

5 Dislocation

Management of recurrent dislocation is one of the most taxing aspects of revision surgery.

In the primary surgery, post-operative dislocation will be avoided by the surgeon's familiarity with the particular technique and the components. In the operative management of dislocation familiarity with all aspects of revision surgery is essential.

Introduction

Except for rare cases of neurological abnormalities, senility or possibly alcoholism, the dislocation of the head of the femoral component out of the socket will be evident to the patient and may be dramatic, bringing the patient to the immediate attention of the surgeon. The complication has been studied on many occasions. Etienne et al. (1978) reviewed 8526 low-friction arthroplasties performed during two consecutive periods. The incidence of post-operative dislocation was reduced from 0.8% to 0.4%. The study indicated that familiarity with the components and the details of the operative technique are the most important aspect in avoiding the complication; the results improve with increasing experience.

In a review of 14 672 Charnley LFAs where the transtrochanteric approach was used routinely the incidence of dislocation was 0.63% (92

cases). Only 16 of these dislocation cases (0.11%) came to revision (Fraser and Wroblewski 1981). In the same study 21 cases revised were analysed in some detail. Five of them (24%) had at least one further dislocation following revision. This patter of high incidence of dislocation following the revision (and previous hip surgery) has been reflected in other studies and has, in some, been the most common complication.

It would appear that with the increasing number of revisions being performed the problem of dislocation following the revision will increase proportionately (Fig. 5.1). The

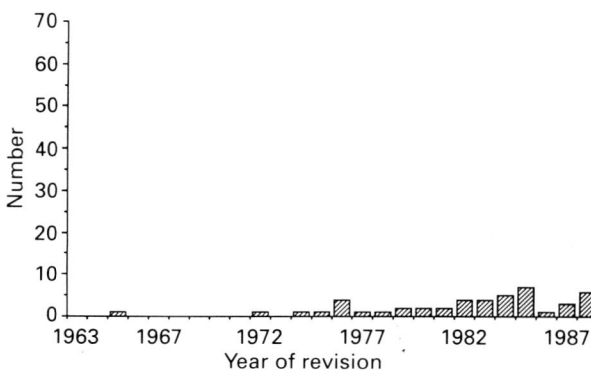

Fig. 5.1. Revisions for dislocation. Not a common problem until 1974, the 12th year of the evolution of the Charnley LFA. Incidence not particularly high but steadily increasing. (All LFAs, primaries, conversions and revisions, are included.)

Table 5.1. Dislocation after total hip replacement

Type of prosthesis	No. of cases	No. of dislocations	% of dislocations
Charnley (after Khan et al. 1981)	4 205	89	2.1
Howse (after Khan et al. 1981)	1 146	21	1.8
McKee (after Khan et al. 1981)	782	16	2.0
Ring (after Khan et al. 1981)	329	7	2.1
Stanmore (after Khan et al. 1981)	312	9	2.9
Charnley (Fraser and Wroblewski 1981)	14 672	92	0.63

study and the development of methods of prevention and management of this complication must, therefore, proceed in pace with revision surgery. Although a single dislocation may not be a problem, once it becomes recurrent it very rapidly undermines a patient's confidence until they learn to avoid it or cope with it.

It is interesting to note that neither the size of the head nor the trochanteric osteotomy used routinely at the time of the exposure are considered as major causes of the complication. It may in fact be argued that the opposite is true, i.e. with an inadequate exposure to allow proper positioning and orientation of the components even a relatively large head of the femoral component or tight reduction is no safeguard against this complication (Table 5.1) (Khan et al. 1981).

The Mechanism of Dislocation

The exact mechanism by which the head of the femoral component loses contact with the bore of the socket has not received detailed attention. Some light may be shed on the subject when the following aspects of the operation are considered.

The components have no mechanism by which joint sensation can be conveyed to the patient. It is therefore in the early post-operative stages that dislocation is likely to occur. With time, as the new capsule forms and grips the neck of the stem, stability is provided to the joint. The new capsule, presumably having some innervation, plus the re-education of the surrounding muscles, does give protection against an excessive range of movements.

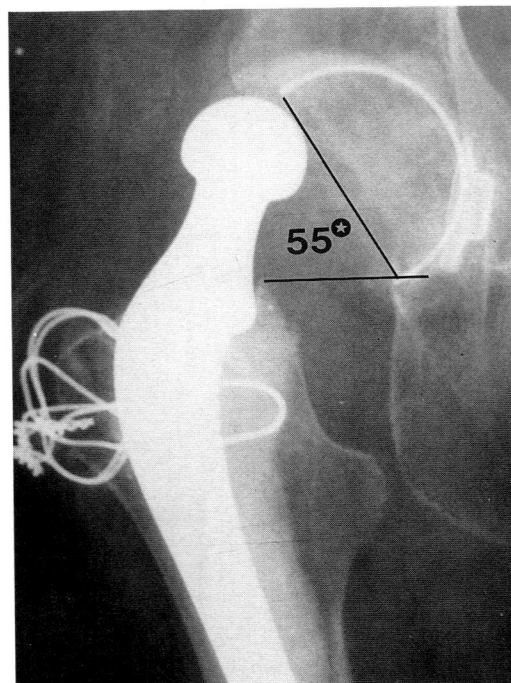

Fig. 5.2. Vertical socket. Angle open laterally measured 55°. The hip dislocated in flexion, adduction and internal rotation.

Impingement

For a dislocation to occur, the range of movement must exceed the limit of the design. The head of the femoral component must come out of the bore of the socket, reach a point of no return and lose contact with the socket bore completely. This is most likely to occur following impingement of the neck of the stem on the rim of the socket. Since the hip functions mainly in flexion, or flexion adduction and internal rotation, it is the retroversion of the socket and/or of the stem that will be the most potent cause of dislocation. In the same context a vertical socket (a socket open excessively laterally) should be considered (Fig. 5.2).

Alternatively, impingement of the neck of the femur on the anterior acetabular rim, on an osteophyte or on extruded cement (Fig. 5.3) is also likely to lead to the same problem. The dislocation in such cases will be posterior. Excessive anteversion of the socket and/or stem will tend to dislocate the hip in extension and external rotation, as when turning away from

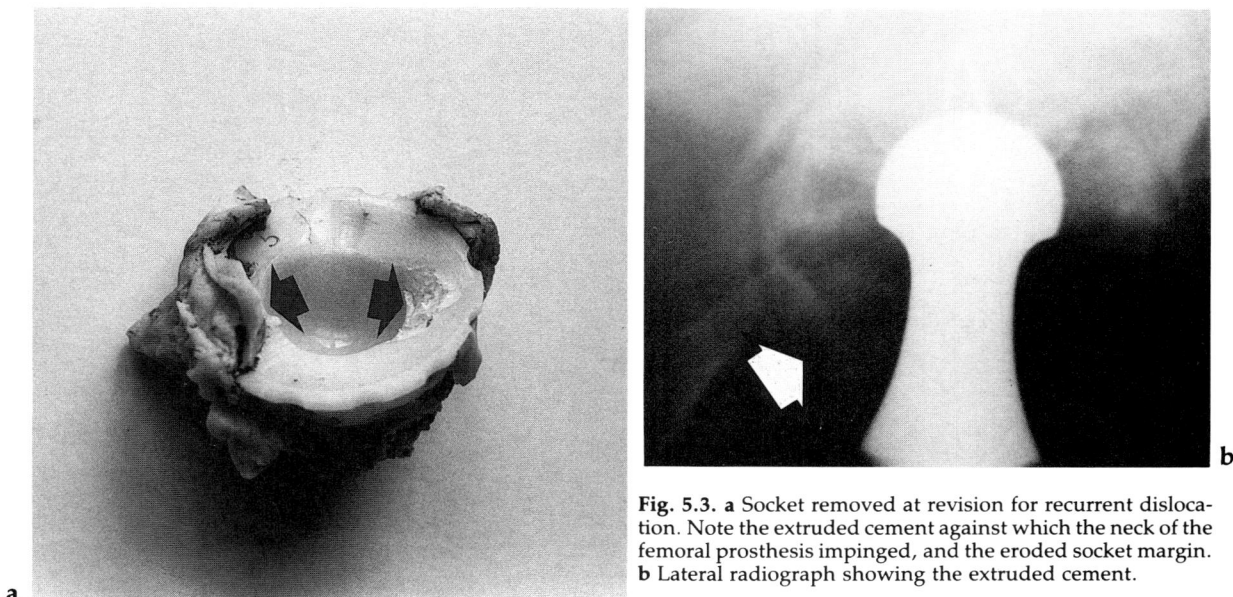

Fig. 5.3. a Socket removed at revision for recurrent dislocation. Note the extruded cement against which the neck of the
femoral prosthesis impinged, and the eroded socket margin.
b Lateral radiograph showing the extruded cement.

the weight-bearing leg, the dislocation this time
being anterior.

Another mechanism comes into play when
the shear bulk of the thigh is able to lever the
head out of the socket without impingement
occurring.

Distraction

In some cases the weight of the limb itself may
allow distraction of the joint. This may be most
obvious when the affected limb is shorter than
the other limb, or when advancing age or disease
result in loss of weight and muscle tone. The
problem presents as a click when walking down
an incline or descending stairs. With the head of
the femoral component subluxed out of the
socket, an unguarded rotation may prevent its
return to the correct position, the dislocation
occurring with remarkable ease. This mechanism resulting in dislocation must be carefully
studied in the cases of proximal femoral replacement and revisions with extensive soft tissue
resection.

Loss of the stabilizing action of the proximal
femoral musculature in general, and the abductors in particular, allows the head to slip out of
the socket by the shear weight of the non-
weight-bearing limb (Fig. 5.4).

Whichever the mechanism, the dislocated
head rides up due to muscle spasm making the
exact mechanism of dislocation difficult to establish. It is in this particular group of cases that the
role played by the diameter of the head of the
femoral component must be carefully studied.

Dislocation Following Primary Surgery

Following primary surgery, mechanical causes
leading to dislocation have been identified as
follows (Fraser and Wroblewski 1981):

1. Loss of the abductor mechanism.
2. Shortening of the limb.
3. Malorientation of components.

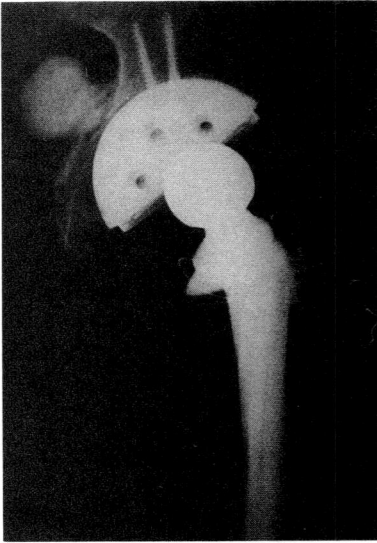

Fig. 5.4. Dislocation by distraction. The weight of the limb is sufficient to distract and dislocate the hip. A common cause in cases of gross shortening and absence of the proximal femoral musculature.

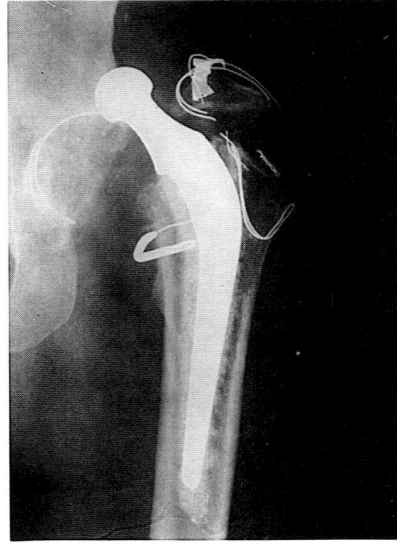

Fig. 5.5. Trochanteric non-union with dislocation. It must not be assumed that the obvious (trochanteric non-union) is the only cause of the problem when revision is being considered.

Loss of the Abductor Mechanism

In cases where trochanteric osteotomy has been used routinely in primary surgery, trochanteric non-union is a potent, albeit comparatively rare, cause of dislocation (Fig. 5.5). Failure of trochanteric union leads to loss of the stabilizing action of the abductors and the lateral part of the capsule, especially in the early post-operative period. With time, formation of the new capsule and "readjustment" of abductors acting through a fibrous union of the trochanter stabilizes the hip and makes it unnecessary to attempt to reattach every un-united trochanter. Provided clear instructions are given to the patient about which movements are to be avoided and about the recommended use of support (sticks or crutches), this is usually all that is required.

The recent upsurge of various approaches based on the original MacFarland–Osborne work has contributed to this problem to some degree. During the exposure, part of the gluteus medius is elevated from the bone with or without a thin shell of the greater trochanter. The fact that that part of the muscle may become replaced by fibrous tissue or involved in gross heterotopic ossification is not readily appreciated. At times it may actually by-pass the greater trochanter and join to the fascia of the vastus lateralis, thus allowing unconstrained rotation and recurrent dislocation (Redfern and Wroblewski 1989).

Shortening of the Limb

This is usually due to high placement of the socket and/or low sectioning of the femoral neck (Fig. 5.6). Charnley introduced the concept of "transverse reaming" and anatomical placement of the socket in relation to the tear drop. This part of the operation is further facilitated by routine exposure of the tear drop both at primary and revision surgery.

It may be of some practical help, if only for the purpose of the placement of the acetabular component, if the problems are considered according to the position of the acetabulum as seen on the pre-operative radiograph. Thus all cases can be divided into three groups: those with a high, with an anatomical or with a low acetabulum (Fig. 5.7).

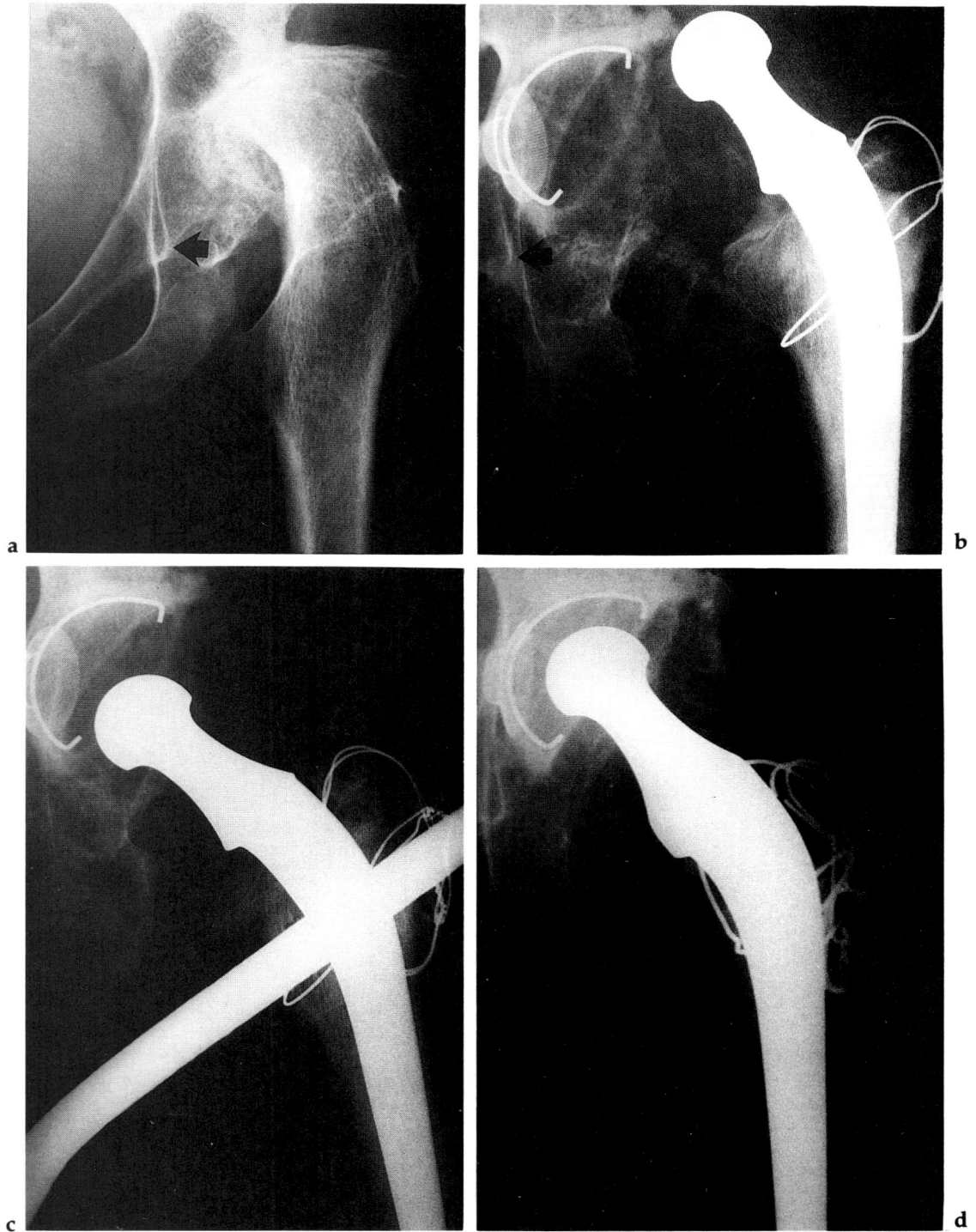

Fig. 5.6. The problem of shortening. **a** Congenital dysplasia with a high-riding femoral head. **b** Socket placed high with respect to the "tear drop"; femoral neck sectioned to the level of the greater trochanter. The result is an immediate post-operative dislocation. **c** Attempt to treat the dislocation on Thomas's splint clearly demonstrates distraction due to shortening. **d** Problem solved, in this case, by the use of the extended neck stem.

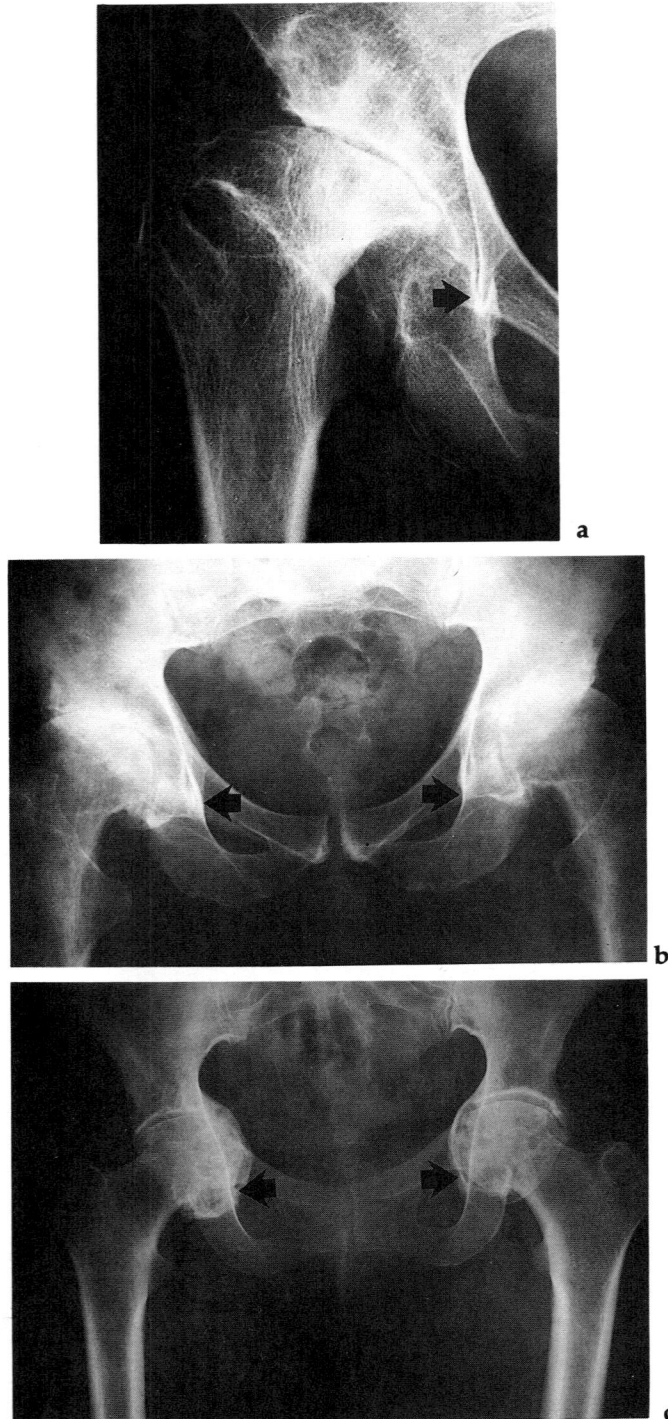

Fig. 5.7a–c. High, anatomical and low acetabuli, with respect to the "tear drop". **a** High acetabulum. Proximal migration of the acetabulum. The hallmark of congenital dysplasia and dislocation. Also a feature of the upper pole grade III arthritic changes. **b** Anatomical acetabulum. Acetabulum remains anatomical in position; the disease process affects the articular surfaces or the femoral neck. Concentric and protrusio type arthritis, fracture of the femoral neck. **c** Low acetabulum. The floor of the acetabulum bulges into the obturator foramen. Arthritis, invariably of the protrusio type.

The High Acetabulum

In this group the acetabulum is higher than the normal anatomical position. This could be due to abnormal development, as in various grades of congenital dysplasia or dislocation, or due to disease processes whereby the roof of the acetabulum is eroded allowing proximal migration of the fermoral head, be it real or artificial.

In such cases the acetabular cup will have to be placed low with respect to the pre-operative position of the acetabulum. If reamers are used then transverse reaming is advocated. In cases of congenital dislocation or dysplasia the Charnley gauges are best used and the acetabulum prepared cautiously using the tear drop as the "bench mark". The reamers are best avoided. It is obvious that in such cases a thick crescent of cement will usually be present above the socket.

The Anatomical Acetabulum

In this group the acetabulum is more-or-less anatomical in position. However, shortening of the limb is due to disease processes involving the articular surfaces or the proximal femur. Included in this group are fracture of the neck of the femur, quadrantic head necrosis, concentric, medial pole type and cases of protrusio. Here the acetabulum usually needs only to be curetted followed by the usual preparation for the cement injection. There is no need to perforate the floor or to use the deepening acetabular reamers.

The Low Acetabulum

This finding is rare and is invariably of the protrusio variety where the floor of the acetabulum actually bulges towards the obturator foramen. The femoral neck is short and in a varus position. Here the acetabulum needs only to be curetted and the neck cut short or a shorter neck stem used to avoid overlengthening.

For practical purposes the identification of the transverse ligament and the tear drop are the most useful aspects of the exposure of the acetabulum, both in primary and revision surgery, and their positions serve as a constant bench mark for the level of the placement of the acetabular component. Identifying the correct level at which to section the femoral neck is made easy by the routine use of the Charnley Adjustable Trial Prosthesis (ATP). Although the design of the ATP may appear complicated the objective is simple; i.e. to centralize the stem within the medullary canal and to maintain that position at trial reduction and definitive stem fixation while allowing correct level of section of the fermoral neck using the appropriate offset and neck length stem. The intramedullary blade maintains the central placement of the stem, the drill guide determines the position of the neck-stem notch which in turn gives the level of the section of the femoral neck and the final position of the stem.

Every effort must be made to achieve stability and to correct leg length. This applies to cases of unilateral hip disease but obviously may not be possible in other cases. In the final analysis, stability of the newly implanted total joint must take priority over leg-length equality. This fact must be made clear to the patient before surgery.

Malorientation of the Components

Correct orientation of the components is essential if stability is to be ensured. Full exposure not only of the hip joint but of the acetabulum, the femoral neck and the canal is essential for the proper alignment of the components. In this respect, a lateral, transtrochanteric approach offers the best possible exposure, more so in difficult and revision cases.

The Socket

When considering the anteversion/retroversion of the socket using the lateral approach the following clinical observations must be taken into account.

With the patient supine the shoulders are square and more-or-less "fixed" to the operating table. At dislocation and exposure of the acetabulum the femur on the operated side lies across the opposite thigh, pinning the opposite hip between the thigh and the operating table. As the second assistant (the leg holder) manipulates and positions the femur, the buttock on the operated side is invariably elevated from the table. (The opposite sacroiliac area is compressed onto the table, hence any pressure areas are usually on the unoperated side.) By doing this the patient is rolled, not uniformly as in rolling a log but asymmetrically. (See Fig. 5.8. The effect is similar to that of turning the right-hand-side page of this book when the top right-hand corner of the page is fixed.) The manoeuvre anteverts

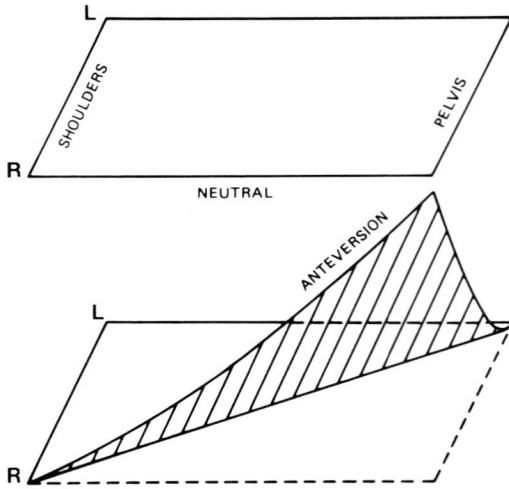

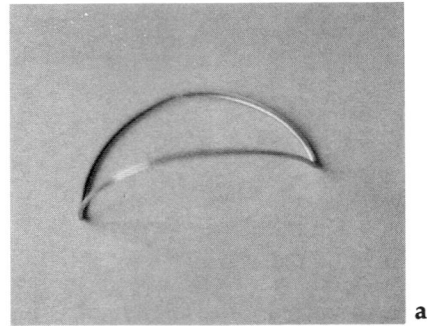

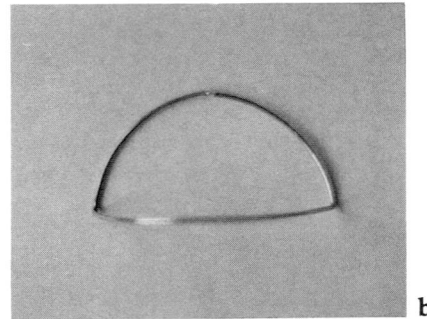

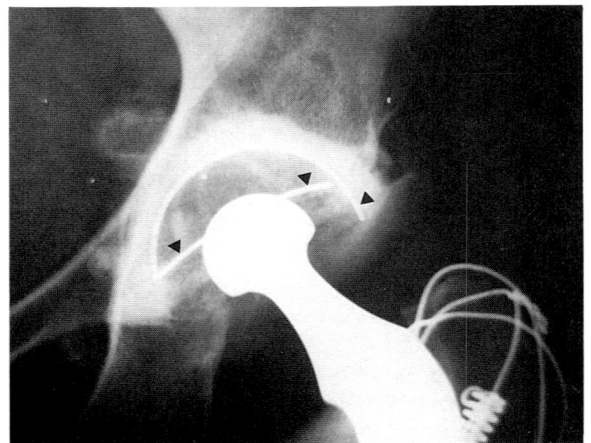

Fig. 5.8. Diagrammatic representation of the concept of acetabular anteversion at surgery. The shoulders and the opposite (left) hip are in a fixed position. Dislocation of the operated (right) hip elevates the right buttock off the operating table while the right hip is moved asymmetrically away from the table towards the opposite shoulder. The net effect is anteversion of the acetabulum with respect to the neutral. The anteversion of the acetabulum caused by the rolling of the pelvis must be compensated for when orientating the socket.

Fig. 5.9. Anteversion wire marker. **a,b** The concept is of two semicircles placed at right angles to each other, the wear marker in the coronal plane and the anteversion marker over the anterior part of the socket and at right angles to the wear marker. **c** Left LFA, socket anteverted about 5°. Lateral wear marker extension denotes left socket in correct side.

the acetabulum and it is more readily performed in slim than in obese patients. These observations must be accounted for when positioning the socket, otherwise when the normal position is restored, the socket, which was placed in neutral, would be retroverted. Thus any method of hip exposure must take this into account and have an element of anterversion built in, though at this stage the exact degree for each case or the method of its estimation is yet to be defined.

The study of orientation of the socket has been made easier by the introduction of the radiographic wire marker (Fig. 5.9) which has allowed reasonably accurate measurements of anteversion to be carried out on AP radiographs only. The marker consists of the standard wear marker placed coronally over the summit of the socket; an additional anteversion marker is then continued over the anterior margin of the socket, at right angles to the wear marker. Thus with the socket in neutral position, i.e. with its face exactly in the line of the x-ray beam, the appearance is that of the wear marker as a semicircle, while the anteversion marker forms a straight line, resembling the string of a bow at rest. The anteversion marker will appear curved towards the wear marker when the socket is anteverted and away from it when the socket is retroverted.

Since the anteversion marker moves across the line of the x-ray beam it is sensitive to changes of the position of the x-ray tube or the patient. (The femoral artery at the groin is a

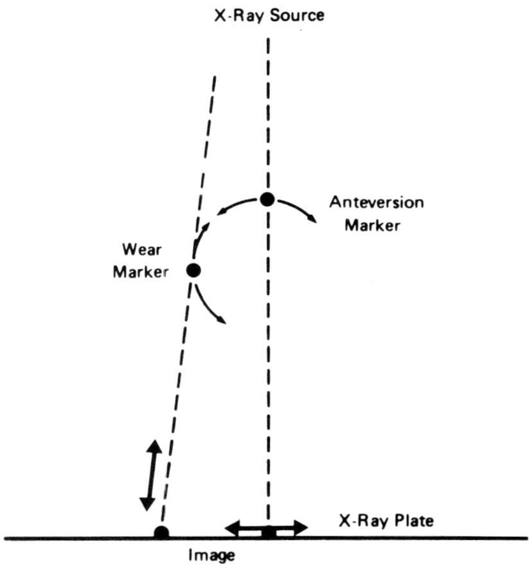

Fig. 5.10. Wear and anteversion markers on the socket: diagrammatic representation of the radiographic appearances. For the wear marker to offer most information it must be placed at the summit of the socket, in the coronal place. Turning the socket into anteversion or retroversion will move the wear marker almost into the line of the x-ray beam, hence its lack of sensitivity until there has been some 15° of change in position in either direction. The anteversion marker, placed on the socket anteriorly, moves across the x-ray beam and is thus very sensitive to changes of the position (anteversion, retroversion) of the socket. This is further magnified by the x-ray plate–marker distance. Being sensitive to the distance and position of the x-ray source, it demands standardization of radiographs.

useful landmark for centring the beam.) By the same token, the wear marker, the movement of which takes place initially more-or-less in the line of the x-ray beam, is less sensitive to the position of the patient or the tube (Fig. 5.10). Extension of the wear marker laterally, past the superior part of the anteversion marker, identifies the correct side (right or left) of the angle-bore socket, giving further information.

The Stem

In order to place the stem correctly and to achieve its sound fixation within the medullary canal, correct exposure is essential. A limited approach through the sectioned femoral neck only directs the tip of the stem laterally and posteriorly because of the anterverted position of the femoral neck (Fig. 5.11).

It is not readily appreciated that when inserting the stem, be it in a hemi or a total hip arthroplasty, the position of the intramedullary portion of the prosthesis should determine the position of the head and neck of the stem. If an attempt is made to introduce the stem through a limited exposure of the femoral neck only, then the head and the neck will determine the position of the intramedullary portion, with obvious consequences (Fig. 5.12).

Unless trochanteric osteotomy is carried out to allow direct access to the medullary canal, the greater trochanter must be excavated at its posterior aspect. In this context trochanteric osteotomy offers unparalleled exposure both for the preparation of the femur and for orientation and fixation of the stem.

Tight Reduction

A suggestion that a tight hip reduction in some way implies stability of the joint is not necessarily correct. Apart from the likelihood of leading to overlengthening and trochanteric detachment, a tight reduction is likely to be counterproductive. Stretching of the muscle fibres is likely to lead to loss of proprioception and tone and to laxity and thus instability. Since muscle tone is regained once the action of the muscle relaxant has worn off, there is no need to fear a trial reduction which is less than tight.

Early Dislocation

Some of the causes of early dislocation have already been discussed. Excluding cases of obvious component malposition or malorientation, the vast majority of cases will settle with conservative treatment. Only those that become recurrent or irreducible will require surgical intervention.

Early Irreducible Dislocation

This usually happens when an early dislocation has been missed for one reason or another, and the patient presents with a high dislocation which it is not possible to reduce by closed manipulation under general anaesthesia and using full muscle relaxants. In this group are also the cases where the head of the femoral component buttonholes through the capsule and the abductor mass. Open reduction is indicated.

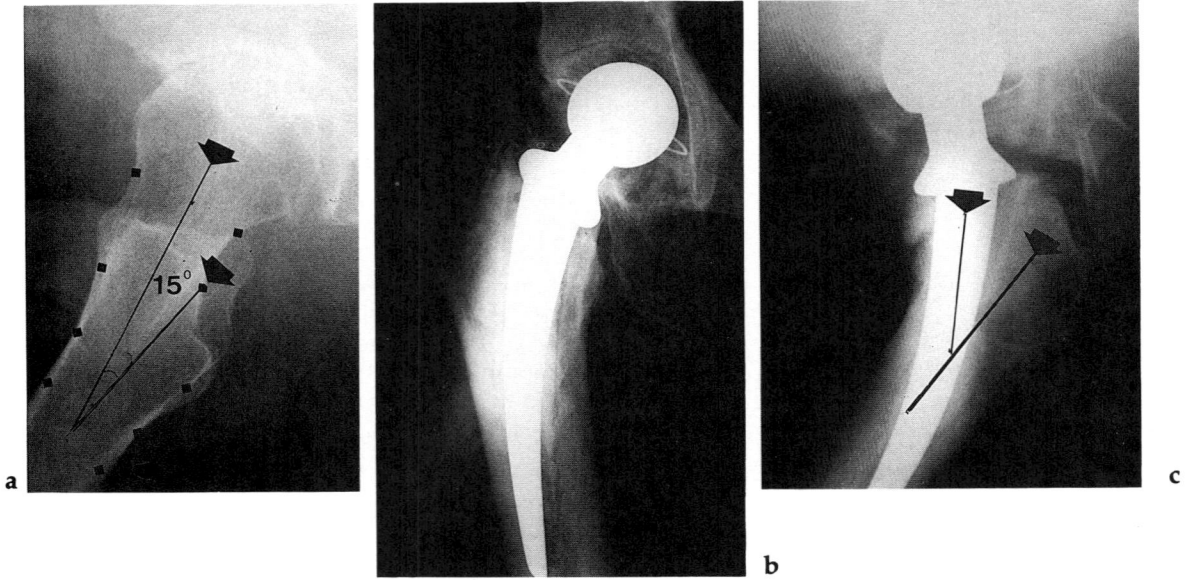

Fig. 5.11. a Lateral radiograph of the hip. Note the relationship between the neck and the shaft of the femur: an anteversion of 15°. Correct direction for stem entry. **b** AP radiograph after total hip replacement. **c** Lateral radiograph clearly shows that the femoral neck was used as the guide for insertion of the stem into the medullary canal. Anteversion of the prosthesis follows anteversion of the femoral neck.

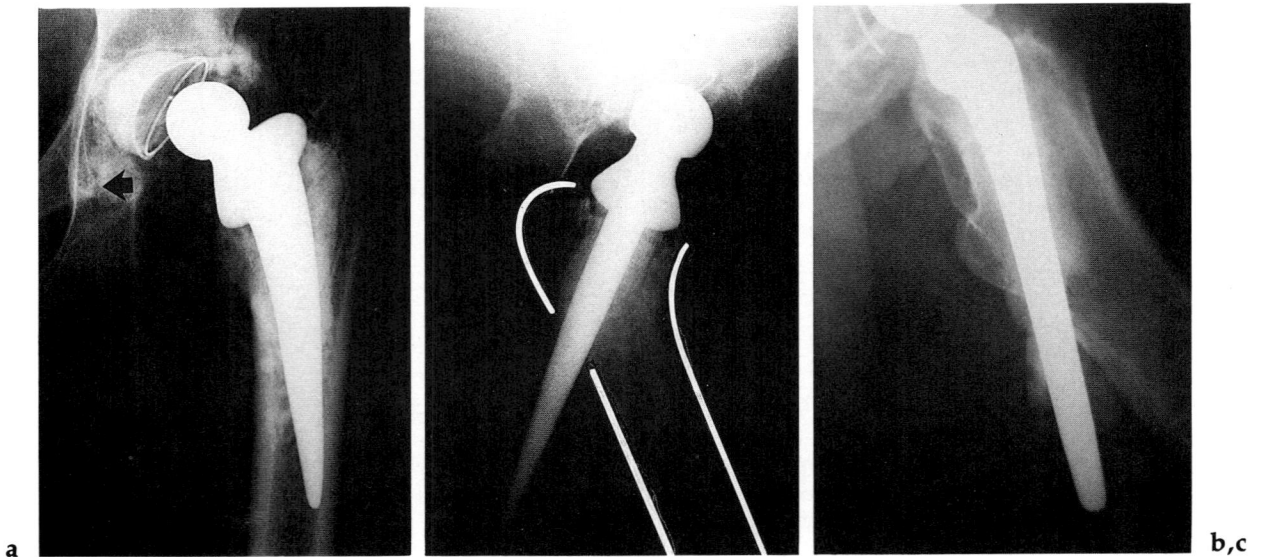

Fig. 5.12. a,b Limited exposure. In this case the anteverted neck of the femur is used as a guide for access to the medullary canal, with obvious consequences. The shaft of the femur is outlined in white. The socket is also placed high with respect to the "tear drop". **c** A further example of a similar problem.

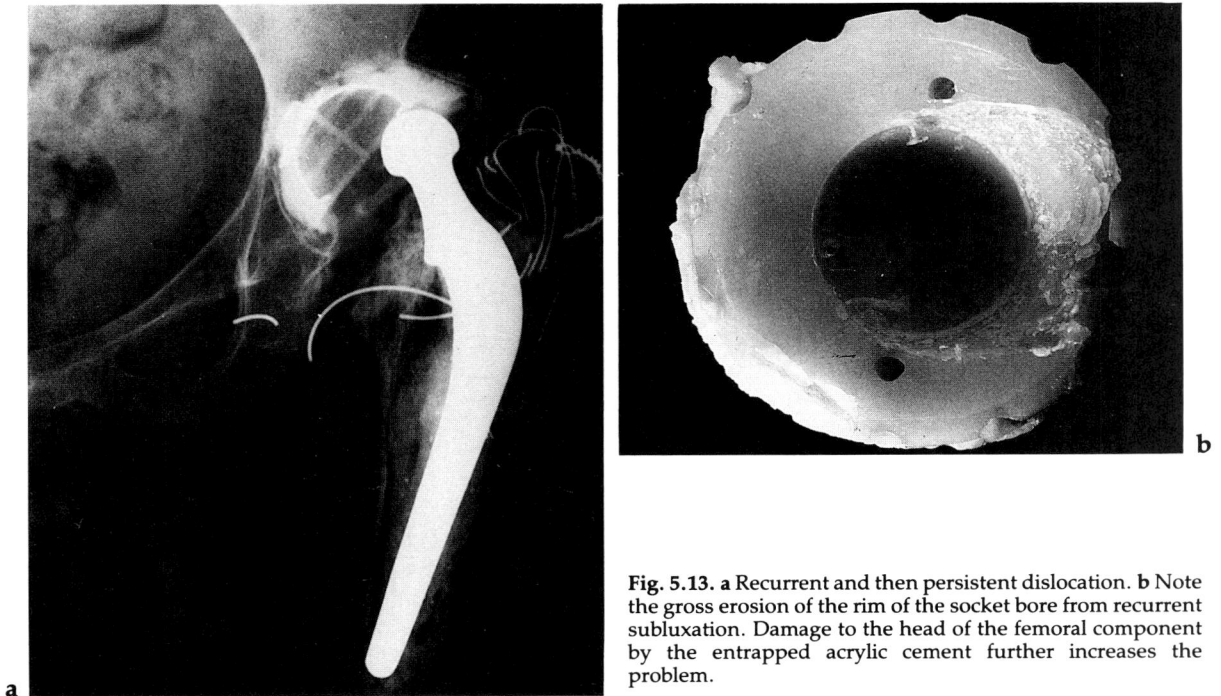

Fig. 5.13. a Recurrent and then persistent dislocation. b Note the gross erosion of the rim of the socket bore from recurrent subluxation. Damage to the head of the femoral component by the entrapped acrylic cement further increases the problem.

Recurrent Dislocation

An obvious abnormality which has led to a dislocation and has not been corrected is likely to lead to recurrent dislocation. Malorientation of the components, loss of the proximal femoral musculature and shortening of the limb are the causes in order of decreasing frequency. With repeated episodes of subluxation or dislocation, erosion of the margin of the socket bore occurs allowing the head to slip in and out on the slightest unguarded movement. The patient can usually reproduce these at will and without too much discomfort. At revision, not only can the socket rim erosion be seen (Fig. 5.13) and the area of impingement of the neck on the socket rim, but also the lax stretched capsule and the voluminous cavity created secondarily by the repeated "escapes" of the head are apparent. The firm sleeve of the capsule gripping the femoral neck is absent.

Late Dislocation

Why some hips dislocate after years of trouble-free function is not immediately obvious (Fig. 5.14). Excluding single traumatic episodes three other possibilities must be considered.

Loss of Muscle Tone. Loss of muscle tone and power and loss of weight for whatever reason will result in laxity of a joint that has hitherto been stable. The head may literally slip out of the socket due to the weight of the limb alone. This appears to be more common in elderly females.

Socket Wear. So far, socket wear has not been identified as a cause of late dislocation. However, the mechanism is simple to imagine. As the socket wears, the head bores for itself a new, roughly cylindrical path. The angular range of movements becomes progressively restricted, the neck impinging on the rim of the socket bore. With time this will lead to socket loosening and change of its position which may lead to dislocation.

Minor Episodes of Subluxation. These may pass unnoticed. The head of the femoral component gradually erodes the rim of the socket bore until it can no longer be contained; dislocation results, sometimes after years of apparently trouble-free function.

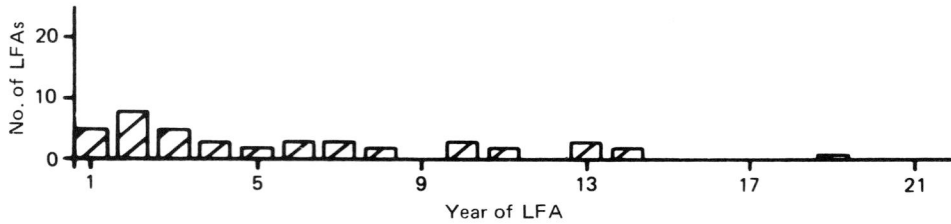

Fig. 5.14. Incidence of revision for dislocation in relation to the post-operative follow-up. Gradual reduction in numbers after the second year. Note some cases presenting many years later.

Dislocation Following Revision Surgery

Following revision surgery, four other potent causes of dislocation must be carefully considered.

1. Excision of the capsule.
2. Loss of tissue turgor.
3. Use of extended neck stems.
4. Absent proximal femur.

Excision of the Capsule. This usually forms part of the procedure in one-stage revisions for deep sepsis. The restraining action of the fibrous capsule is lost. The muscles around the hip joint, being more elastic, will not prevent over-distraction except by "active action". The laxity of the arthroplasty at trial reduction may be an obvious feature. It is for this reason alone that the arthroplasty should be protected for some weeks until the new capsule has formed. Bed rest, avoidance of excessive movement and use of support are advocated.

Loss of Tissue Turgor. Tissue oedema around the arthroplasty is an obvious feature especially in cases where the patient's function has been poor for some time, and is very evident in cases of deep sepsis and persistent dislocation. Following successful revision and bed rest the oedema settles quite rapidly and what was a stable joint at trial reduction may become a very lax and unstable joint some days later. A 3-week bed rest following revision for deep sepsis or persistent dislocation is the recommended minimum and even then use of external splints should be considered.

Use of Extended Neck Prosthesis. It is not often realized that the use of extended neck stems may be a potent cause of dislocation. Although the neck length is increased thus increasing the limb length and apparently improving the stability, the available design demands an increase in the neck–shaft angle in order to maintain or even to reduce the offset and thus compensate for the effect of increasing the length of the extra-femoral unsupported part of the stem.

Let us examine this in detail. A conventional stem design has three integral parts: (a) the head and neck, (b) the relatively straight intramedullary portion and (c) the curved part connecting the two.

Accepting that the angle between the head and neck and the straight portion of the stem remains unaltered then the length of the connecting curved portion will determine the offset (the longer the portion the greater the offset). Increase of the neck length will increase the offset thus increasing the bending moment and effectively weakening the stem. To reduce the effect of this and then further reduce the offset the neck–shaft angle must be increased. This has a twofold effect: it brings the shaft of the femur close to the pelvis and it alters the relationship between the socket and the angle of inclination of the femoral component. The first is more likely to lever the head out of the socket, particularly if the thigh is bulky which is especially the case in obese patients; the second makes the socket relatively more vertical with respect to the head of the femoral component.

All these problems can be further compounded by insistence on a valgus orientation of the stem. Any malorientation of the component

Table 5.2. Incidence of post-operative dislocations in various series

Operation	No. of LFAs	No. of dislocations	% dislocations	Reference
Primary				
Charnley LFA	14 672	92	0.63	Fraser and Wroblewski (1981)
Revision				
Fractured stem	120	6	5.0	Wroblewski (1982b)
Deep infection (one stage)	102	13	12.7	Wroblewski (1986b)
Dislocation	21	5	24	Fraser and Wroblewski (1981)

will further add to the problem. In such a situation internal rotation of the femur will effectively completely eliminate the offset of the stem. All the above, plus flexion, are likely to lead to dislocation.

Absent Proximal Femur. This, unfortunately, is an increasingly common problem. Delayed and repeated revisions result in the loss of the proximal femoral bone stock, and very often in loss of the abductor muscles. In such cases proximal femoral replacement may have to be considered. The absence of the abductors results in uncontrolled and excessive rotation and the possibility of joint distraction. (Excessive and uncontrolled rotation "winds up" the capsule around the extramedullary portion of the stem thus stretching it and making it lax.) Both of these are very potent causes of dislocation. No solution is as yet forthcoming though some aspects are discussed on pages 42–45. It may be of practical interest to record here the incidence of post-operative dislocation in various groups studied, following both primary and revision surgery (Table 5.2). The problem is clearly highlighted by the increasing incidence from primary surgery to revision for recurrent dislocation.

Deep Haematoma

Recently, new information has come to light and is worth noting. It concerns the finding reported by Woo and Morrey (1982) and then confirmed by Coventry (1985): "the pseudocapsule was so stretched out that it offered no intrinsic support". Although this may be considered to be secondary to recurrent dislocation this is not necessarily the case; there may be an alternative explanation.

An opportunity presented itself to explore two cases of dislocation which occurred within 3 months of revision surgery. It was striking that there was not only a complete absence of capsule which "gripped" the neck of the stem but also that the whole cavity containing the implant was grossly distended with what was obviously a resolving deep haematoma. The cavity extended from the pelvic brim to below the lesser trochanter with some ramifications between the various muscle planes. The cavity was lined with a thin layer of shining, smooth granulation tissue which had extended to all the areas of the cavity including the bony surfaces of the un-united trochanter and its bed.

The finding almost certainly represents an encapsulated deep haematoma which distends the joint cavity, prevents formation of the capsule and allows the joint to dislocate by the same mechanism as does the collection of pus in septic arthritis.

Practical Approach to Dislocation: Non-operative Methods

It is essential to make a positive diagnosis of dislocation before embarking on treatment and in this context radiological evidence is mandatory. In the majority of cases the diagnosis is never in doubt – the patient presents with a dislocated total hip. A "click" or description of a single subluxation followed by the dramatic relief of spontaneous reduction and several days of discomfort are worthy of notice, as in the movement that had caused it. It is not however an indication for revision. In fact very few dislocations come to revision surgery, fortunately. At manipulation of the dislocation under general anaesthesia opportunity must be taken to assess the position or movement which led to this problem.

Until such time as revision is deemed inevitable it is essential that all the following non-operative measures are tried, unless an obvious cause is present which demands surgery:

1. Three weeks bed rest with an abduction mattress, avoiding flexion but carrying out muscle-strengthening exercises under the supervision of a physiotherapist.
2. Traction is best avoided but use of an anti-rotation tibial pin is of benefit. This may be followed by a 6-week period in plaster spica. Not all patients can or will tolerate this and it may not be practical in the obese or the elderly. In the case of the obese and elderly one of the following three methods may be appropriate.
3. The use of various bespoke or custom-made movement-blocking splints has a lot to commend.
4. The use of a back splint for the knee to avoid knee and thus hip flexion has been suggested before. This in association with early mobilization under careful supervision of a physiotherapist is worth a try.
5. Very occasionally manipulation and closed reduction followed by an adductor tenotomy, 3 weeks bed rest or use of a tibial pin to control external rotation may be of benefit.

Operative Procedures

At revision surgery all the causes of recurrent dislocation must be looked for and corrected if present. It is obvious that such an exploration cannot be carried out without dislocating the joint. It must not be assumed that a single factor, e.g. trochanteric detachment, is the cause, nor that the use of a longer neck stem will correct the problem.

When the opportunity is taken, as it must be, to check the components for impingement, loosening or wear it becomes obvious that what started off as a mere exploration may end up as a full-scale revision with the consequent risk of a further dislocation post-operatively. It is therefore essential to be prepared for a full-scale revision when exploring a total hip arthroplasty for dislocation.

Only a summary of the operative approach to dislocation will be given here to avoid repetition of details already outlined in other parts of this volume.

Limited exposure of the hip without trochanteric osteotomy is acceptable where open reduction has to be performed and where no further action is considered necessary. The opportunity must be taken, however, to identify and correct the cause of dislocation and to check the components. The various stages are summarized as follows:

1. Adequate incision to expose every part of the joint.
2. Removal of trochanteric wires, if present.
3. Biplane trochanteric osteotomy.
4. Mobilization of the upper end of the femur.
5. Careful assessment of the position of instability.
6. Dislocation of the hip and the examination of the components for position, orientation and loosening.
7. Check of the rim of the socket bore for any evidence of impingement and erosion.
8. Check for damage of the socket bore and head of the femoral component by trapped particles of acrylic cement.
9. Correction of *all* factors thought to have contributed to dislocation, as well as all the other abnormalities found incidentally.
10. Bacteriological cultures to exclude infection.
11. Secure reattachment of the greater trochanter.
12. Consider adductor tenotomy if adduction deformity is present.
13. Insert tibial pin to correct tendency to external rotation. (Essential if the abductor muscles are poor or absent.)
14. Bed rest and careful physiotherapy.
15. Slow mobilization, with the use of splints if indicated.
16. Detailed instructions to the patient on the movements and positions to be avoided.
17. More frequent follow-up, if only to keep a careful eye on the rate of the patient's progress.

Recent Advances

In the management and prevention of post-operative dislocation some recent advances have been made. Although at the time of writing results have not yet been evaluated in detail, use of the following is considered advantageous:

1. The angle-bore socket.
2. Compression fixation of the greater trochanter.
3. Use of a reduced diameter neck stem.
4. Attachment of a stabilizer to the socket rim.
5. Extended neck stems of new design.
6. The "Lotus" hip.

Angle-Bore Socket

This socket, by its design, simulates the anatomy and thus the range of movements and stability of the normal acetabulum. It moves away from the design of the standard socket which, by its symmetry, allows equal movements in all directions.

The hip naturally functions mainly in flexion, or flexion adduction and internal rotation; it does not possess the same degree of movements in extension. The natural acetabulum is deficient anteriorly and inferiorly, but offers the greatest cover to the femoral head posteriorly and superiorly. The angle-bore socket takes into account this asymmetry of movement and the need for stability in flexion adduction and internal rotation.

In the manufacture of the socket, the centre of the solid high-density polyethylene (HDP) hemisphere is approached by the drill at a predetermined angle (less than 90°) to the face. This part having been completed the socket is rotated backwards through 30° and the chamfer is cut anteriorly. The socket thus made becomes lateralized for side and cannot be reversed (Fig. 5.15). Because of the asymmetry of the bore, cover for the head of the femoral component is offered over its posterior and superior aspect. The head must be distracted by some 4 mm before dislocation will occur. The detailed analysis of the results obtained with this design is outside the scope of this work and will be presented in due course. Suffice it to say that, excluding cases where the replacement of the proximal femur has proved necessary, the incidence of post-operative dislocation in revision surgery over 4 years and 400 cases has been

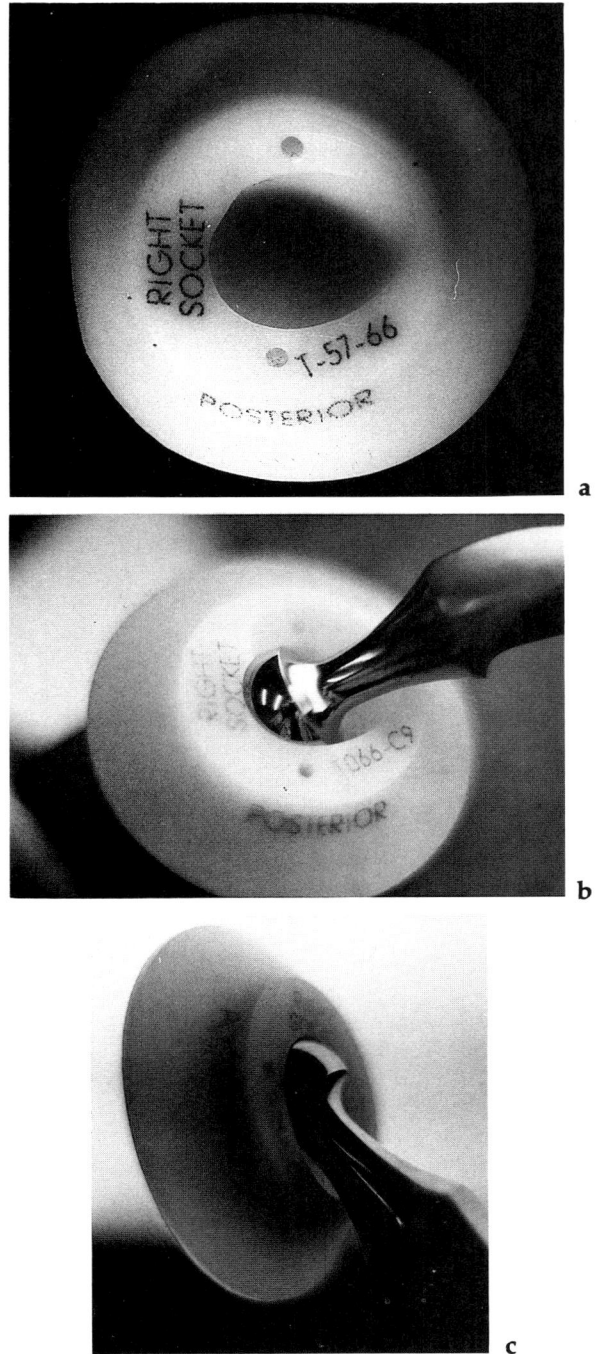

Fig. 5.15a–c. The angle-bore socket. The concept of asymmetry of socket design to simulate the anatomy of the normal acetabulum with freedom of flexion, adduction and internal rotation while maintaining stability by providing cover for the head of the femoral component postero-superiorly. The socket thus becomes "sided" for the hip and cannot be reversed. Note the stability without dislocation: the socket does not "fall off" the head when free.

reduced from 15% to 2%. The fact that using this socket gives such excellent stability at trial reduction must not be taken for granted; attention to every detail is still essential.

Compression Fixation of the Greater Trochanter

A detailed description of the technique and the results from a prospective study have already been published (Wroblewski and Shelley 1985). The technique is relatively simple but, like all cases of fixation, demands attention to detail. The incidence of non-union of the trochanter using this technique is the lowest achieved so far and has no doubt contributed in some measure to the reduction in post-operative dislocations coming to revision surgery.

The same method of trochanteric fixation (though obviously not of osteotomy) has been used in cases of revision with trochanteric non-union. Careful preparation of the trochanter and the trochanteric bed is essential.

Reduced Diameter Neck Stem

The standard Charnley stainless steel stem had a neck diameter of 12.5 mm and a head diameter of 22.25 mm; the head–neck ratio was therefore 1.78 : 1. With this system the angular range of movements possible is 90° before the neck impinges on the socket rim.

With the introduction of high-nitrogen-content stainless steel and the cold forming process for stem manufacture, a very tough stainless steel (Ortron, Chas. F. Thackray Ltd.) has been produced. Sir John Charnley was the first to recognize its potential for allowing the reduction of the diameter of the neck from 12.5 to 10 mm in order to reduce still further the incidence of dislocation. The head–neck ratio was now increased to 2.25 : 1 which is comparable to those with a larger head diameter. The stem was introduced into clinical practice in Octobesr 1983 and has been used routinely since. Its exact contribution to the reduction of post-operative dislocation in revision surgery cannot, as yet, be fully assessed because other measures are often part of the management. However, the absence of impingement of the reduced neck on the rim of the socket at trial reduction is impressive. The greatest value of the reduced diameter neck stem is probably in the long-term results where socket

wear, restriction of angular movement, impingement and socket loosening are the likely problems. This aspect is discussed in detail in Chap. 10.

Attachment of a Stabilizer to the Socket Rim

Sven Olerud was the first to point out the technique of fixing part of the socket to the socket rim to avoid recurrent dislocation (Olerud and Karlstrom 1985). This plus the natural extension of the work with the angle-bore socket has resulted in the evolution of a formal stabilizer – a separate attachment to the standard socket. It is a part of the face of the angle-bore socket and forms the posterior and superior parts. It can be fixed with two screws onto the part of the socket face where the dislocation occurs (Fig. 5.16).

The stabilizer is held on its holder and apposed to that part of the socket face where the dislocation is thought to be occurring, as judged by erosion of the rim. The joint is tested for stability and impingement and once the correct position is found a gentle tap with the mallet onto the stabilizer holder will mark the face of the socket. Two holes are cautiously drilled, using the punch marks, through the plastic and cement and into the bone. The depth is measured with a depth gauge and the appropriate length screw is used to hold the stabilizer in place. The hip is reduced, the second screw introduced and both screws then tightened. Range of movement, stability and freedom from impingement are checked. If impingement occurs anteriorly then obviously that part of the socket should be cut away with a sharp scalpel, otherwise with time the stabilizer is likely to be dislodged or the screws fractured. Care must taken to avoid creating a captive head system which is likely to lead to socket loosening.

Extended Neck Stems of New Design

The possible disadvantages of the extended neck femoral prostheses have been pointed out. Reduced offset and increased neck–shaft angle bring the femur close to the pelvis and effectively increase the "angle open laterally" of the socket. The new design incorporates the standard 40-mm offset stem. The neck length is effectively increased by bringing the flange down the shaft of the stem (Fig. 5.17). This design maintains the

Fig. 5.16. a The stabilizer; extension of the concept of the angle-bore socket. The postero-superior part of the angle-bore socket available as a separate piece, the stabilizer. **b** The two-prong stabilizer holder allows handling, correct positioning of the stabilizer and marking of the socket for drilling of the screw holes for the stabilizer attachment. **c** Eroded socket. **d** Stabilizer in place.

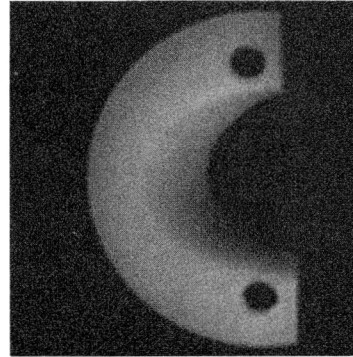

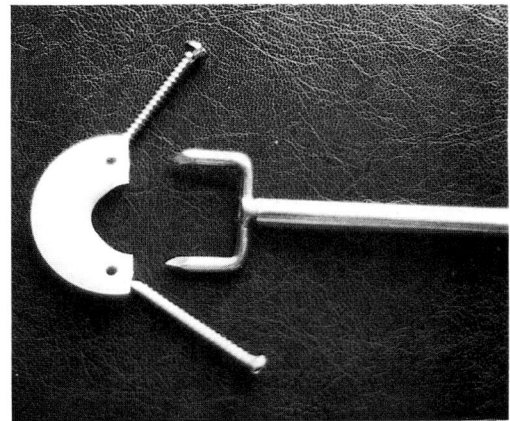

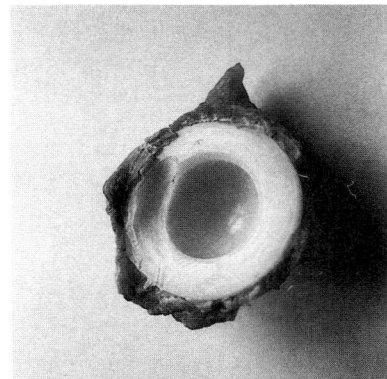

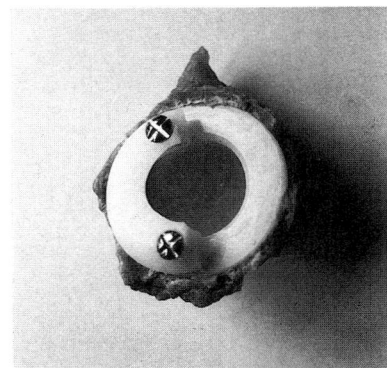

──────────────────────────────➤

a

b

c

d

offset and the configuration of the established and tested flanged series. It effectively increases the length of the neck without altering the offset or the neck–shaft angle. The gain in neck length is along the neck–shaft portion of the stem; the extramedullary portion of the stem is thus effectively reduced compared with previous designs. The same principle has been used in the design of the modular stem for proximal femoral replacement: the head–neck configuration remains constant and the effective length of the extramedullary portion is decided along the shaft of the stem.

The "Lotus" Hip

The "Lotus" hip has been designed to improve stability and prevent recurrent dislocation. In cases of loss of proximal musculature in general, and proximal femoral replacement in particular, post-operative dislocation is a serious problem. Loss of the stabilizing action of the abductors, excessive rotation and the readiness with which the hip can be distracted by gravity alone all contribute to the problem. No ideal solution exists and any attempt to solve the problem is likely to have its limitations and must prove itself in clinical practice. In such situations both the "captive head" system and the larger diameter head (28 mm) have been tried, without consistent success.

The "captive head" system invites impingement, loosening of the socket and levering out of the head, while the larger head diameter is of little benefit until it has exceeded 30 mm (an increase from 22.25 to 28 mm adds less than 3 mm only) and at the same time introduces the problem of loosening associated with the larger heads.

The new "Lotus" design (Fig. 5.18) attempts to combine the advantages of the low-frictional torque inherent in the small-diameter head (essential when under load) and the stability of the large captive head while at the same time

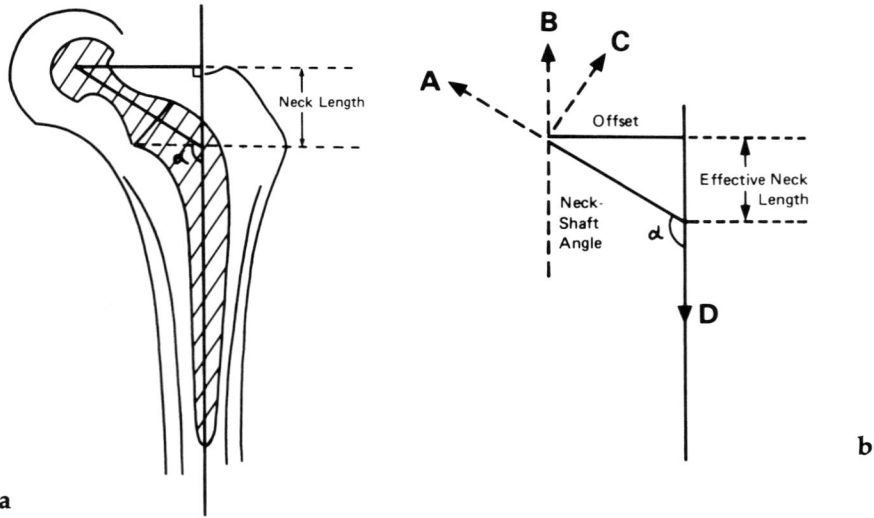

Fig. 5.17. The effective neck length. **a** Template of the femoral stem superimposed on the proximal femur. Note the effective neck length and the neck–shaft angle α. **b** Diagrammatic representation of the effect of increasing the neck length in various directions and the resulting changes in the offset and neck–shaft angles. *A*, neck–shaft angle unchanged, offset increased; *B*, offset unchanged, neck–shaft angle increased; *C*, neck–shaft angle increased, offset reduced; *D*, neck–shaft angle maintained, offset maintained, neck length increased most effectively. (The concept for revision stem design.)

having the benefit of the range of movements of a combination of the two. Thus a 22.25-mm Charnley head is combined with a 36-mm diameter hemi-arthroplasty which is in turn sited in a cemented captive HDP socket. The stability is obvious, the impingement is taken advantage of when the larger head diameter comes into function and there is an increase in the range of movements to 125° (Fig. 5.19).

The design has produced most encouraging results in cases where other methods have failed.

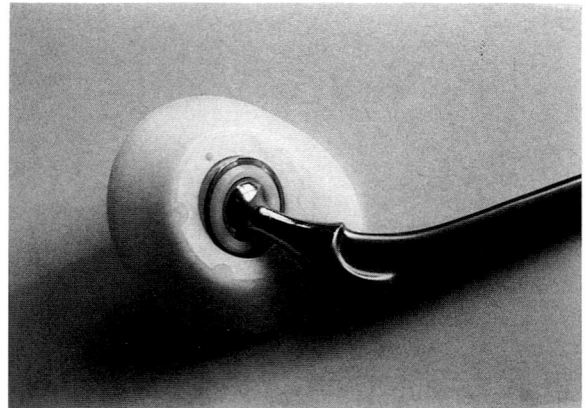

Fig. 5.18. The "Lotus" hip. A new concept to improve stability in the management of problem cases.

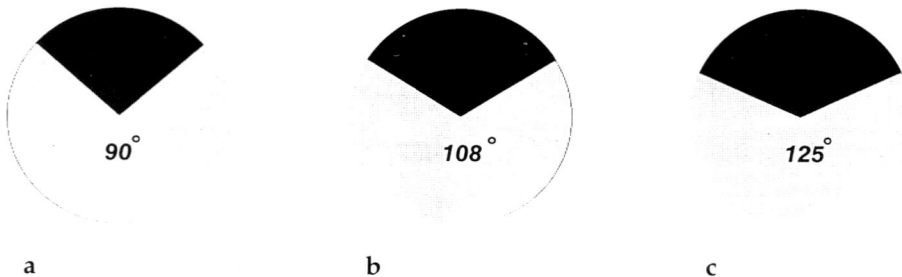

Fig. 5.19. The range of angular movements. **a** Standard Charnley design, 90°. **b** Reduced diameter neck stem, 108°. **c** The "Lotus" hip, 125°.

6 Infection

Introduction

Excluding fatal complications, deep infection is rightly considered to be the most serious complication of total hip arthroplasty. It may lead to prolonged hospital stay, repeated operations, discharging sinuses, protracted mobilization and the need for support during ambulation as well as to leg shortening, telescoping and lack of control over the hip and possibly even to pain, and is sufficient to affect the patient adversely and to disappoint the surgeon.

There exists for this subject a vast collection of references on clinical presentation, diagnostic tests, methods of management, operative procedures and results. The collective work edited by Eftekhar (1984) is a valuable contribution in this sphere, while the work of Buchholz et al. (1984) on the various aspects of practical management using antibiotic-loaded acrylic cement is second to none.

Very early on in his work Charnley realized that implant surgery on the scale of total hip arthroplasty was not practical if the deep infection rate was to remain at its original level of over 7%. Following introduction of the concept of clean air enclosure, the deep sepsis rate was gradually reduced as the number of air changes per hour was increased. It was not until this reached 300 per hour and total body exhaust suits were introduced that the infection rate was reduced to below 1% (Fig. 6.1), and that without antibiotics used either locally, systemically or in the acrylic cement.

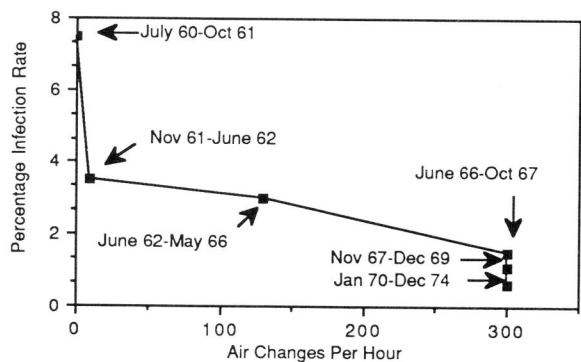

Fig. 6.1. Deep infection rate in the various stages of evolution of the clean air enclosure and the total body exhaust suits (after Charnley 1979).

In order to investigate the possible sources of deep sepsis still further there was need for a systematic study of various aspects of patient selection, surgical methods, wound contamination at the time of surgery and the efficacy of gowns and drapes as well as for a methodical review of infected cases.

Incidence of Deep Infection

When discussing the incidence of deep sepsis two other aspects must be taken into account: the size of the sample studied and the length of the follow-up.

The Size of the Sample Studied

Once every effort was being made to reduce the incidence of deep infections it gradually fell to around 1%. It is obvious that with such a low incidence vast numbers of cases must be studied making it an almost impossible task for a single unit yet alone an individual. However, multi-centre studies bring with them the problem of variation in patient selection, environment, surgical technique, prophylaxis, the length of follow-up and the criteria used to establish the diagnosis.

No case of sepsis is likely to be diagnosed and recorded more than once. In fact the opposite is more likely – cases may be missed for whatever reason. This will obviously result in an under-estimation of the problem. If the number of infected cases is not particularly great, then a single case may lead to wide variations of the results.

The Length of the Follow-up

That the incidence of deep infection recorded is likely to increase with an increasing length of follow-up is probably obvious. An interesting insight into the problem is provided by Eche-verri et al. (1988) and will be outlined briefly in this chapter.

When one also needs to consider the problems with selection of criteria for defining deep sepsis, the inherent difficulties with collection, transportation and culturing of samples plus any losses of the case material over time, the magnitude of the problem and the difficulty of interpretation become apparent.

Deep Sepsis in Osteoarthritis

Van Niekerk and Charnley (1979) reviewed the cases of 2154 patients operated upon between January 1974 and January 1976. They established a deep infection rate following primary surgery for osteoarthritis of 0.3%. This figure may be questionable because of the way in which the bacteriology of the infected cases was presented; also, the study obviously did not take into account cases that have not yet come to revision. With a relatively short follow-up the figure of 0.3% must be considered as a likely underestimate.

Lynch et al. (1987) reviewed 1542 LFAs carried out by the author over an 8-year period beginning 2 years after the last operation had been carried out. The diagnosis of deep infection was made either at revision or radiologically if the revision had not been carried out at the time of the review. In this way they hoped to minimize the loss of cases. The incidence of deep sepsis in patients with osteoarthritis undergoing primary LFA was 1.5%.

Deep Sepsis in Rheumatoid Arthritis

In the same study (Lynch et al. 1987) a small group of 41 cases of rheumatoid arthritis were included, and in these the deep infection rate was found to be 4.9% if plain acrylic cement was used and 3.5% if antibiotic-loaded acrylic cement was used. This compares unfavourably with a rate of 1.2% reported by Van Niekerk and Charnley (1979) for patients with rheumatoid arthritis.

Deep Sepsis Following Previous Hip Surgery

In patients who have had previous hip surgery the deep infection rate is really unpredictable since it depends on the nature of the hip surgery. Dupont and Charnley (1972) reviewing 217 cases have found the deep sepsis rate to be 3.7%. The follow-up period was relatively short.

Echeverri et al. (1988) continued the type of work carried out by Dupont and Charnley (1972). They reviewed 119 patients (127 hips) who had had the Charnley LFA carried out for failures of previous hip surgery. The average follow-up was 10.4 years (range 0.6 to 23.1 years). The infection rate was found to be 11.8% as compared with the 3.7% reported by Dupont and Charnley (1972).

Patients at Risk for Deep Sepsis

In order to extend our knowledge of this very complex subject and to identify patients at risk for deep sepsis a number of prospective and retrospective studies have been undertaken. The results are summarized as follows.

Males with Post-operative Urinary Retention, Catheterization and Prostatectomy (Wroblewski and del Sel 1980)

One hundred and ninety-five males who had had hip surgery and who had post-operative urinary retention required catheterization. Seventy of them needed prostatectomy. The overall deep infection rate was 6.2%. A direct relationship between urethral instrumentation and deep infection of the implant could only be assumed from the study; similar organisms were isolated from four out of 12 cases.

Diabetics

Menon et al. (1983) reviewed 16 113 LFAs carried out between January 1967 and December 1980. Forty-eight diabetics were identified. Between them, they had 66 Charnley LFAs. Four hips (6.0%) had deep infection. Although the number of diabetic patients is small, the study reflects the inherent difficulty of such a review.

Patients with Psoriasis

Menon and Wroblewski (1983), reviewing the series previously reported (see *Diabetics*), identified 38 patients with psoriasis. Between them they had 55 Charnley LFAs. Deep infection occurred in three hips (5.5%) suggesting that psoriatic patients are at higher risk for postoperative deep sepsis.

Table 6.1. Incidence of deep infection after LFA in various groups of patients

Diagnosis	No. of cases	Deep infection %	Reference
Osteoarthritis	994	1.5	Lynch et al. (1987)
Rheumatoid arthritis	70	4.8	Lynch et al. (1987)
Psoriasis	55	5.5	Menon and Wroblewski (1983)
Diabetes	66	6.0	Menon et al. (1983)
Urinary retention; urethral instrumentation	195	6.2	Wroblewski and del Sel (1980)
Previous hip surgery	127	11.8	Echeverri et al. (1988)

All the above results were obtained from studies where plain acrylic cement was used. They are summarized in Table 6.1.

Prevention of Deep Infection

The value of clean air enclosure and total body exhaust suits has already been outlined briefly.

Buchholz introduced the concept of antibiotic-loaded acrylic cement (ALAC) in total hip arthroplasty. Using this method he reduced the infection rate from 7.5% to less than 1%. This very low rate showed a tendency to increase with longer follow-up (Buchholz et al. 1984).

Josefsson et al. (1981) compared the results using plain acrylic cement, systemic antibiotics and ALAC in a series of 1685 hip replacements. The results suggested that ALAC was more effective in preventing deep infection (0.4%) as compared with plain cement and systemic antibiotics (1.6%).

Lidwell et al. (1982) in an extensive, prospective, multicentre study compared the efficacy of various methods of prevention of deep sepsis. This monumental research must be studied in detail by all. Antibiotics used together with clean air enclosure reduced the deep infection rate to 0.7%. When total body exhaust suits were also used the deep infection rate was further reduced to 0.06%. From the correspondence that followed it became apparent that with progressively longer follow-up times further cases of deep sepsis came to light, making the eventual deep infection rates higher than found initially. Similar observations were made in other studies.

Lynch et al. (1987) reviewed 1542 LFAs carried out by the author over an 8-year period, beginning 2 years after closure of the trial. The results of this retrospective review comparing use of plain and gentamicin-containing acrylic cement (Palacos with 0.5 g of gentamicin per 40-g pack) are summarized in Table 6.2.

Statistical analysis suggests that use of antibiotic-loaded acrylic cement in cases of secondary operative interventions (conversion and revision surgery) offers significant benefit ($0.05 < P < 0.01$). In primary surgery this benefit is less obvious.

Table 6.2. Comparison of results using plain and antibiotic-containing acrylic cement

	CMW	Palacos + 0.5 g gentamicin
Total no. of LFAs	871	671
No. of infections (%)	19 (2.18%)	9 (1.34%)
1. Osteoarthritis, no previous surgery	599	395
No. of infections	9 (1.50%)	6 (1.52%)
2. All diagnoses previous hip surgery other than THA or endoprosthesis	125	55
No. of infections	5 (4%)	1 (1.82%)
3. All diagnoses previous total hip arthroplasty or endoprosthesis	106	192
No. of infections	3 (2.83%)	1 (0.52%)
4. Rheumatoid arthritis, no previous surgery	41	29
No. of infections	2 (4.88%)	1 (3.45%)
1 and 4 combined	640	424
No. of infections	11 (1.72%)	5 (1.18%)
2 and 3 combined	231	247
No. of infections	8 (3.46%)	2 (0.81%)

Review of the Use of ALAC in Total Hip Arthroplasty

The literature on the subject of ALAC, both clinical and experimental, is so vast that it would be an impossible task even to attempt to summarize the major publications. The reader must refer to the original work. The author's own views have evolved over the years and over a number of studies, both clinical and experimental. The results are summarized briefly here.

Leaching out from Acrylic Bone Cement

In an experimental evaluation the author (Wroblewski 1977), using common salt to simulate the behaviour of a water-soluble antibiotic mixed with the acrylic cement, has confirmed that the amount released is proportional to the surface area of the acrylic cement. This is most likely to be a purely surface phenomenon.

Revisions for Deep Sepsis Using Plain Acrylic Cement (Wroblewski 1980)

In a short series of 40 one-stage revisions for deep sepsis using plain acrylic cement (CMW) the success rate achieved was 75% (30 out of 40 cases) with an average follow-up of 38 months. Great reliance was placed on thorough debridement, systemic antibiotics, local antiseptics and sound fixation of the components.

Revisions for Deep Sepsis Using ALAC (Palacos plus 0.5 g Gentamicin) (Wroblewski 1986b)

Following the experimental findings and the clinical results of the one-stage revisions for deep infection presented above, the author carried out a prospective study of one-stage revisons of infected cemented total hip arthroplasties in 102 consecutive cases. The success rate was 91%, with an average follow-up of 38 months, indicating the obvious benefits of ALAC in this type of surgery.

Release of Gentamicin from Acrylic Cement: Ex Vivo Study (Wroblewski et al. 1986)

Unlike so many other studies, the author and his colleagues studied the amount of gentamicin that had been *retained* in the acrylic cement in patients undergoing revision surgery between 1

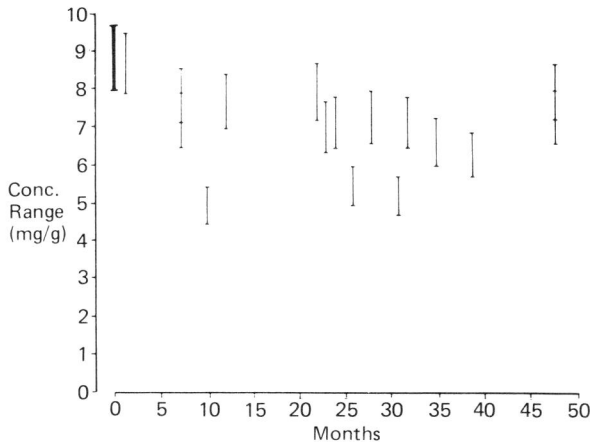

Fig. 6.2. Concentration of gentamicin remaining in the acrylic cement as found at various stages from 1 to 48 months after surgery, compared to a freshly mixed sample. The release of the antibiotic is neither continuous nor complete.

and 48 months after primary surgery. On average, 78% of the gentamicin was retained within the acrylic cement. The release of the antibiotic was neither continuous nor a complete process (Fig. 6.2).

Comparison of Plain CMW Acrylic Cement and ALAC (Palacos plus 0.5 g Gentamicin) (Lynch et al. 1987)

This aspect has already been mentioned above. Antibiotic-loaded acrylic cement does not appear to be of benefit as a prophylactic measure in cases of primary total hip arthroplasty when clean air enclosure and total body exhaust suits have been used, though it is of obvious benefit in secondary operative interventions. In fact, if the antibiotic starts to be released at some stage during the operation, it can be argued that, by definition, it is not a prophylactic.

The author's views on the use of ALAC are summarized as follows:

1. Release of an antibiotic from the acrylic cement is purely a surface phenomenon.
2. The amount released is proportional to the surface area of the cement.

3. The process of antibiotic release is completed early, probably within days rather than weeks or months.
4. The release is neither continuous over a long period of time nor complete.
5. Although between 2% and 45% of the antibiotic may be released, on average 78% remains within the acrylic cement.
6. In primary surgery, and excluding cases known to be at risk, ALAC probably has little to offer over and above the protection given by use of clean air enclosure and total body exhaust suits.
7. In secondary operations ALAC offers a distinct advantage.
8. In one-stage revisions of infected total hip arthroplasties ALAC is essential and increases the success rate from 75% to 90% in cases where ALAC has not been previously used.
9. ALAC is not a long-term prophylactic against systemic infection.
10. Any antibiotic included in the acrylic cement must be clearly recorded in patient's records.
11. In cases where ALAC has been used at the primary total hip arthroplasty the success of one-stage revisions for deep infection is likely to be lower.
12. Emergence of resistant organisms is to be expected, demanding the use of larger doses and multiple antibiotics.
13. At revision surgery break up of ALAC will result in release of antibiotic. This may affect bacteriological studies.

Diagnosis of Deep Infection

There is no single method of preventing deep infection. Careful patient selection, attention to the details of tissue handling at surgery and use of clean air enclosure, total body exhaust suits and antibiotics (either systemically or in the acrylic cement) all have their place.

Despite the large amount of literature on the subject of infection there is no agreement on its definition in the context of total hip arthroplasty. Appearance of a sinus is not a constant feature and cultures need not be positive as determined by the common bacteriological methods. (Even if positive their value may be in doubt in the presence of a sinus.) It is obvious that no single finding is diagnostic in itself; it is a collection of findings and exclusion of other causes of failure that make the diagnosis possible.

In this context a collection of good-quality serial radiographs is indispensable. The radiographs must include the whole of the prosthesis and the cement must be radio-opaque. (It cannot be stressed strongly enough that in the study of the long-term results of total hip arthroplasty, radiographic appearances must take precedence over the clinical findings.) A review of the radiographs of the infected cases in the study by Lynch et al. (1987) has shown that retrospectively *all* cases of deep sepsis could have been diagnosed radiologically within 1 year of the surgery.

A well-carried out total hip arthroplasty so consistently produces spectacular clinical results that a problem should be suspected in a patient who is less than mildly enthusiastic. Although there may be many reasons for a less than perfect result, an open mind and careful follow-up will eventually reveal the cause of the problem. It is for that reason that the diagnosis of deep infection will often be made retrospectively.

There is no single feature that will lead to the diagnosis being made beyond a doubt, although it can be argued that a collection of symptoms, clinical signs and radiographic changes in the presence of positive bacteriological cultures will clinch the diagnosis.

History

Previous operative procedures, a history of haematoma, delayed wound healing, repeated application of dressings and courses of antibiotics all indicate the possibility of deep infection.

Pain

Although relieved of the arthritic pain, the patient has never been pain free. At times the pain can be quite severe and often referred to the front of the thigh.

Clinical Progress

This may be slow and the patient continues to use support. This information may be readily volunteered by the patient with bilateral total hip arthroplasty when one of them has failed.

Use of Support

The patient may never have discarded sticks or crutches and without them will walk with a typical lurching gait in an attempt to unload the hip by "throwing" the body over the affected side. This gait is by no means diagnostic of deep sepsis only. Any painful mobile hip will function in an abducted position; this is the mechanism by which the load on the hip joint is reduced, thus reducing the pain.

Examination

The scar may show evidence of delayed wound healing, induration or puckered areas from a healed sinus. When there is a collection of pus locally the diagnosis becomes obvious.

Investigations

Availability of any investigation is not an indication for its performance unless as a research tool, to establish its practical value or to help in planning treatment. It must not be used as a delaying tactic in order to put off the decision-making day.

Plain Radiography

Infection has a tendency to present itself at the weakest part of the arthroplasty. This is true of sepsis anywhere, which tends to follow tissue planes or seek the easiest exit.

On the acetabular side, early demarcation of the outer third of the bone–cement junction rapidly progresses to full demarcation. By the time tilting or migration occurs the infection has been well established for some time and the fixation of the socket has been lost (Fig. 6.3).

On the femoral side excavation of the medial portion of the femoral neck may be the earliest sign. This is almost certainly caused by the mechanical effect of the changing pressure caused by the deflection of the stem as well as pus and pyogenic granulation tissue (Fig. 6.3).

Periostitis may be difficult to spot in the very early stages. On radiography it can be seen as no

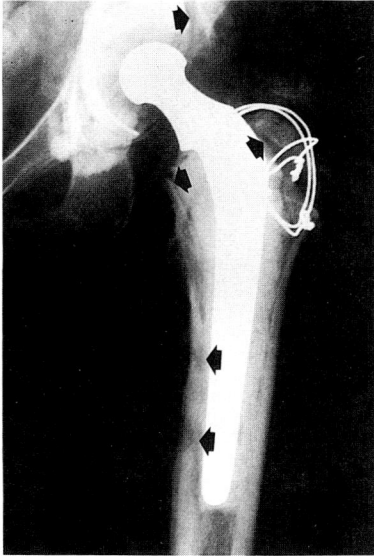

Fig. 6.3. A clear example of severe deep infection, showing fibrous union of the greater trochanter, complete socket demarcation, socket tilting into a vertical position, gross thinning of the medial femoral neck at the bone–cement junction and cloacae in the medial femoral cortex with early endosteal cavitation. (Patient on steroids for total body atopic eczema. *Staphylococcus aureus* was the infecting organism.)

more than a thin, very feint line of periosteal elevation, usually near the lower portion of the stem, and more often medially than laterally (Fig. 6.3).

Endosteal cavitation (Fig. 6.3) of the femur indicates that a certain proportion of the bone mass must have been lost for it to "show through" the femoral cortex. Experimental evidence suggests that a change in bone density close to 20% must occur before the changes are obvious to the naked eye.

Cloacae in the femoral shaft, with their smoothed off edges, are typical but appear rather late (Fig. 6.3).

If trochanteric osteotomy has been part of the exposure then trochanteric non-union and rarefaction of bone round the trochanteric wires, a fibrous (Fig. 6.3) greater trochanter may be observed.

Special Investigations

These are discussed in some detail in the chapter on assessment of the patient (Chap. 18).

Classification of Infection

Infection can be classified as early or late. Early infection can be further subclassified into superficial or deep infection and late infection into delayed or latent infection.

Superficial Infection

By definition, superficial infection is superficial to the deep fascia and has no connection with the implant. Although simple to define it is less simple to diagnose. It is probably correct to state that a fair proportion of cases of superficial infection are in fact superficial presentations of deep infection. The distinction between the two will become obvious with the passage of time.

Deep Infection

Deep infection involves the implant. Clinically there are two basic types of deep infection: the bone–cement junction type and the osteitis–osteomyelitis type.

Bone–Cement Junction Type. Demarcation of the bone–cement junction is the main radiological finding together with positive bacteriological specimens. There is very little or no evidence of bony involvement but changes associated with component loosening are usually present (Fig. 6.4).

Osteitis–Osteomyelitis Type. The involvement of the bone in the infective process is obvious. Periostitis, osteitis and osteomyelitis are clear features and cloacae are usually present (Fig. 6.5; see also Fig. 6.3).

A review of 100 infected cemented total hip arthroplasties has confirmed the presence of the two types of deep infection. The osteomyelitis type, especially with a sinus, carried a poorer prognosis.

Late Infection

The question of late or latent infection in total hip arthroplasty has often been discussed. Though the existence of this clinical entity

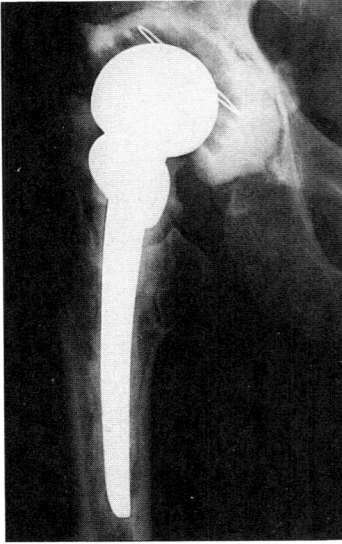

Fig. 6.4. "Bone–cement junction" type of deep infection. Appearances of bone–cement demarcation of both components without any obvious bone involvement.

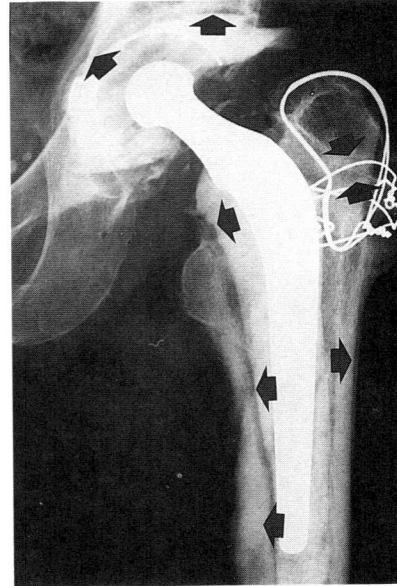

Fig. 6.5. "Osteomyelitis" type of deep infection. Bone involvement presenting as periostitis laterally, distal to the greater trochanter, femoral cortical thickening and cloacae medially. Bone rarefaction around the trochanteric wires. Complete socket demarcation.

cannot be denied it is essential that it be viewed objectively. It is all too easy to dismiss the problem as "late sepsis" rather than attempt to examine each case in detail in order to establish the sequence of events leading up to it if not the cause itself. This is due partly to a lack of adequate records, but mostly to a natural reluctance to accept that something could possibly affect adversely the outcome of the operation and that the problem may in fact be deep infection. There are really only three possibilities:

1. The infection occurs late.
2. The infection is diagnosed late.
3. The infection presents late clinically.

The Infection Occurs Late

This would imply that following a straightforward total hip arthroplasty carried out under ideal conditions and not involving conversion or revision surgery, in a patient known not to be "at risk" for deep sepsis, there were no postoperative complications likely to be manifestations of deep infection or to lead to deep

infection. This to be followed by a period of not less than 1 year of complete freedom from pain and with normal function. All this in the presence of normal sequential radiographs.

To accept all the above is to accept that the infection has been seeded from some other source, thus indicating genuine septicaemic/bacteraemic infection, the source of which is known or suspected and preferably confirmed bacteriologically. The diagnosis can often only be made retrospectively and may be based on incomplete evidence. The author has had one such case out of 1542 operations over an 8-year period (Fig. 6.6).

The Infection is Diagnosed Late

This is probably the commonest scenario. The patient is not aware of what is to be expected in the way of pain relief or improvement in function; the surgeon may not be alert to the possibility of infection; and the records may be incomplete. With time the diagnosis becomes obvious, usually when loosening of the components supervenes or a sinus appears.

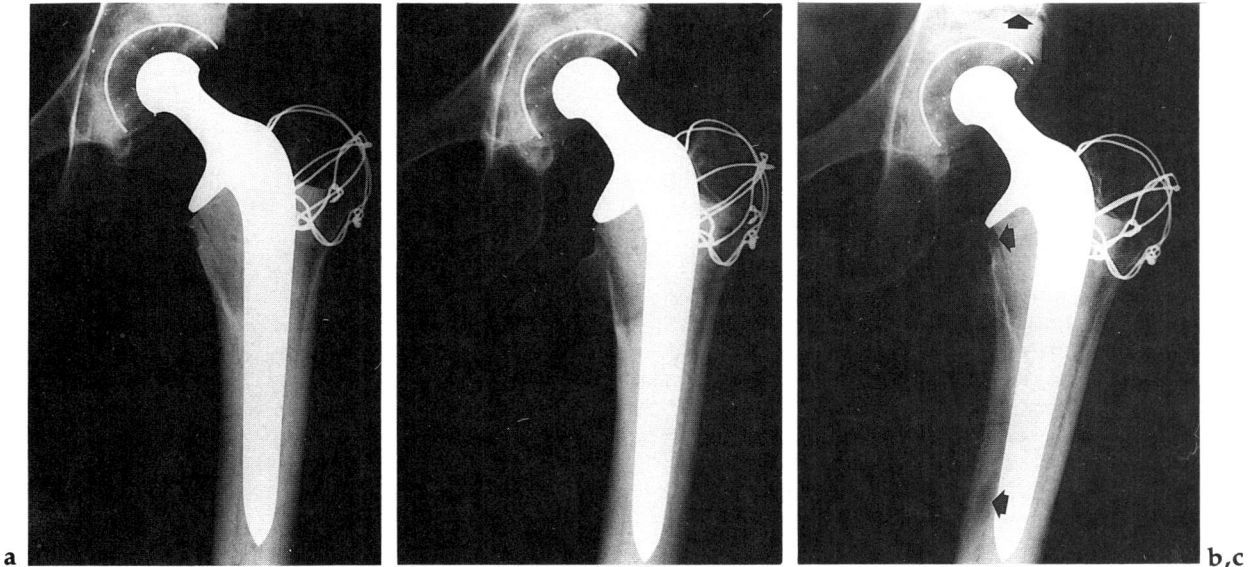

Fig. 6.6. Late infection. **a** Post-operative appearance at 2 weeks. **b** Appearance at 3½ years. Patient pain-free with normal function. **c** Radiographic appearances 6 weeks after **b**, showing demarcation of socket, erosion of medial femoral neck, periostitis of the medial femoral cortex and endosteal cavitation medially. (Local steroid cream applied to a long-standing rash on the ipsilateral leg followed, within hours, by systemic symptoms of infection and painful left total hip arthroplasty.) (Photograph by courtesy of Mr. M. Lynch.)

The Infection Presents Late

Colonization of the implant by bacteria, as opposed to an overt clinical problem, is the possibility being considered here. The implant may be colonized by bacteria without presenting as a clinical or a mechanical problem. If a mechanical problem, i.e. loosening, does occur then infection may become obvious. Clinical and long-term implications both for the individual patients and the method in general are too frightening to contemplate.

If implants can become colonized by bacteria then the relationships between the quality of component fixation, the area of contact between the implant and the bone and the use of antibiotics will have far-reaching implications in clinical practice.

The better the component fixation the later will the loosening due to sepsis occur, thus suggesting late onset of infection. Slow and incomplete release of antibiotics included in the acrylic cement may lead to a similar conclusion. On the other hand sound component fixation could possibly allow deep infection to heal, or delay its clinical presentation. This fascinating theory merits study in depth.

Management of Deep Infection

Conservative

In cases where early or superficial infection is the problem an intensive course of antibiotics may save the arthroplasty or at least reduce the severity of the local or systemic effects. The antibiotic and the dosage to be used will depend on the bacteriology and the sensitivity of the organisms. The treatment may have to be continued for weeks or even months, and may include enforced rest of the patient. Any superficial collection of pus must be formally explored and drained and treated by secondary sutures if the situation warrants it. Provided the local and the systemic effects of infection are controlled and the integrity of the components remains unaffected, no further action need be taken. Careful follow-up *must* be continued. Such cases are rarities.

Although in some cases a "cure" may be achieved by such a method, more often than not the infection continues and loosening of the components supervenes. In such cases revision must not be delayed.

Operative – One- or Two-Stage Revision?

Whether a one- or two-stage revision is carried out will depend to a great extent on the surgeon and his views on the subject. It must be pointed out that in a two-stage revision, the first stage of the operation, the pseudarthrosis, must leave the area ready for implant of the new components, either immediately or at some later date. The cavities created by this stage of the revision collect haematoma which is an excellent culture medium. These cavities can be adequately filled with the prosthesis and the antibiotic-loaded acrylic cement, thus also giving rest to the otherwise grossly unstable excision arthroplasty. If the latter procedure is carried out at the same time as the pseudarthrosis, this now becomes a one-stage revision. It must be questioned whether a two-stage procedure offers better results or whether there is higher morbidity and mortality associated with two major operations. The arguments appear to be in favour of one-stage revisions, except in some special cases.

The Principles of One-Stage Revision for Deep Infection

In carrying out the procedure a demand is placed on the surgeon to perform the operation in a series of clearly defined stages. All these stages should be performed relatively quickly using full exposure, not just of the joint itself but of every part of the arthroplasty. Although the principles are the same for all cases each one should still be regarded and tackled as an individual entity. The essential steps are:

1. Full exposure.
2. Removal of the components and all the acrylic cement.
3. Excision of the synovium and capsule.
4. Preparation of the bony bed.
5. Systemic antibiotics.
6. Local antiseptics.
7. Antibiotic-loaded acrylic cement.
8. Sound fixation of new components.
9. Bed rest and slow mobilization.
10. Antibiotics.

Full Exposure

This is essential. Trochanteric wires, if present, should be identified and carefully removed. Trochanteric osteotomy is mandatory. Before attempting dislocation, the upper end of the femur must be carefully mobilized in order to bring it away from the pelvis.

Removal of the Components and all the Acrylic Cement

This aspect is dealt with in Chap. 23. It must be stressed that when dealing with deep infection we are hoping to eradicate a hidden or invisible problem by attempting to remove what is visible and may indicate infection.

Full exposure, adequate illumination, patience and attention to detail at every stage are essential. It is wrong to imagine that only one side of the arthroplasty is affected. There is no justification for changing one component unless the diagnosis of deep infection has been missed for whatever reason. It must be admitted, however, that such cases do exist in the author's practice, and with apparently continuing good clinical and radiological results (Fig. 6.7).

Excision of the Synovium and Capsule

This must obviously be part of the debridement. Cutting diathermy is favoured as it reduces bleeding. Various ramifications of such tissue must be carefully sought out and excised completely. The capsule between the greater trochanter and the superior acetabular margin must not be forgotten. The posterior capsule should be excised *after* the removal of the north–south retractor. Until that moment, the posterior capsule serves as a useful protection for the sciatic nerve from the teeth of the retractor.

Preparation of the Bony Bed

This is carried out by meticulous curettage of all the areas containing pyogenic granulation tissue. To fail to do this adequately is to risk almost immediate failure of component fixation and continuation of the infection. This part of the revision is very time consuming.

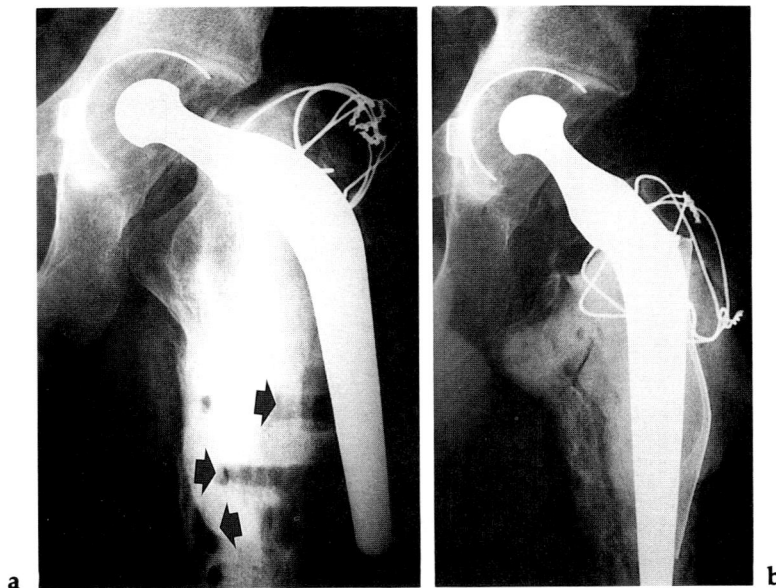

Fig. 6.7. Changing one component (the stem) in the presence of deep sepsis. **a** Fracture of the femoral neck; severe previous operations including the LFA. After severe trauma, stem jutting out laterally. Attempts at fixation with HDP straps has failed. **b** Change of the stem only using wire mesh to contain the cement. Although all cultures proved positive (Coagulase-negative staphylococcus) and the socket was not changed, there is no evidence of extension of the infection to the bone–cement junction of the socket 3 years later.

Systemic Antibiotics

The use of systemic antibiotics in this type of surgery is logical although was not accepted initially. Buchholz relied exclusively on ALAC, no doubt in an attempt to prove the efficacy of the method. The author always used systemic antibiotics since ALAC was not used initially; greater emphasis was therefore placed on the more mechanical aspects of the procedure. Systemic antibiotic use has now been accepted as integral to the method. The type of antibiotic and the dosage will depend on the infecting organism. A good stand-by is cephradine 1 g intravenously 6–8 hourly, starting either at the time of induction if the sensitivities are known, or immediately bacteriological cultures have been collected. After 24 hours the patient can usually tolerate oral antibiotics. If sensitivities are not available then cephradine is continued until such a time that results indicate which antibiotic is to be used. The usual practice is to continue the antibiotics for 6 weeks though the real value of this cannot be accurately assessed. It is conceded that patients' compliance with such treatment may, at times, not be total.

Local Antiseptics

The use of antiseptics in surgery has been accepted practice for a long time now, and it is only logical that their topical use in revision for deep sepsis should be advocated. Initially 2% tincture of iodine was used (beware of diathermy!). Now pure Betadine antiseptic solution, a swab for packing cavities or a 10% solution with normal saline is used for irrigation. What effect this has on the results cannot be quantified since so many variables are involved in each case as to make any prospective study not only impossible but probably also unnecessary.

Antibiotic-Loaded Acrylic Cement (ALAC)

There is little doubt that the introduction by Buchholz and his colleagues of the concept of ALAC has revolutionized the treatment of deep sepsis. Until ALAC the only possible treatment was repeated courses of antibiotics and repeated exploration and debridement, all in the hope that the infection would settle and the components would remain in situ. Failing all that, pseudarthrosis was, and still at times is the only and the ultimate solution to the problem.

The literature on ALAC is so vast that the reader *must* refer to the original publications. The author's views on the subject are briefly summarized on p. 51. The amount of the antibiotic released is proportional to the surface area of the cement. It is of significant benefit in secondary operative interventions. (ALAC must not be used to the exclusion of sound fixation of the components.)

Sound Fixation of the Components

This concept is not new and was no doubt originally the basis of operative (rather than conservative) fracture treatment. It is based on the belief that avoidance of movement of the components, limb or the patient should promote healing. This has often been demonstrated in the treatment of infected compound fractures.

What constitutes sound fixation of the components is difficult to define or describe. It is probably correct to state that the closer the soft tissues and bone resemble those in primary surgery the nearer the surgeon is to achieving what he has set out to do. The opposite is equally true: if sound fixation of the components cannot be achieved then the revision is doomed to failure, if not by continuation of sepsis then certainly because of loosening of the components. Inadequate bone stock for component fixation has always been regarded by the author as an absolute indication for pseudarthrosis.

On the practical side of the procedure, excavation of the lesser trochanter to expose its strong cancellous bone offers an excellent support for the stem where it is most needed, i.e. postero-medially.

Bed Rest and Slow Mobilization with Support

The axiom of prolonged, uninterrupted rest as advocated by Hugh Owen Thomas holds true in the post-operative management of deep infection. Whether this actually affects the "clinical" result is not possible to assess with any certainty. The author's original practice was to mobilize the patient at 2 days, as after primary surgery. Although the incidence of continuation of deep sepsis was probably no higher, the trochanteric non-union rate was 12.5% and the

dislocation rate 15%. All this has changed dramatically since 3 weeks' bed rest became routine. (It must be pointed out, however, that at the same time a better method of trochanteric fixation and the angle-bore socket were introduced.) This period of bed rest does not seem to produce any nursing problems for once the first week is over the patient is independent in bed (with the abduction pillow) and is usually ready for discharge during the fourth post-operative week. (The fear of increased risk of pulmonary emboli appears to be unfounded see Chap. 28.) It is also prudent to recommend continuing use of support. In the revision for deep infection we are using a salvage procedure, rather than attempting to achieve results comparable with those of primary surgery. With time, loosening of components is to be expected.

Antibiotics

Oral antibiotics should probably be continued for some time, though it is difficult to set a logical time limit. The author's practice is an arbitrary 6 weeks, probably more in line with the treatment of fractures than of infection.

Results of Revisions for Deep Infection

The revision for deep infection in total hip arthroplasty has evolved over a number of years and through several stages. Although the basic mechanical concepts have remained unaltered there has been a gradual change of thought on the use of ALAC.

The Use of Plain Acrylic Cement

In the early stages it was considered that ALAC had probably very little, if anything, to contribute to the success of this type of surgery. This

Fig. 6.8. One-stage revision for deep infection using plain acrylic cement and systemic antibiotics. **a,b** McKee–Farrar arthroplasty with radiolucent cement. History of a sinus, now healed. Note the changes in the femoral cortex indicating infection. **c** One-stage revision using plain acrylic cement and systemic antibiotics. **d** Appearances at 10½ years. Socket fully demarcated. **e** Prolapse of socket following a severe fall. **f** Revision using uncemented socket. Stem was also changed in order to facilitate the exposure. All cultures were negative.

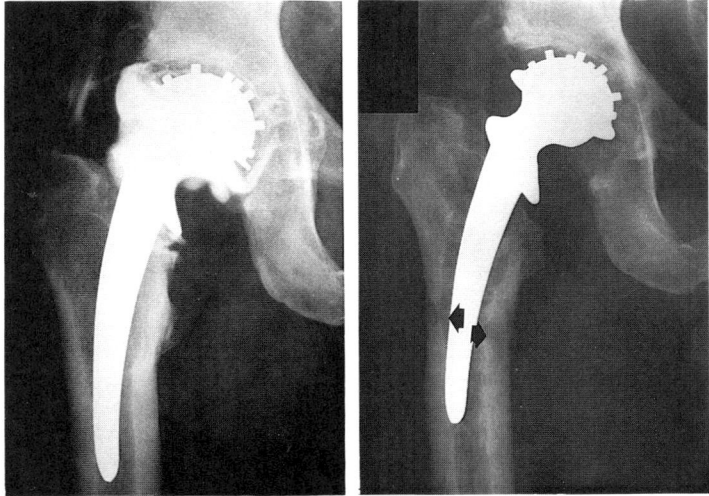

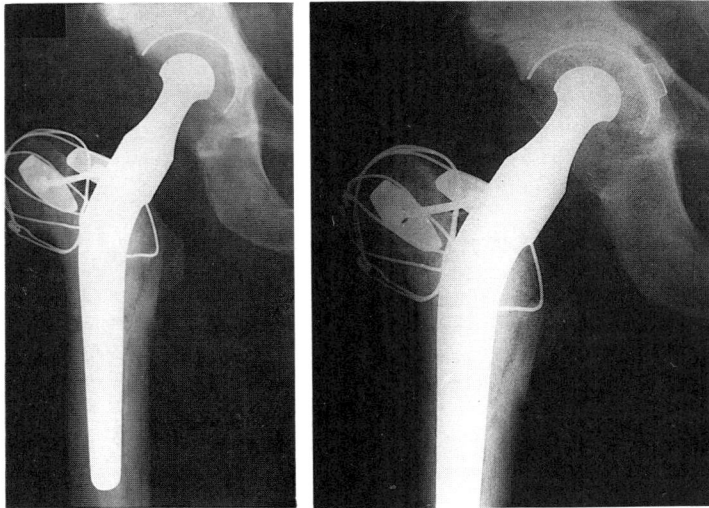

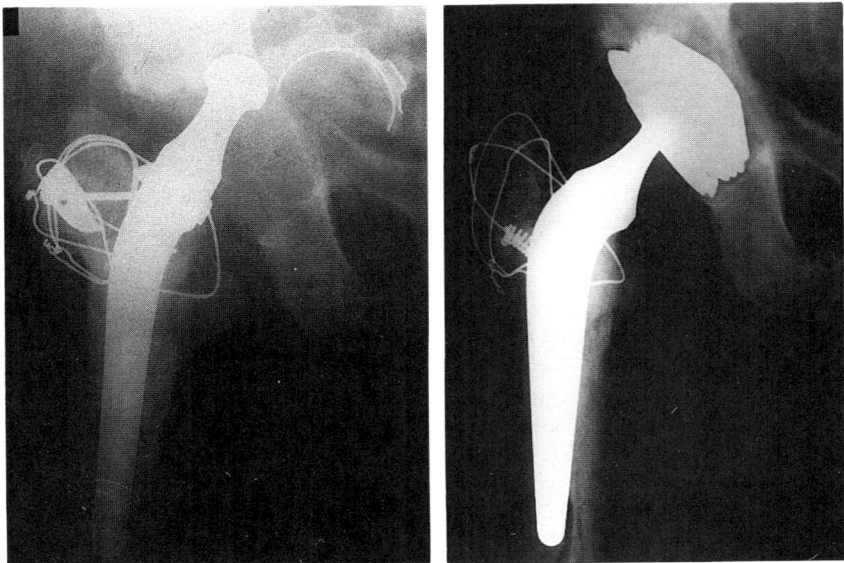

was based on experimental evidence (Wroblewski 1977), the fear of allergic reactions which may demand pseudarthrosis and the possibility of the emergence of gentamicin-resistant organisms. A purely mechanical approach was therefore used as outlined on p. 50 and 40 cases of one-stage revision were carried out using plain acrylic cement. The most common infecting organism was coagulase-negative *Staphylococcus*. The revision was successful in 30 cases with an average follow-up of 38 months (range 24–65 months). Although the series was relatively small the results were encouraging and indicated a success rate of 75% at 3½-year follow-up (Wroblewski 1980) (Fig. 6.8).

Palacos with Gentamicin

Following this series the number of revision cases referred increased quite dramatically and a 25% failure rate was not thought to be acceptable if large numbers were to be treated. It was therefore postulated that if ALAC were to have any role to play in this type of surgery, if would be necessary to show a greater success rate using it than was previously obtained without it (i.e. 75%). Without changing the basic technique or patient selection a prospective series was carried out using ALAC (Palacos with 0.5 g gentamicin). The early results were as follows:

1. In 104 cases thus revised the success rate was over 90% (Wroblewski 1983).

2. A series using ALAC in a study comparable to the 1983 one was reported (Wroblewski 1986b). This was a continuation of the study using the method already outlined but using Palacos acrylic cement with 0.5 g gentamicin in a one-stage revision for deep sepsis. (In only four cases was extra antibiotic added.) In this group only cemented total hip arthroplasties were included.

The average follow-up was 3 years and 2 months and 102 consecutive cemented total hip arthroplasties were studied. The commonest infecting organism was coagulase-negative *Staphylococcus* either as a pure growth or in combination with other organisms. The success rate was 91%. This study highlighted certain aspects of this type of surgery. Almost a third of cases had had a sinus at some stage between the

total hip arthroplasty and the revision. In 17.6% of cases the revision was carried out in the presence of a discharging sinus. The vast majority of patients (88%) received antibiotics between total hip arthroplasty and the revision. Loosening of one or both components was found in all cases. Delay in establishing the diagnosis or carrying out the revision is likely to lead to loss of bone stock making adequate fixation of the components difficult if not impossible, hence there should be no delay in carrying out the revision once the diagnosis has been made and the acute cellulitic phase has been treated adequately.

In both the series quoted no attempt was made to identify the organisms though in some cases the information was available from cultures from pre-revision wound discharge or a sinus.

Use of Extra Antibiotics in the Acrylic Cement

With time certain aspects of this type of revision surgery became apparent. First, success was not always achieved, even with an apparently adequate procedure and in the presence of gentamicin-sensitive organisms. Second, these failed cases, and the ones where ALAC had been used in primary surgery and where infection had occurred, were obviously unlikely to succeed with repetition of the same method of revision. During this period a steady trickle of failed revision cases appeared, ALAC having already been used at least once, possibly twice.

At this stage, therefore, the ideal would be to prepare a suitable antibiotic mixture specific to each case as determined by accurate bacteriological studies. This type of surgery places a heavy burden on the surgeon, bacteriologist and the pharmacist. The surgeon must document clearly if and what ALAC has been used at primary surgery. This information must be readily available to anyone having to undertake revision surgery. Collection of bacteriological specimens must be carried out with this information in mind. Any fragmentation of the ALAC will release some of the antibiotic which will obviously affect the results. The bacteriologist should really form part of the team and be clinically involved in every case to be treated so that the best possible methods of specimen collection, transportation and culture and antibiotic selection can be made available to the patient.

Two-Stage Revision

There are probably very good reasons for a two-stage revision other than fashion or length of the operation. It may be that staging of the revision will allow healing or eradication of resistant organisms. If so then this should be seriously investigated. Developments in this type of surgery are constantly being made. Newer antibiotics and improved methods and designs may make the two-stage procedure more acceptable, more so for a patient who for one reason or another cannot cope with a pseudarthrosis and whose life expectancy would allow the timing of the two procedures.

The Use of Antibiotic-Loaded Acrylic Beads

For those interested in this method of management of sepsis the excellent work of Walenkamp (1983) is recommended. The concept and clinical use of the method will be briefly discussed here.

The Concept

As the amount of antibiotic released from the acrylic cement is proportional to the surface area of the cement it can be argued effectively that a sphere is the wrong shape to allow maximum release of the antibiotic. (A sphere offers the minimum of surface area with the maximum of volume.) What is really required is a thin disc with an irregular surface. The use of such a shape would obviously create problems at introduction and removal.

Clinical Use

The author's use of gentamicin beads is restricted to only a handful of cases. The beads were used exclusively in cases where sinuses, because of their position or extent, did not allow their full excision. Thus the gentamicin beads were used where the sinus was in the area of the femoral triangle, the groin, the area of the sciatic nerve or so close to the wound that the excision would mitigate against primary closure of the skin incision. Considering the type of cases tackled the beads have proved extremely successful in eradicating deep sepsis and ensuring soft-tissue healing.

Two aspects warrant further comment – the insertion and removal of the beads. The insertion of the beads into a deep sinus produces a problem equivalent to pushing a piece of string. A simple instrument has been designed by the author to overcome this. The beads are placed into the introducer which can now be inserted down to the depth of any sinus. Once in place the push-out rod expels the beads as the introducer is withdrawn. The need for careful and progressive removal of the beads has already been pointed out by others. They should be gradually removed over 7 to 10 days following the operation, several beads each day. Delay in doing this may lead to the beads breaking off or to excessive bleeding, especially if the beads were originally in the area of the femoral triangle.

It is obvious that this type of surgery is not for an occasional operator and must be concentrated in units backed by technical and bacteriological expertise. Multiple operations, diminishing bone stock, resistant organisms and technically difficult procedures are not things that should form part of the routine practice of a busy orthopaedic surgeon. Revision surgery in general and revision for deep sepsis in particular cannot be undertaken in a schedule which is frequently interrupted by call to emergencies.

7 Loosening of the Components

Introduction

In order to understand why fixation of the components has failed we must understand what is required at primary surgery. The study and management of loose components in total hip arthroplasty are complex issues. Some of the complexity stems from a lack of understanding of the problem, some from conflicting and inaccurate definitions and most of it from the failure to separate clearly and objectively two important aspects of this method of treatment – the clinical success of the operation for an individual patient and the long-term success of the method of total hip arthroplasty being used.

The clinical success of an operation for the individual patient is an integral part of any type of clinical practice. Here the objective is to relieve a patient's symptoms and improve mobility. Accepting, however, that this is the indication for the operation in the first place, little else needs to be added. Having achieved this objective, there may be a tendency to go no further. From then onwards the follow-up, if any, is restricted to inquiry into symptoms and examination of the range of movements. The study of serial radiographs is not undertaken, the clinical picture taking precedence over everything (Fig. 7.1).

The long-term success of the method of total hip arthroplasty directs the attention towards detailed study of every aspect of the arthroplasty; its design, materials, the method of surgery, long-term clinical results, radiological and ex-vivo studies of the components and the "living/non-living" interface, all this directed towards constant improvement in the light of long-term results and past experiences. The aim is to develop a method with predictable long-term results, at least for some groups, if not for all patients in general. Thus if long-term success of the method is achieved, it will give the surgeon better knowledge, understanding and confidence when dealing with individual problems. Clinical success will inevitably follow. Individual short-term clinical success cannot give confidence in the long-term results of the method used.

Since absolute rigidity does not exist in nature, loosening of the components in the context of total hip arthroplasty cannot be defined in terms which can be generally agreed or which uniformly reflect the mechanical state of the arthroplasty. Even grossly loose and migrating components can be compatible with some level of function, which may even be considered normal (Fig. 7.1). In such cases the apparent clinical success cannot be considered an indication for its continued use or for non-intervention.

For practical purposes loosening of the components can be said to be present if sequential radiographs show failure of fixation, be it partial or complete, resulting in change of position or orientation either at the bone–cement or at the cement–component interfaces, indicating excessive movement at that level leading to a progressive loss of bone stock. The clinical result of the operation is not a part of this definition. It

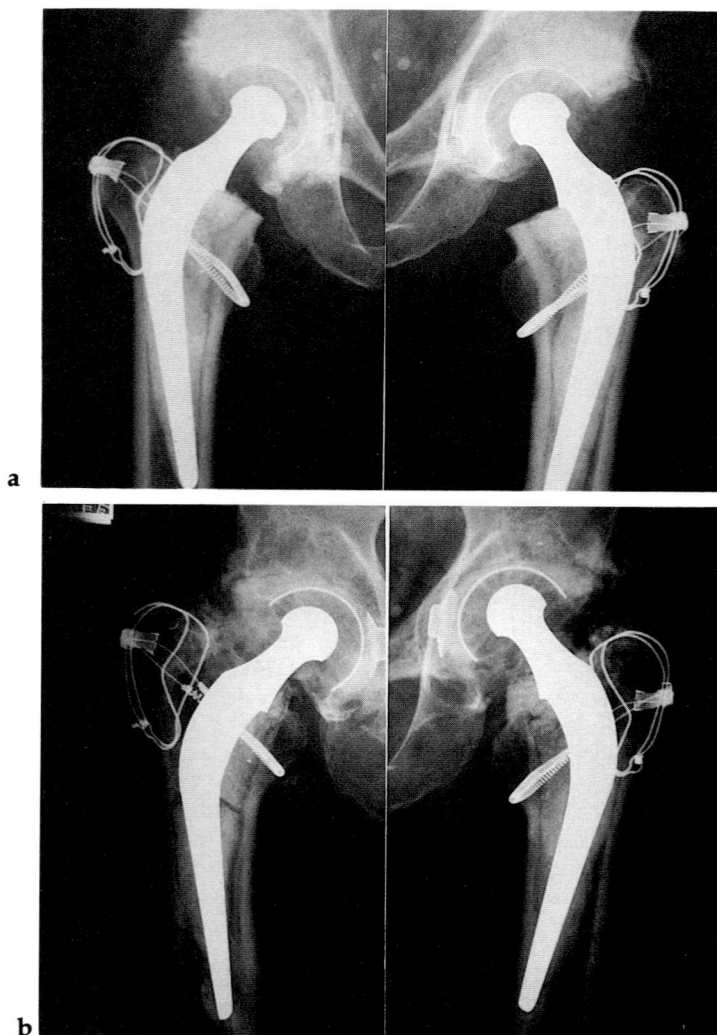

Fig. 7.1. Clinical success of the operation for an individual patient. **a** Bilateral low-friction arthroplasties: post-operative appearance. **b** Appearances at 15 years. The patient has occasional discomfort only.

is obvious that various appearances will inspire various descriptive terms which should not be considered contradictory or mutually exclusive. What we are really attempting to define and describe is a radiological appearance which is undesirable and which, given time and function, will eventually become an indication for revision. The long-term success of component fixation can be defined as normal and unchanging radiological appearances in the presence of normal clinical function.

The study and management of loose components must be undertaken objectively and with a clear understanding of the following:

1. Sound or adequate fixation is a relative term.
2. The clinical result does not necessarily reflect the mechanical state of the arthroplasty.
3. Radiological changes indicating failure usually precede clinical symptoms.
4. Fixation having failed, the radiographic appearances do not improve with time.
5. Some changes are related to time and function.
6. Any total hip arthroplasty must be considered as a potential risk for complications and no patient can be formally discharged from the follow-up.

1. That sound and adequate fixation of the components is a relative term has already been pointed out. In carrying out the operative procedure there has been a growing tendency in the direction of careful preparation of the cancellous bone and the use of the water pick and low-viscosity pressurized cement, be it by pressurizing devices or flanges incorporated in the components. All this is based on a simple yet sound principle: if loosening of the components is a problem the first thing to do is to fix them better. Yet how many surgeons test the quality of socket fixation at primary surgery?

2. The clinical result does not necessarily reflect the mechanical state of the arthroplasty. It is probably correct to say that failure to appreciate this fact has led to the delays in revision surgery. Far too often reliance is placed on the patient's performance rather than on radiological appearance. All patients should have access to follow-up facilities on a routine and individual basis, not only if symptoms arise.

3. Radiological changes often precede clinical symptoms. It has been pointed out that in a large proportion of the cases that come to revision for fracture or loosening of the stem, the changes putting them at risk for the complication can be seen radiologically within 1 year of surgery. Most, if not all, cases of deep sepsis can be diagnosed within the same period of time. Loosening of the socket appears to be related to wear to a greater degree and obviously long-term follow-up is essential. This aspect is discussed in the section on Socket Wear. Radiographic appearances at 1 year are a very useful prognostic guide to the eventual outcome of the operation.

4. Fixation having failed the radiological appearances do not improve with time. Loss of bone stock resulting from progressive loosening makes future revision surgery difficult. Thus it is inevitable that in some cases revision may have to be suggested to the patient if only to preserve the bone stock, offer a better mechanical solution or avoid further complications. This aspect must be understood and accepted by the patient and the surgeon before primary surgery.

5. Some changes affecting the eventual outcome of the operation are related to time and function. Of these the wear and loosening of the socket are most obvious. The sequence of events is as follows: the head bores for itself a new roughly cylindrical path; the angular range of movements becomes restricted; and impingement of the neck on the rim of the socket leads to shock loading and socket loosening. The incidence of socket loosening will thus be related to the depth of socket penetration.

6. Since total hip arthroplasty is a mechanical procedure it must be considered to be at risk for a mechanical complication at a future date. This type of surgery must not be equated with "soft-tissue surgery". What can be termed humorously as "after sales service" must be available to all patients undergoing total hip replacement or in fact any implant surgery.

What is Required for Component Fixation?

Component fixation relies on the grouting effect of the acrylic cement, the cement being injected into the cancellous bone of the femur and the acetabulum. The quality of the fixation will thus depend on the intimacy and area of the contact, the strength of the cancellous bone, the quality of the cement, the design of the components and the load imposed on the system. In practice, therefore, preservation of the strong cancellous bone is desirable. The bone must be cleaned to remove fat, fragments of bone and fibro-fatty marrow. Reaming of the medullary canal as far as the cortex is doomed to failure.

The cement must be devoid of laminations and there must be no admixture of blood and air with it. Although theoretically desirable, this may not always be possible in practice. Injecting the cement into the cancellous bone must improve the quality of fixation, whichever method is used. Care must be taken to avoid the escape of the cement into areas where it is not required.

Containment and Pressurization of Cement

It is a drawback at this stage of the procedure that bleeding of the cancellous bone cannot be even momentarily arrested or reduced by means other than hypotensive anaesthesia and by maintaining the pressure on the polymerizing cement. The effect of these measures is probably more obvious at the bone–cement junction than

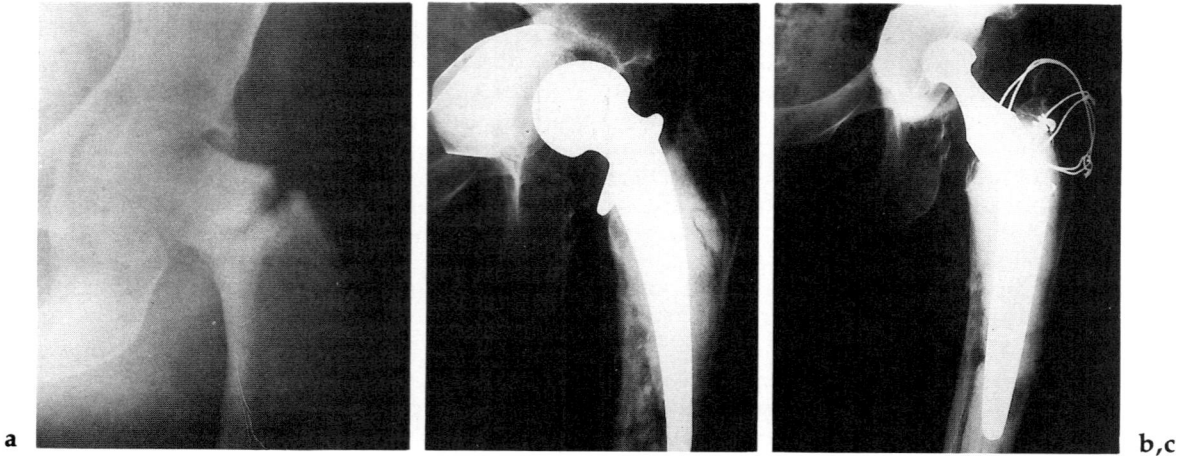

Fig. 7.2. Absence of the acetabular floor for socket support. **a** Fracture of the femoral neck. **b** Total hip arthroplasty. Note the wire mesh used to cover the acetabular defect and the position of the stem. **c** Four years after revision: flanged socket supported on the rim; wire mesh covering the central acetabular defect.

within the body of the cement itself, provided of course that the cement is well contained.

The femoral component must be devoid of stress risers and must take up a proportion of the medullary canal leaving a layer of well-injected cement which is thick and strong enough to support the load, yet thin enough to allow the transfer of it onto the femoral shaft. This load transfer must be aimed at the proximal femur and jamming of the stem too far distally within the medullary canal is to be avoided. A narrower or even a slightly shorter stem is to be preferred. The size of the head of the femoral component must be such as to give the lowest possible frictional torque without creating instability. In the study of the long-term results the original 22.25 mm (7/8″) Charnley design has been shown to have withstood the test of time.

The socket must be as thick as possible. This is to give it some rigidity and to offer a reasonable thickness of plastic for wear. A flange should be an integral part of the socket. When trimmed to size and shape it will further allow cement containment and pressurization. Metal backing of the socket has been advocated for some time now. Charnley was the first to use this type of socket in 1962–1964, albeit uncemented. Its recent re-introduction was based on interesting

experimental evidence. However, the clinical results have so far not fulfilled the expectations (Harris and Penenberg, personal communication). The importance for metal backing may be more obvious in cases of thin plastic sockets with a thin layer of cement. It must be accepted with their use that some of the bone–cement junction changes will become obscured by the metal and accurate radiological measurements of socket wear may not always be possible. The concept is discussed in more detail in Chap. 12.

Socket Fixation

In practice, fixation of the socket depends upon injection of the acrylic cement into the cancellous bone of the acetabulum using either the multiple drill hole technique or exposure of the cancellous bone deep to the subchondral plate or more often a combination of the two.

Preservation of the strong, load-bearing subchondral plate, if present, appears to be logical. (Its function could probably be compared to that of the femoral cortex.) The load is now transmitted across the joint, into the body of the plastic socket, into the cement and onto the hemi-pelvis. By the very nature of the concentricity of the socket design and its fixation, and due to the fact that the socket is hardly ever loaded exactly symmetrically, the superior part of the socket will be under compression while the inferior part is under tension. The turning moment thus applied to the socket will tend to move the socket into a vertical (open laterally) and ante-verted (open anteriorly) position.

The floor of the acetabulum by itself is prob-ably incapable of transferring anything more than a partial load and can be seen to fail under certain circumstances, be they natural or artifi-cial; witness the failure of the floor in protrusio, femoral head replacement and prolapse of the socket in total hip replacement. Thus it can be argued that in the design of the component and the method of its implantation, transfer of the full load onto the floor of the acetabulum is to be avoided. Preferably the load should be trans-ferred through the rim of the acetabulum while full cover of the socket is maintained. Failure of the acetabular rim does not occur except occasionally if the disease process is of the grossly destructive variety, or if the large superior margin cysts collapse or following trauma.

A sufficient number of cases of revision have now been carried out, and with a reasonably long follow-up, to suggest that a socket securely supported on the rim, even in the absence of the acetabular floor, is compatible with excellent clinical results (Fig. 7.2). And yet is socket fixation really essential for the clinical success of the operation? Probably not. A handful of Charnley uncemented press-fit sockets are still functioning 25 years later. A loose socket is asymptomatic and this point has been missed by those who advocate cement-free systems. Free-dom from symptoms is equated with clinical success which in turn is taken as an indicator of socket fixation by bony ingrowth!

"In order to achieve clinical success in total hip arthroplasty fixation of the socket is not essential – but a change in position of the socket is likely to lead to a clinical failure" (Wroblewski 1987).

The Femur

The femoral side of the operation is based on a common engineering principle – that of male (stem) and female (cement) tapers engaging under load. For the system to become load bearing the stem must slip within the cement. (For the cement to slip within the femur would very likely indicate a mechanical and a clinical failure but there are exceptions.) From experi-ments, McLeish (1977) estimated that slip with the early flat-back Charnley stem was about 0.5 mm and probably occurred in the very early stages of weight bearing. Loudon and Charnley (1980) also studied this slip, taking accurate measurements from radiographs. The advan-tage of the slip of the stem within the cement mantle is also an integral part of the design and implantation of the Exeter prosthesis. This slip and its consequences must be examined in the light of the surgical technique and the com-ponent design.

If cement injection leaves a poorly supported area of cement proximally then slip of the stem will result in splitting of the cement mantle, as pointed out by Stauffer (1982). If the cement is well injected, giving excellent support for the stem, then the stem may slip within the cement mantle, its integrity being preserved. This is the most likely explanation for the success of implantation of the Exeter prosthesis, but it can only succeed if the stem is unsupported distally.

The stem design will obviously play a part as well. The greater the offset the more extensive is the proximal cement disruption likely to be. The smaller the taper the greater the slip. Thus a combination of a relatively straight stem with a small offset, a narrow taper and a polished finish is likely to give the greatest slip and the mini-mum of medial femoral destruction.

In clinical practice this slip of the stem within the cement mantle is associated with fracture of the cement at the tip of the stem and separation of the lateral aspect of the stem from the cement. The significance of this becomes apparent if in the process the proximal support of the stem is lost while its distal portion becomes tightly fixed within the cement mantle. Increased leverage of the proximal unsupported part of the stem will result in an increased deflection of the stem and stress concentration between the fixed and the unsupported parts of the stem, thus increasing the "functional offset". Deflection of the stem under load will lead to very small movements between the stem and the cement and between the cement and bone at its proximal part, and this in turn will lead to micro fractures of the cancellous bone and fragmentation of the cement. Repeated mechanical pumping action of the "synovial" (actually bursal) fluid and its

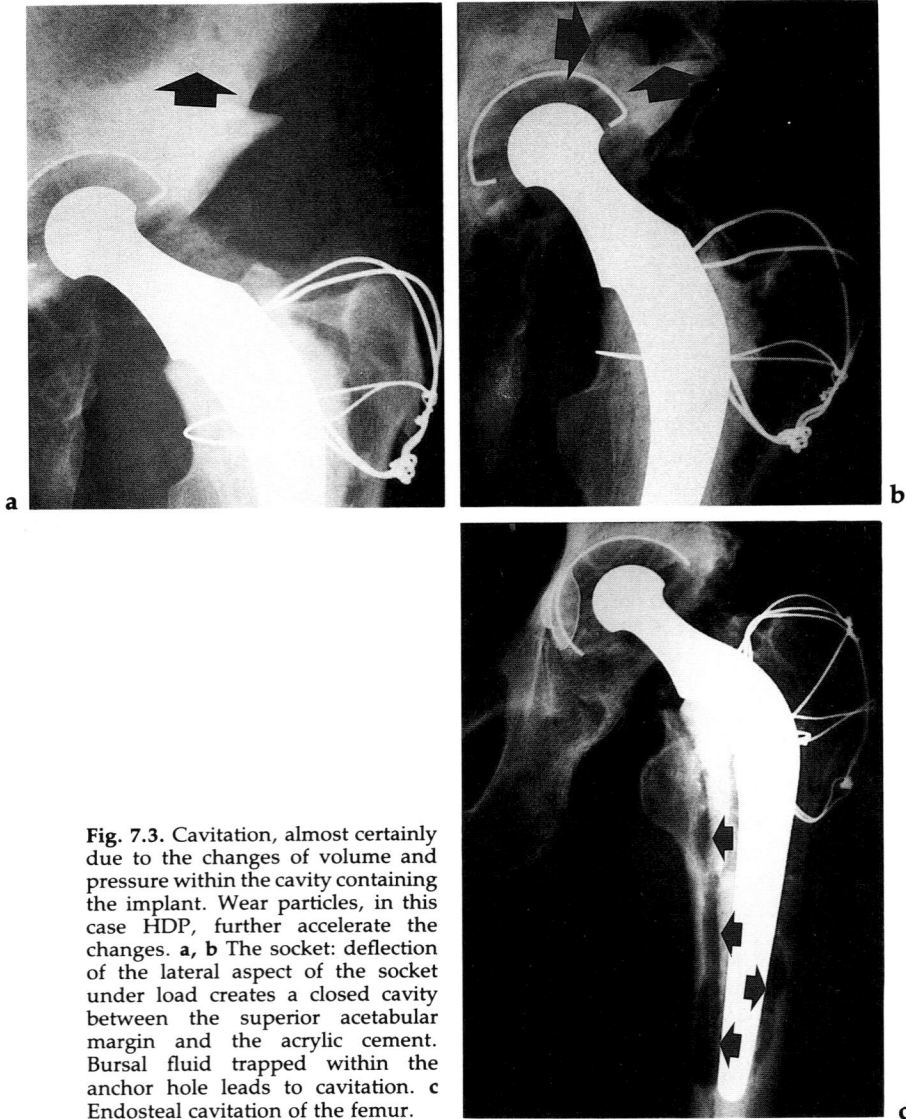

Fig. 7.3. Cavitation, almost certainly due to the changes of volume and pressure within the cavity containing the implant. Wear particles, in this case HDP, further accelerate the changes. **a, b** The socket: deflection of the lateral aspect of the socket under load creates a closed cavity between the superior acetabular margin and the acrylic cement. Bursal fluid trapped within the anchor hole leads to cavitation. **c** Endosteal cavitation of the femur.

contents will lead to gradual erosion of the cancellous and cortical bone and to endosteal cavitation (Fig. 7.3) because of the changes in the volume and pressure within the joint cavity. Fracture of the stem is likely to follow.

Thus on the femoral side there can be two sites of failure: between the stem and the cement and between cement and bone. Furthermore, on the femoral side the load is transferred through the stem to the cement and then through the cancellous bone of the endosteum to the femoral cortex (as hoop stress) and not in a physiological manner through the proximal femoral cortex. This in itself may defunction part of the proximal femur, transferring the stress onto its more distal part. In this context the anatomy of the proximal femur must be considered. In the development of the proximal femur the lesser trochanter is

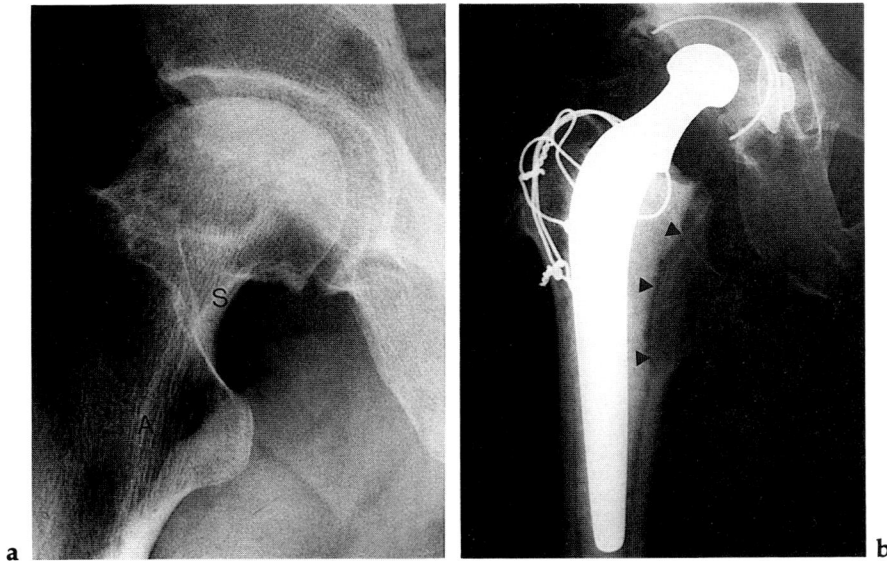

Fig. 7.4. The calcar. **a** *A*, the anatomical calcar; *S* the surgical calcar. **b** The position of the anatomical calcar clearly shown on the post-operative radiograph by the lack of cement injection into its cortical-like structure.

formed by the traction of the ilio-psoas which separates the femoral cortex into two layers, the outer cortex and the inner calcar (or calcar femorale) (Fig. 7.4). The two join proximally to form the medial portion of the femoral neck, erroneously called "calcar". With advancing years the calcar (the anatomical one) is thinned out and eventually lost, in some measure no doubt contributing to the increasing incidence of fractures of the femoral neck. This anatomical calcar, if poor in quality, should be removed at primary surgery to allow cement injection into the strong cancellous bone of the lesser trochanter, thus offering postero-medial support of the proximal part of the stem.

In the design and technique of total hip arthroplasty the objective is to transfer the load from the head and neck of the stem to the most proximal part of the femur in a physiologically feasible way. Two things become immediately clear. First, the intramedullary portion of the stem serves as an anchor for the head and neck. Second, the head and the neck, being of necessity extrafemoral and therefore unsupported, now serve to clear the femur away from the pelvis which allows a certain range of movements. The head and neck act as a counterlever beam and there will therefore always be the

potential for failure at the junction of the fixed stem and the unsupported head and neck.

In the design of the stem and in its surgical fixation all the aspects discussed must be taken into account. Because stem fracture has been such as dramatic complication and stem loosening an early symptom-producing problem, most work on component fixation concentrated initially on the stem. Use of a larger, longer stem, closure of the distal portion of the medullary canal and pressurization of low-viscosity cement were advocated. Experimental work suggests that a 10-cm intramedullary portion of the stem, provided it is well supported, is sufficient. If the segment is shorter then the great increase of the stress within the cement at the tip of the stem is likely to lead to failure of the cement.

In the context of total hip arthroplasty the function of the collar of the femoral stem appears at this stage to be an unresolved issue. A prospective study has been completed but the detailed analysis is outside the scope of this work.

The thickness of the cement layer within the various areas of the medullary canal has been the subject of much discussion and many publications. It is largely irrelevant however, and only distracts attention from the real issue. Even a piece of tissue paper is capable of supporting the weight of an elephant provided the tissue paper itself is well supported, and stress risers and sheering stress are avoided. Our attention must accordingly be directed to the preparation of bone, cement injection, stem design, load and function, bone changes occurring with age and repeated or accidental stresses. The cement will look after itself provided it has been used properly at primary surgery. It is the use of the cement that is equated with the surgical technique. The latter is a commodity that cannot be sold by a manufacturer but must be learned by the surgeon. Successful surgery requires an understandiing of the technique and the design and attention to detail at every stage of the procedure. To blame cement for failures is to blame surgical technique in the majority of cases.

It is fascinating to contemplate what attention each one of us would pay to acrylic cement and the technique of component fixation if our own freedom from pain and mobility depended on two "bags of cement", not just for a short period, but for many years to come.

8 The Socket: Changes at the Bone–Cement Interface

Appearances of the implant–bone interface of a cemented socket have been the subject of many studies and publications. The description and recording of radiographic images are bound to be associated with variations in terminology and differences between observers or between the same observer on different occasions. Even if a classification did become universally acceptable it would have to bear some relation to clinical practice and long-term management. In this context the systematic studies of Hodgkinson et al. (1989a) are most valuable.

Since almost all cases of failure of the cemented socket occur at the bone–cement interface, it may be of interest to consider the likely reasons as well as the sequence for the various radiographic appearances. Whether or not the changes at the bone–cement junction are obvious on a radiograph will depend on the intimacy of the contact and the angle of incidence of the x-ray beam. Thus direct contact between intact, strong, load-bearing, subchondral bone of the roof of the acetabulum and the cement may give an appearance of demarcation, yet multiple drill holes into the same plate, with cement injected, may obscure that picture. Is this more desirable in the long term? Extensions of cement into soft cancellous bone may give an impression of good fixation in the early cases, but is that synonymous with long-term success?

We must direct our attention to the behaviour of the implant under load, to the direction and magnitude of that load, to load transmission from the implant to the skeleton and to the mechanical changes resulting from wear. Meanwhile uniformity of descriptive terms, correlation between radiographic appearances and operative findings and definition of prognostic signs would go a long way towards improving our understanding of this complex subject.

Any discussion of the appearances of the bone–cement junction of the socket is best carried out under separate headings, and the terminology should be standardized. This almost compartmental logic may appear rigid yet it serves a very useful purpose when attempting to understand radiographic appearances, operative findings, clinical outcome and the long-term results.

Demarcation of the Socket

Whether or not an obvious junction between the bone and the cement is seen on a radiograph will depend on the intimacy of contact and the degree of ramification between the two as well as on the angle of incidence of the x-ray beam, exposure and no doubt on the availability of serial radiographs for comparison. Traditionally it has been accepted that the extent of demarcation should be measured according to segments as seen on an AP radiograph. Although very convenient, this approach is immediately limiting. It suggests that a demarcation increasing from the outer third of the socket to affect the

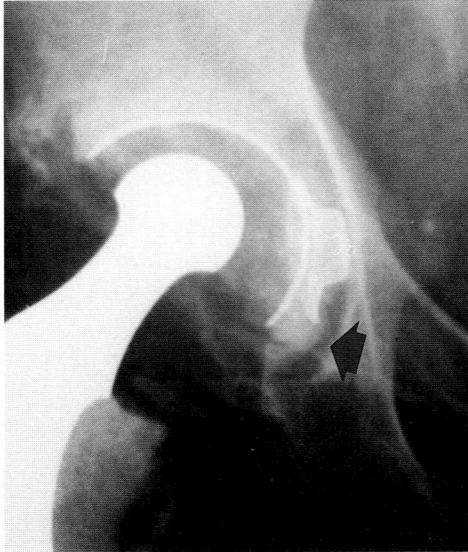

Fig. 8.1. Collection of wear debris at the inferior margin of the bone–cement junction of the socket. The appearance superiorly is deceptively "benign". The socket was in fact loose.

Table 8.1. Indications for revision in the group of cases studied

Indications for revision	No. of cases
Fractured stem	89
Loose stem	32
Loose socket and stem	26
Infection	22
Loose socket	17
Recurrent dislocation	14
Total	200

complete socket is a continuous progression of the same process, and it completely disregards the lateral radiograph which is often more informative. The two-thirds demarcation of the socket is difficult to diagnose with confidence and as such may be of limited value. Attempts to measure accurately this often very irregular space may be misleading; it is probably correct to accept a division into two categories: (a) 1 mm or less and (b) more than 1 mm. Finally, in order to be able to diagnose socket migration with certainty, good quality serial radiographs must be available.

Socket Migration

The term socket migration is used to define a change in position of the socket (usually the socket–cement complex). The degree of socket migration is best determined on good quality serial radiographs by using various anatomical points in the area for comparison. (Watch out for the collection of wear products at the inferior margin of socket, see Fig. 8.1.) It is easy to diagnose when obvious but more difficult when the changes are only minor or are the result of the socket rotating only a few degrees on its

central axis. There are bound to be "grey areas" when the test is applied to clinical situations. The immediately obvious questions which must be asked are: Is movement or rotation of the implant synonymous with migration? Does the migration have to be in a particular direction (upwards, inwards or outwards)? How does complete demarcation correlate with migration? Although the answers to the questions may be essential, they are best viewed in isolation so as not to detract from the essential problem, i.e. progressive loss of bone stock.

Thus demarcation of the outer third of the socket may be obvious on the immediate post-operative radiograph and if so is probably the result of the surgical technique. It needs to be watched. Although it may not progress, if it does it will lead to socket migration. A socket which is fully demarcated by 1 year will eventually migrate. A socket showing no demarcation will maintain this appearance until the penetration due to wear reaches a certain depth; demarcation and migration will almost certainly follow.

Table 8.2. Classification of radiographic demarcation irrespective of the gap size

Type 0 = No demarcation
Type 1 = Demarcation of outer third only
Type 2 = Demarcation of outer and middle third
Type 3 = Complete demarcation
Type 4 = Socket migration, change of position as judged on serial radiographs

Table 8.3. Correlation between radiographic appearances and operative findings

	Demarcation				Socket migration
	None	Outer third	Outer and middle thirds	Complete	
No. of cases	24	68	28	52	28
Socket loose at revision	0	5	20	49	28
Per cent loose sockets	0	7	71	94	100

Correlation Between Radiographic Appearances and the Clinical Results

There is no clear correlation between the radiographic appearances of the bone–cement junction and the clinical results. This fact is not appreciated often enough. Surgeons are at times in strong disagreement as to the need for operative intervention for radiographic changes alone, demanding that revision should be carried out only in the presence of symptoms. But then, what are the symptoms of a fully demarcated socket? To await symptoms may mean having to retrieve the socket from inside the pelvis. Papers have been published mentioning "symptomatic socket loosening" but these failed to define the entity – a sad omission. Allan et al. (in press) studied all the cases of socket revision of the Charnley LFA carried out by the author. Symptoms other than discomfort were exceptional. More common were comments on changes in function.

Correlation Between Radiographic Appearances and the Operative Findings

This correlation has been studied in some detail by Hodgkinson et al. (1989a) in a review of 200 consecutive revisions of the Charnley LFA (Table 8.1) carried out by the author. The appearances on the pre-operative radiograph were classified according to the extent of bone–cement demarcation (Table 8.2) and without the knowledge of the operative findings. Only then was the correlation between the radiographic appearances and operative findings assessed. The results have been tabulated (Table 8.3) and are probably more obvious when presented

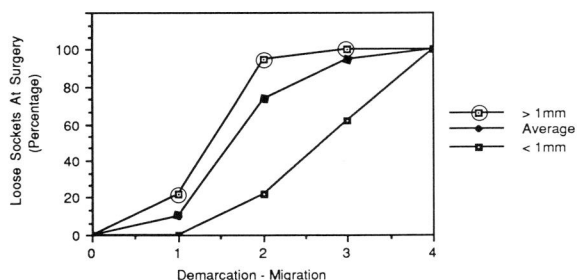

Fig. 8.2. Correlation between the radiographic appearance of demarcation (both in extent and depth) and the incidence of socket migration (after Hodgkinson et al. 1989a).

graphically (Fig. 8.2). The study has also shown that sockets that were fully demarcated at 1 year had migrated by the time of revision. No attempt was made to correlate the appearance with symptoms or the need for revisions. However, this study has been criticized even before publication, the strongest objection being that conclusions were drawn from revisions and not from unrevised cases. This objection is unfounded. Testing of sockets at primary and revision surgery gave a good indication of the difference between successful and failed cases. On the acetabular side radiographic findings were not always an indication for revision as in cases of fractured or loose stems. The mere fact that a total hip arthroplasty has not come to revision and thus has offered no opportunity to test the socket surely cannot imply that the socket is firmly fixed. What the Hodgkinson study has given is an excellent example of a simple and reproducible method which is of practical value in assessing radiographic appearances and in planning any future management.

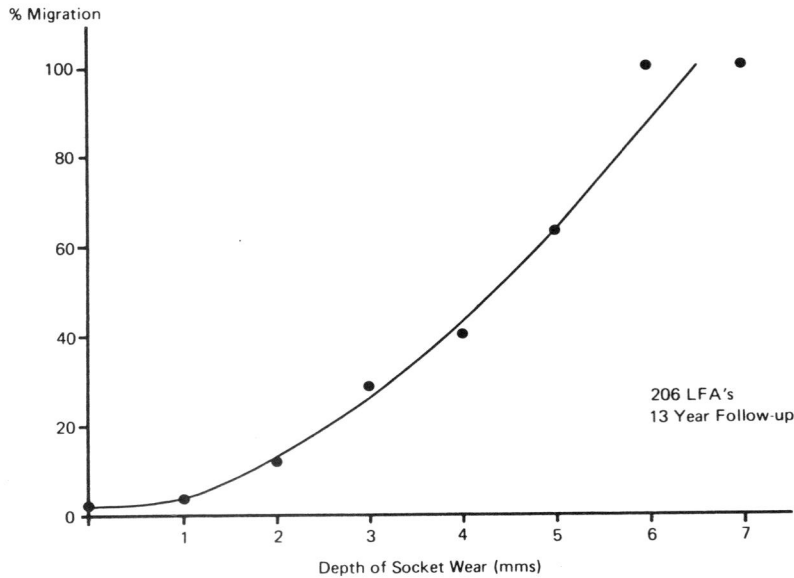

Fig. 8.3. The correlation between the depth of socket wear and the incidence of socket migration. Based on 206 LFAs with an average follow-up of 13 years.

Correlation Between the Depth of Socket Wear and the Incidence of Socket Migration

This rather unexpected correlation between the depth of socket wear and the incidence of socket migration was discovered accidentally when reviewing a group of 104 Charnley LFAs in 71 patients under the age of 40 (Wroblewski 1985a) and was confirmed when the results of a 15–21-year follow-up of Charnley LFAs were analysed in similar manner (Wroblewski 1986a). The second group was in fact reviewed first but correlation between the depth of wear and the incidence of socket migration was not sought at the initial review.

The results of the two studies are shown graphically in Fig. 8.3. The implication appears to be obvious: progressive wear will result in socket migration. Study of wear, friction and impingement of the neck of the stem on socket rim is thus considered to be more important than attempts to fix the socket by bony ingrowth; the first addresses the cause, the second attempts to solve the effect but disregards the cause.

Correlation Between Radiographic Appearances and Long-Term Clinical Results

It may be of interest to point out at the outset that "long-term" is an expression used loosely and no attempt is made to quantify the period of time involved. It may imply time to revision or time to radiological or clinical failure or the longest follow-up available with normal clinical function, or may be concerned with clinical results and radiographic appearances in a group of patients with the longest follow-up to date. Since socket demarcation and even migration is compatible with apparently normal clinical function, it must not be assumed that normal function is synonymous with long-term success. Regular follow-up and careful radiographic study are essential if gross loss of bone stock is to be avoided. This aspect of the operation must be understood by the patient and surgeon alike. To assume otherwise is to practice in ignorance of the real problem.

That a loose socket is often asymptomatic is probably the result of the fact that such a situation does not produce a "closed system" which would generate changes in the pressure within the bone. The socket being loaded asymmetrically must relieve pressure at the bone–cement junction almost automatically, unlike on the femoral side where the "one-way non-return value" of the stem–cement complex operates. Witness the symptomatic nature of a loose stem and the frequency of endosteal cavitation which results from the consequent pressure and volume changes.

Socket Demarcation and Loosening

This very important subject has not received sufficient theoretical and experimental evaluation. Excluding cases of deep sepsis and disregarding the inherent variations in component design there are probably three basic mechanisms that are likely to result in socket demarcation and loosening. These are surgical technique, socket wear and the long-term response of bone to the implant in the context of the natural history of the hip condition demanding total hip arthroplasty.

Surgical Technique

Excessive Reaming

Historically this was the result, in some cases, of attempts to restore the lever ratios by total hip arthroplasty. It was not only bone of the medial wall that was lost but often subchondral bone as well. When combined with lack of rim support, this sometimes resulted in socket loosening.

Inadequate Fixation

A socket implanted in the usual orientation of 45° open laterally and neutral or a few degrees open anteriorly (anteversion) will be subject to a load which is probably never exactly directed through the centre of the socket, and may even be lateral to the vertical drawn from the centre of the head of the femoral component.

When under load, the socket, if given the opportunity to spin in any direction, will tend to tilt into a vertical and anteverted position (open

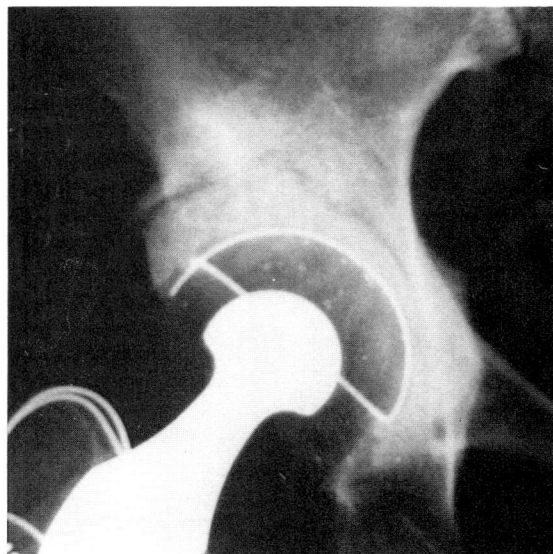

Fig. 8.4. Poor cement injection. Low-viscosity cement was used but was apparently neither fully contained nor adequately pressurized. Two-thirds of the socket demarcated by 3 months. Patient asymptomatic.

laterally and anteriorly). (Witness the mechanism of the stem fracture, slipped upper femoral epiphysis and fractures of the femoral neck.) The superior part of the socket will be in compression, the inferior part under tension. The bone–cement junction will be affected likewise. This basic mechanism will obviously not vary according to the surgical technique of socket implantation but will be merely a reflection of the load and its direction.

Thus a surgical technique which results in the collection of blood and debris at the cement–bone junction or poor cement injection will lead to early demarcation (Fig. 8.4). When the socket is under load, the tendency will be for the gap to be reduced superiorly, but for it to be increased inferiorly and medially. If attention is directed to the usual outer third of the socket it may appear that the superior demarcation is decreasing, but this would be misleading.

It may be of interest to note that in the vast majority of cases with the longest follow-up (15–21 years) there was an extrusion of cement through the pilot hole. This extruded cement possibly acted as a collar stud and reduced the likelihood of socket tilting (Fig. 8.5). In the early years of the Charnley technique this acetabular cement restrictor was not available.

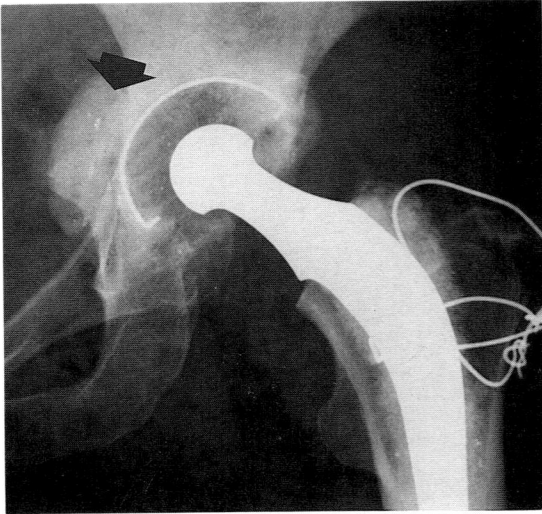

Fig. 8.5. The typical appearance of the longest follow-up cases of the Charnley LFA. Acetabular pilot hole, not covered by the wire mesh cement restrictor, allowed intra-pelvic intrusion of the cement. Could this have been one reason why the socket did not tilt?

Inadequate Lateral Support

If the supero-lateral part of the acetabulum is not prepared accurately, if the cement is not properly injected, if the socket is not fully covered superio-laterally or if during socket insertion the socket is allowed to tilt into a transverse position then a gap may develop at the bone–cement junction leaving the implant partly unsupported. Under load there are bound to be changes in volume and pressure within that space leading to wear and to entry of bursal fluid and other debris. This progressive supero-lateral cavitation may be quite spectacular (Fig. 8.6) and may even occasionally lead to fracture of the unsupported socket (Fig. 8.7). The effect is almost certainly purely mechanical; any histological effects of the high-density polyethylene (HDP) or cement particles are almost certainly secondary to the loosening. With a large head and a thin HDP shell fracture is probably a combination of wear and fatigue (Fig. 8.8) and is a relatively common finding.

Socket Wear

This is the result of repeated shock loading of the rim of the socket by the neck of the stem as the

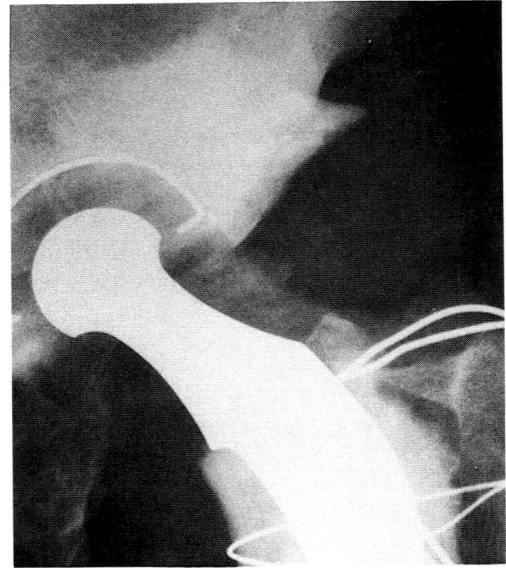

a

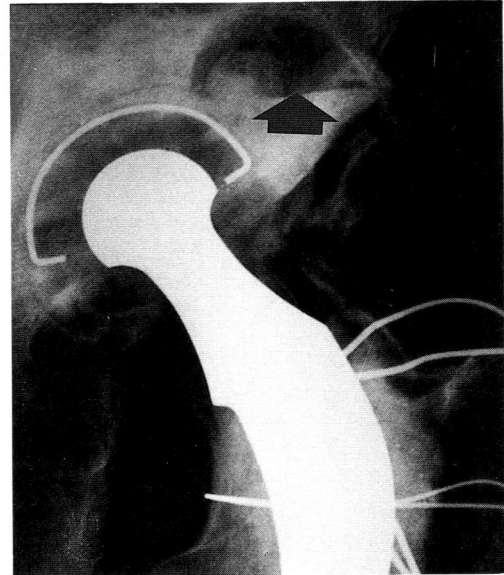

b

Fig. 8.6. Supero-lateral cavitation around the anchoring cement peg. **a** Post-operative radiograph. **b** Cavitation around the anchoring cement peg 7½ years after surgery. Clinically asymptomatic.

depth of socket penetration increases with wear and restricts the range of movement. Since the socket rim erosion is invariably in the same direction as the socket penetration, i.e. in the coronal plane, and since the area eroded is almost always symmetrical in outline and does not exceed the initial bore diameter in the sagittal plane, the conclusion drawn is that it is the

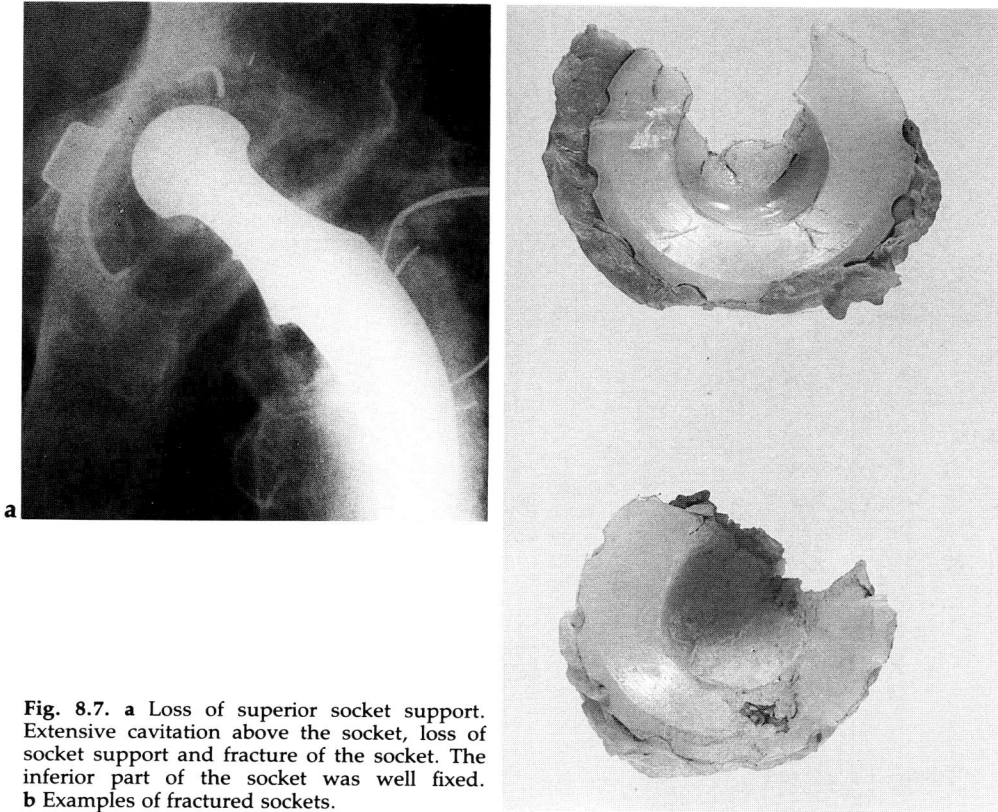

Fig. 8.7. a Loss of superior socket support. Extensive cavitation above the socket, loss of socket support and fracture of the socket. The inferior part of the socket was well fixed. **b** Examples of fractured sockets.

coronal movement of the pelvis rather than the sagittal movement of the limb which is responsible for this impingement and loosening (Fig. 8.9). Impingement in the sagittal plane, as in flexion–extension, would be expected to lead to an asymmetrical erosion, being more extensive anteriorly and exceeding the size of the initial bore diameter. The net effect must be progressive separation of the socket–cement complex from the underlying bone following deformation of the plastic, and compression superiorly and tension and separation from the bone inferiorly. Obviously in any particular case several processes are likely to be occurring simultaneously.

Natural History of the Hip Condition

This aspect has not been studied in detail. It is clear that various types of arthritis can produce cysts, osteophytes, subarticular sclerosis, protrusio or bone destruction which are all visible on radiographs. It is probably not correct to assume that all cases will respond uniformly to a cemented total hip arthroplasty. In fact it is probably more likely that the long-term result will, to a degree, depend on the natural history of the hip condition. Why is it that three series, those of Charnley (1979a), Wroblewski (1986a) and Fowler et al. (1988), have recorded an almost identical incidence of long-term socket loosening of around 25% (Table 8.4)? Could it be that the incidences are a reflection of clinical selection of patients and the natural history of the arthritic hip rather than the effect of surgical technique or of component design? What about the effect of drugs?

It is apparent that socket demarcation, migration and wear are very complex issues. When component design, surgical technique, length of follow-up and clinical results are also taken into consideration the complexity becomes even more obvious. Any variations in definition or observer description will further add to the problem. Thus it is futile to use one descriptive

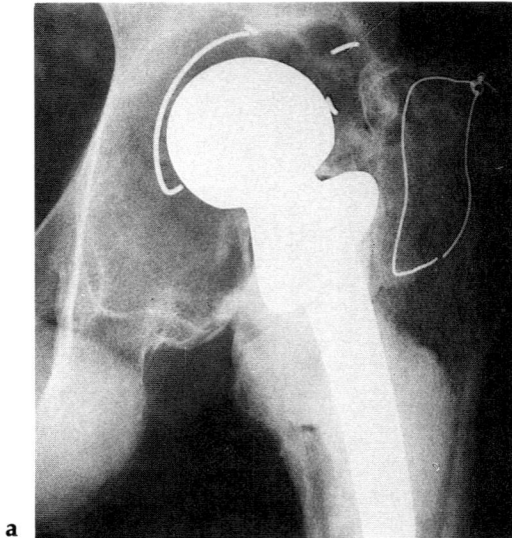

Fig. 8.8. The problem of wear, loosening, large head of the femoral component and thin HDP socket. **a** Wear, loosening and fracture of HDP socket. **b** Examples of fractured sockets.

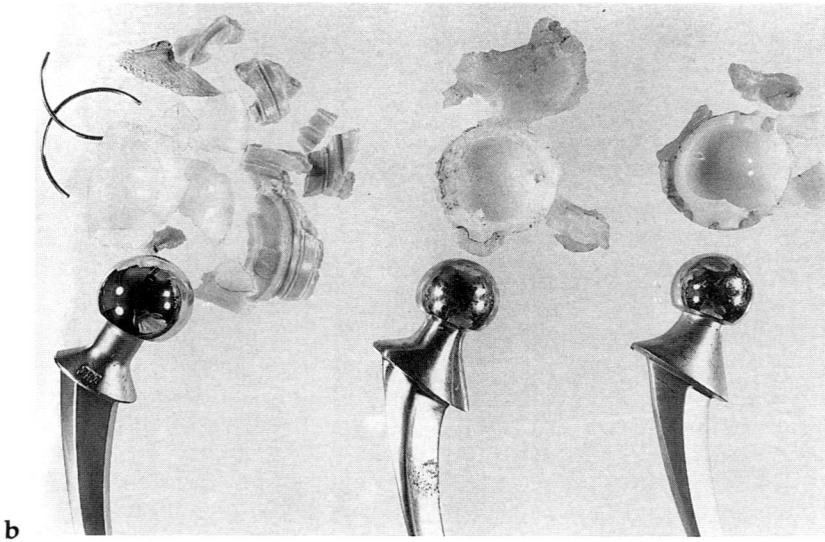

Table 8.4. Socket loosening: the long-term problem. Comparison of results of various series

Total hip arthroplasty	Follow-up period years	Complete socket demarcation, migration, loosening (%)	Reference
Charnley LFA	11–15	24.0	Charnley (1979)
Charnley LFA	15–21	22.5	Wroblewski (1987)
Exeter			
Pressurization satisfactory	5–10 10–16	1.96 24.5	Fowler et al. (1988)
Pressurization unsatisfactory or not used	5–10 10–16	12 22.4	

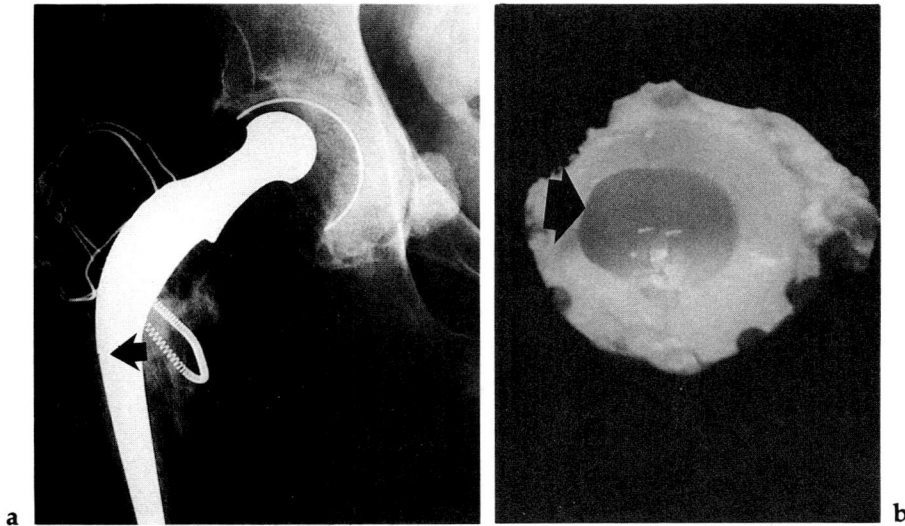

Fig. 8.9. Direction of impingement with socket wear. **a** Gross wear and grade 3 demarcation of the socket in a very active male. Asymptomatic until the stem fractured. **b** Photograph of the socket rim (due to the impingement of the neck of the stem) was exactly in the coronal plane.

term in an attempt to convey the many aspects of the possible problems. Descriptions of radiographic appearances must be simple and easily recognizable, socket wear must be measurable and the clinical result must not overshadow the radiographic changes. Socket fixation does not improve with time and function, and bone stock is readily lost. Function, not as a clinical result, but as a reflection of load and sliding distance at the hip level, is something that is yet to be quantified, and yet it must be if progress is to be made in this type of surgery.

In any study, and for any surgical procedure, the surgeon must be aware of the various aspects of the appearance of the bone–cement junction as a reflection of component design, surgical technique, function and wear. In order to do this long-term follow-up is essential.

9 Loosening of the Socket

Introduction

Study of the socket in the context of total hip arthroplasty is a complex subject. No single aspect can be viewed in isolation. Any review must take into account the state of the art and science as applied to primary surgery and interpret them as clinical and radiological results some years later. Thus the longest follow-up results will invariably be based on the earliest designs and surgical techniques. It is also necessary to take into account the time lag between the primary operation and the revision; the correlation, or lack of it, between the radiographic appearances, the clinical function and the operative findings; the mechanical and histological effects of socket wear; and the various attempts to improve the long-term success by changes in the technique or component design.

Thus it is not possible to have the latest component design, the most up-to-date surgical technique and the longest follow-up all at the same time. All this is made even more complex by the varieties of designs and surgical techniques, the length of the follow-up, the variations in terminology and in the clinical or radiological interpretation of the results.

When it is appreciated that in order to achieve clinical success fixation of the socket is not essential, but that changes at the implant–bone interface may lead to failure, the whole aspect of the socket in total hip arthroplasty may appear incomprehensible.

In order to understand the problem of socket loosening in total hip arthroplasty in general, and in the low-friction arthroplasty in particular, it may be of interest to review briefly the evolution of the technique and of the component design of the Charnley low-friction arthroplasty. The central theme of the arthroplasty is the low-frictional torque with a small femoral head and a thick plastic socket. In the execution of the operation, the teachings of Pauwels were followed. Every attempt was made to restore, or even to improve, the lever ratios. The acetabulum was reamed deep and proximally. The "bench mark" was the thickness of the floor remaining rather than its quality or the degree of socket cover. The subchondral plate, if present, was often removed. The socket was invariably placed deep and proximally. Preparation of the acetabular bone for cement injection was basic. No washing or brushing was carried out. Usually no more than two (ilium and ischium) and only sometimes three (ilium, ischium and pubis) 12.5-mm (1/2") anchor holes were made for cement injection. The cement was used relatively late and the scalloped socket was usually much smaller than the cavity it was being fitted into. (The flanged socket and the ogee-flanged socket were very much later additions designed specifically to improve cement containment and pressurization.) Cement was not always allowed to polymerize before the next stage of the operation, i.e. the preparation of the medullary canal, was undertaken. It must be appreciated

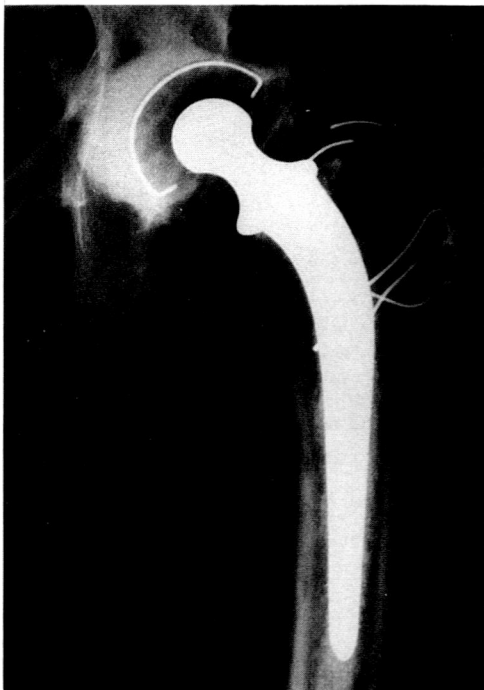

Fig. 9.1. Over 20-year follow-up. There is nothing to distinguish the latest appearance from the post-operative radiograph. The design of the stem indicates the stage of evolution of the LFA.

The Time Lag Between Primary and Revision Surgery

Charnley was the first to point out that loosening of the socket was going to be the most likely long-term problem. His views on the subject are probably accurately summarized in the following statement: "An important observation derived from a 12–15 year study, was that migration [of the socket] appeared to accelerate after about 10 years" (Charnley 1979a). In the theoretical considerations as well as practical execution of the operation, this was the problem uppermost in his mind. And yet, because of the asymptomatic nature of loose sockets the problem was not studied in great depth. This, in a way, has no doubt contributed to some delay in the advancement of socket design and of the technique of socket fixation. It was not until Charnley presented his 12–15-year results that the magnitude of the problem likely to present itself with time became obvious.

In his review of 396 cases, Charnley (1979a) pointed out that some 25% of sockets were considered to be likely to need revision in the future because of loosening. This was probably the statement that has led to the explosion in the use of uncemented arthroplasty, judging by the frequency with which the reference has been quoted.

A review of all revisions of low-friction arthroplasties carried out at the Centre for Hip Surgery, Wrightington Hospital, has brought some interesting facts to light. The first revision for loosening of the socket was carried out in 1968, 6 years after the introduction of the low-friction arthroplasty into routine clinical practice (Fig. 9.2). At that stage some 2500 operations had already been carried out. Two conclusions can be drawn from this finding. First, that at any stage a number of cases may be potential candidates for revision because of loosening of the socket. The second conclusion is that a minimum, of 6 years of clinical experience and some 2500 cases are needed before any meaningful pronouncement can be made on the likelihood of success or failure of any new method aimed at improving socket fixation. Shorter follow-up may be of interest but only if the aim is specifically to study certain radiological features that may appear earlier.

The findings also showed that with time the number of cases being revised for loosening of the socket is increasing. This is probably also a

that in the early days of the low-friction arthroplasty the restoration of the lever ratios combined with the surgical technique of the acetabular preparation led at times to loosening of the socket.

Even though the technique was unsophisticated and the components had not reached their full design potential, many of the early cases have enjoyed normal function for more than 20 years (Fig. 9.1). This must surely be a tribute to the correctness of the concept of low-frictional torque in its clinical application.

Three further observations make the study and management of socket loosening of the utmost importance:

1. The time lag between primary and revision surgery.
2. The correlation between the clinical, the radiological and the operative findings.
3. The wear of the HDP socket and the resultant mechanical and histological changes.

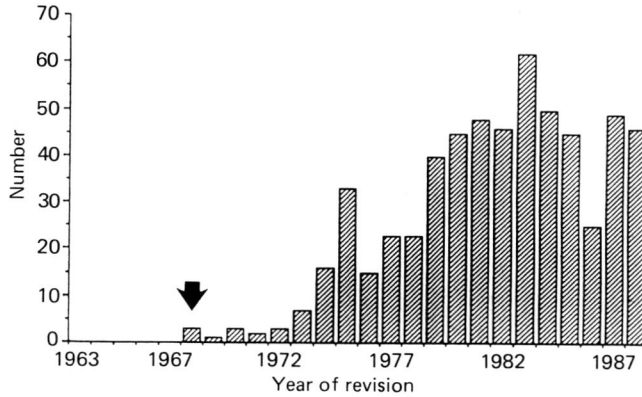

Fig. 9.2. The time lag between introduction of the LFA into clinical practice and revision for socket loosening. The 6-year period, November 1962–1968, was free from revisions for socket loosening.

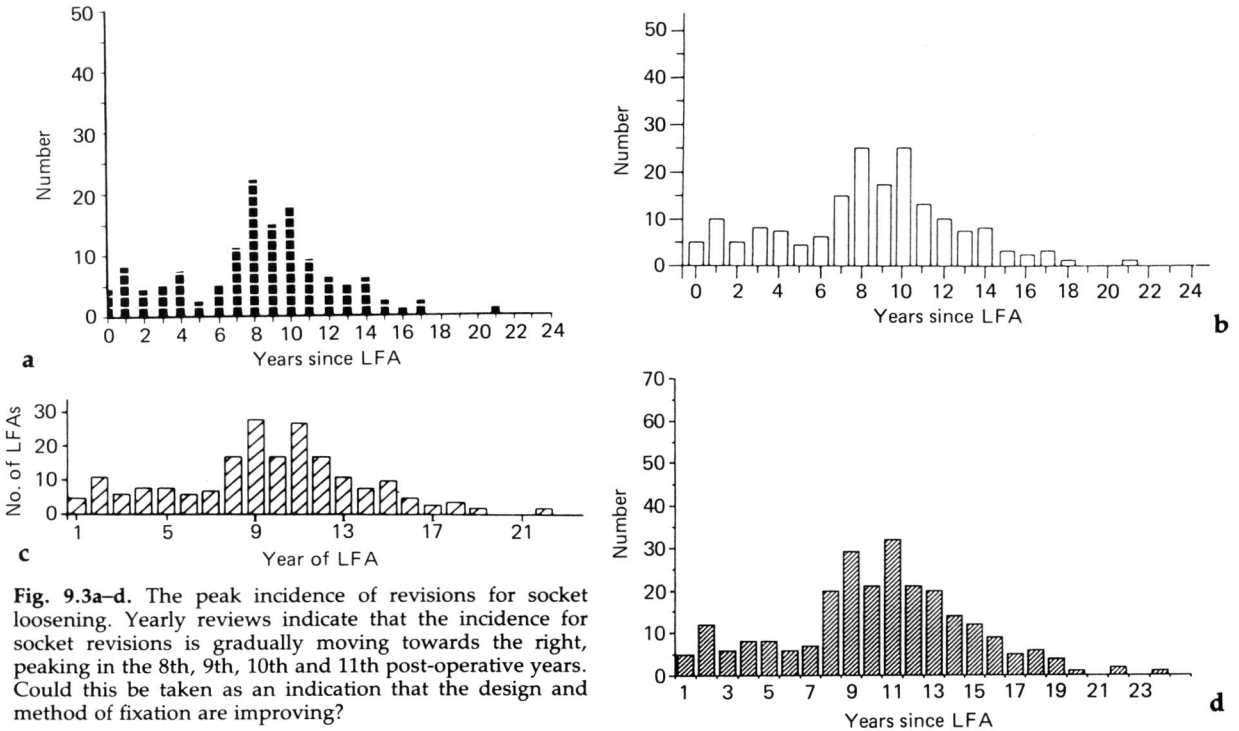

Fig. 9.3a–d. The peak incidence of revisions for socket loosening. Yearly reviews indicate that the incidence for socket revisions is gradually moving towards the right, peaking in the 8th, 9th, 10th and 11th post-operative years. Could this be taken as an indication that the design and method of fixation are improving?

reflection of the increasing follow-up time and the realization that revisions should be carried out at an earlier stage. Detailed analysis shows that wear of the socket plays an ever-increasing role in this problem.

Although some sockets have been revised as early as 2 years post-operatively the problem really peaks in the eleventh post-operative year (Fig. 9.3). This finding once again stresses the need for long-term follow-up.

The Correlation Between the Clinical, the Radiological and the Operative Findings

Although radiological reviews have always formed a part of the study of results of the Charnley low-friction arthroplasty it was not until recently appreciated that the radiological

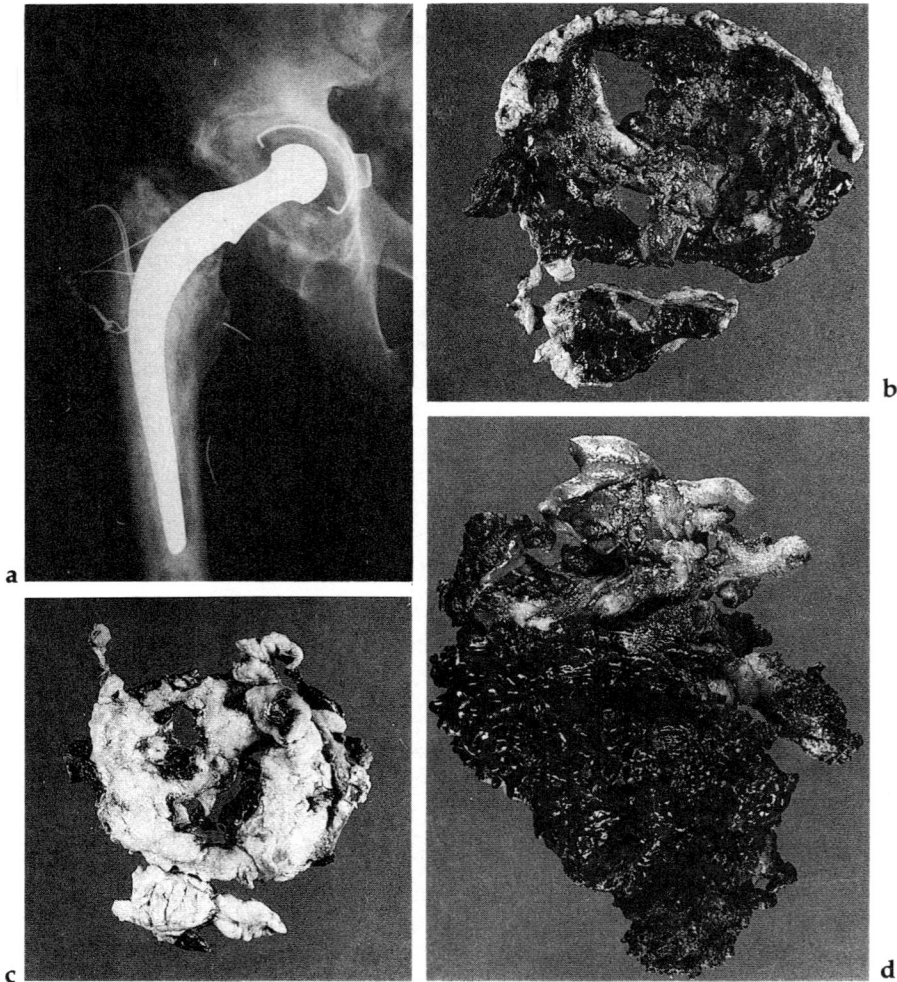

Fig. 9.4. The extent of granulation tissue at the bone–cement junction. Comparison of the pre-operative radiograph and the operative findings. **a** Pre-revision radiograph. **b,c** Granulation tissue from the acetabulum. (Note the difference in colour between the areas of contact with cement (*black*) and bone (*white*). **d** Granulation tissue from the medullary canal.

changes at the bone–cement junction need not necessarily be reflected in clinical function. This was forcefully brought home in the 12–15-year study: "Thus gross demarcation together with migration affected a total of 25% of sockets, though at the time of review none of these patients showed any clinical defect" (Charnley 1979a p. 45).

The incidental finding of a loose socket in cases of revision for a fractured stem was often surprising. This discrepancy between the radiological appearances and the clinical function has no doubt contributed largely to the delays in carrying out revisions as well as to the lack of

studies of the causes of socket demarcation, migration and wear.

The extent of the fibrous membrane at the bone–cement junction of the socket can only be appreciated at revision surgery; it is always more extensive than anticipated from the radiological appearances (Fig. 9.4). In order to establish the correlation between the radiological appearances of the bone–cement junction of the socket and the operative findings in the Charnley low-friction arthroplasty Hodgkinson et al. (1989a) studied 200 consecutive revisions of low-friction arthroplasty carried out by the author. In each case the socket was tested with a socket tester

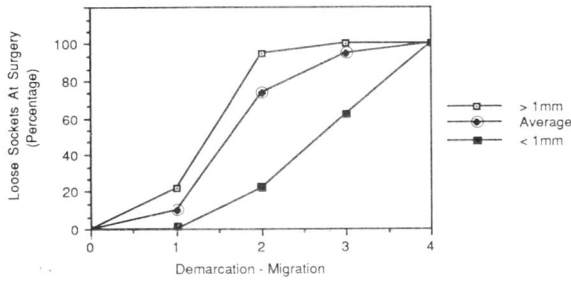

Fig. 9.5. The correlation between demarcation (both in the extent and depth) and the incidence of socket loosening and migration (after Hodgkinson et al. 1989a).

Table 9.1. Correlation between the radiological appearances of the bone–cement interface of the socket and the operative findings in the Charnley low-friction arthroplasty (Hodgkinson et al. 1989a)

Socket demarcation	No. of cases	Loose at revision	% of loose sockets
Nil	24	0	0
Outer third	68	5	7
Outer third and Middle third	28	20	71
Complete	52	49	94
Socket migration	28	28	100

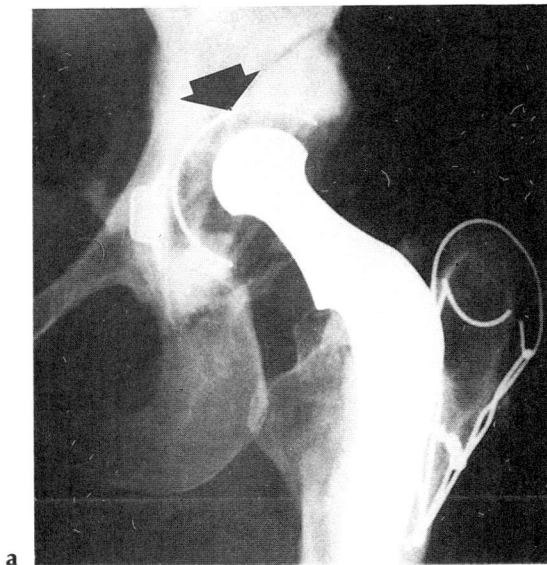

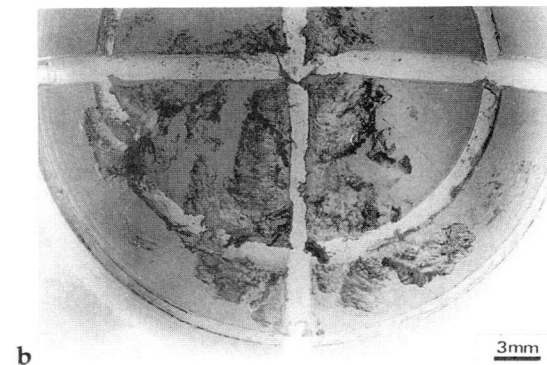

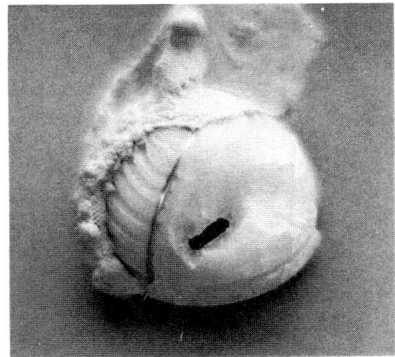

Fig. 9.6. Wear of the outside of the socket. **a** An area of the socket where bone–HDP contact can readily occur if the acetabulum is not prepared correctly. **b** Typical appearance of the socket's external surface pitted by wear against the bone. **c** Gross wear by contact with and movement of socket against bone.

after the bone–cement junction over part of the socket had been exposed. The results are briefly summarized in Table 9.1 (see also Fig. 9.5). The study has shown that in socket fixation the demarcation of the bone–cement junction is to be avoided.

Wear of the Socket: The Mechanical and Histological Changes Resulting from It

Wear of the socket is such an important subject that it is discussed in some detail (Chap. 10).

Initially Teflon sockets were used but were found to wear rapidly. In November 1962 high-density polyethylene sockets were introduced. Early experience with HDP showed that wear was unlikely to be a serious problem, although a suggestion was made that socket loosening was likely to occur if the wear was more than 5 mm. The most important mechanical effects of socket wear are the progressive restriction of angular movements, impingement of the neck of the stem on the rim of the bore of the socket, shock loading and socket loosening. The abrasive effect of the to and fro movement of the loose socket leads to progressive excavation of the bone of the acetabulum and to socket migration. Any part of the HDP socket in direct contact with the bone will wear against it (Fig. 9.6) producing HDP granuloma and the changes associated with it. Because of the loosening of the socket the effective joint cavity becomes extended to the bone–cement junction of the socket. Any particles of HDP or cement present within the capsule can migrate freely to that area because of the repeated pressure and volume changes which occur during activity. Some of the HDP particles are generated locally, others migrate with the wear debris from the socket bore. Many of the changes at the bone–cement junction are purely secondary to the effects of mechanical loosening of the components in general and the socket in particular. The presence of the HDP particles is almost certainly an effect and not the cause of loosening.

10 Wear of the Socket

In studies of the long-term results of the Charnley low-friction arthroplasty, and of other total hip arthroplasties, wear of the socket will be seen to be increasingly important.

Introduction

Teflon was the first plastic to be used for the acetabular components. Initially the acetabular components were uncemented, but later they were fixed with acrylic cement. The plastic wore rapidly, lasting only about 2–3 years. Socket migration and teflon granuloma resulted in extensive loss of bone stock (Fig. 10.1). The use of Teflon was obviously abandoned but certain important lessons were learned. The short-term-clinical results were spectacular, proving that the concept of the design and the surgical technique were correct. What was lacking was a suitable material for the socket.

Charnley et al. (1969) studied the wear of the Teflon socket in some detail. Their findings can be summarized as follows:

1. The plastic socket did not wear in a random fashion by enlarging and deepening the socket bore. The head bored for itself a new, roughly cylindrical channel, the diameter being determined by the size of the head.
2. The volume of plastic lost was proportional to the diameter of the head and the depth of the penetration ($\pi r^2 \times$ depth of penetration) (Fig. 10.2).

3. The depth of socket penetration was considered to be inversely proportional to the diameter of the head of the femoral component.
4. It became apparent that in any design using metal on plastic there had to be a compromise between the depth of socket penetration and the volume of plastic likely to be shed into the tissues and between the diameter of the head of the femoral component and the thickness of the socket wall.
5. Friction between the articulating surfaces of an arthroplasty depends on the materials used, their surface finish and the load applied to that system and is independent of the area of contact. Achieving the lowest possible frictional torque was considered to pay better long-term dividends because it reduced the incidence of socket loosening, hence use of the smallest possible head diameter (7/8", 22.25 mm) together with a thick-walled socket. The concept embraced the possibility of deeper socket penetration but was aimed at lowering the incidence of component loosening and reducing the volume of plastic being shed into the tissues. This new design was a result of the early experiences with Teflon.

In November 1962 high-density polyethylene was used for the first time for socket manufacture. This material has become the standard for the majority of total joint replacements. Within days of the first few operations it became obvious that valuable information would be lost unless the acrylic cement was rendered radio-opaque. It was also realized that socket wear

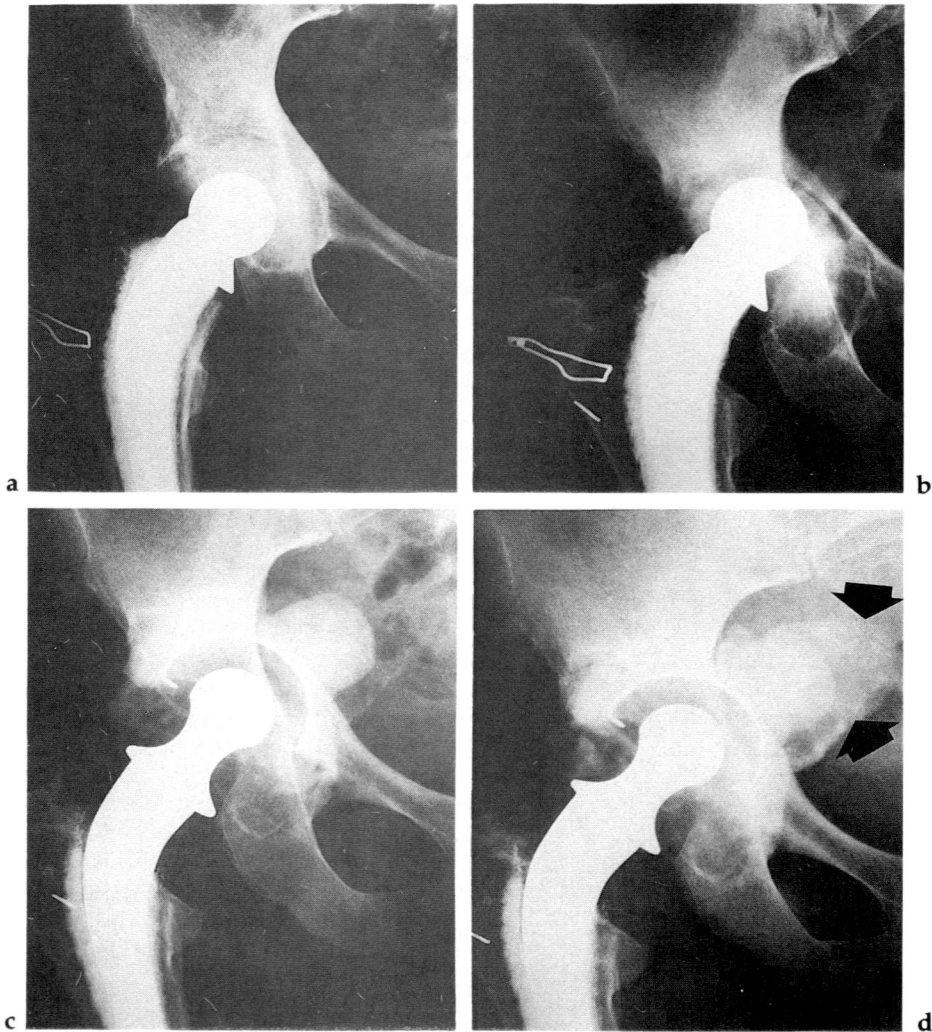

Fig. 10.1. Teflon arthroplasty of the hip. **a** Uncemented teflon socket, cemented stem. **b** Appearances some 3 years later, showing socket completely worn, erosion of the acetabulum and erosion of the medial femoral neck down to the lesser trochanter. **c** Revision to cemented HDP socket. Note the extrusion of cement through the defect in the acetabular floor. Stem not changed. **d** Five years after the revision. Note the calcification of the intrapelvic granuloma around the extruded cement.

could not be measured radiographically (Fig. 10.3). To render the acrylic cement radio-opaque, barium sulphate was added to it. In order to allow radiographic measurement of wear a wire marker was added that ran in a recess of the HDP socket in a coronal plane. The wisdom of the decision to incorporate these additions is more obvious 25 years later than

ever before. Sadly, designs or techniques not having these facilities mean that valuable information is lost.

With increasing clinical experience of HDP it was becoming apparent that the socket wear seen with Teflon was not presenting as an immediate clinical problem. Although various studies of socket wear were being carried out it is

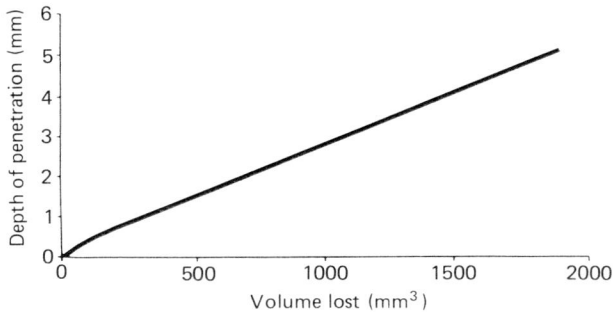

Fig. 10.2. Volume of plastic lost in relation to the depth of socket penetration with the 22.25-mm diameter head. After 1 mm penetration there is a straight-line relationship between the depth of penetration (mm) and the volume (mm^3) of HDP lost.

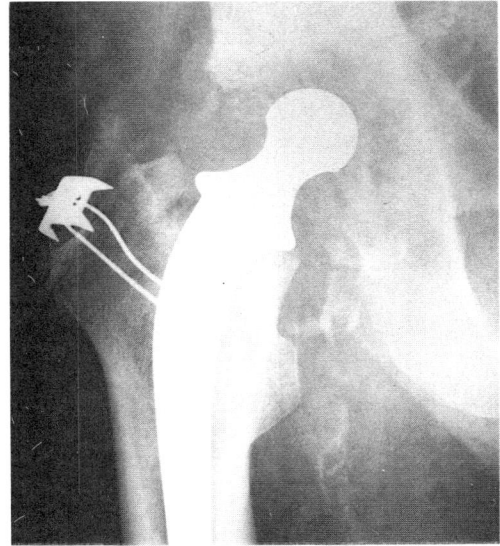

Fig. 10.3 Charnley LFA, 7 January 1963. Radiolucent cement. The socket has no wire marker. Note the potential loss of information.

probably correct to say that socket loosening in relation to socket wear, although mentioned, was not seriously considered. Initially, what was considered was fracture of the stem and then loosening of the socket but not in the context of wear. Loosening of the stem, per se, was never considered to be a serious problem numerically.

Radiographic Measurement of Socket Wear

Charnley and Cupic (1973) studied wear of the HDP socket in the low-friction arthroplasty after 9–10 years. The average depth of penetration was 0.12 mm in 1 year with a range of 0.09 to 0.3 mm. This study did not take radiographic magnification fully into account.

Charnley and Halley (1975) measured socket wear comparing the most recent with the post-operative radiographs all measurements being corrected for magnification. Three groups of patients were studied:

1. Those patients included in the Charnley and Cupic (1973) study.
2. A group of patients under the age of 30. (Although young they were limited in their activities by the involvement of other joints. This was in keeping with the criteria for patient selection with a "built-in restraint".)
3. Four patients under the age of 50 whose function was considered normal after surgery.

The average rate of wear was 0.15 mm per year, but in some 15% this was 0.25 mm per year. There was a decrease in the rate of wear with the passage of time. Body weight and physical activity did not appear to affect the wear. The sockets of the grossly disabled patients under the age of 30 wore rather more than the average while the sockets of three of the four patients considered normal wore less than the average. (The reader must refer to the original study in order not to loose the meaning of the detail.) It must be pointed out that although the activity level of the patients was charted in some detail according to the accepted clinical method it in no way took into the account the more detailed and thus more important parameter, that of the actual distance walked by individual patients over a period of time, expressed as a sliding distance at the level of the articulation. The important finding of the study is the scatter of the results. This clearly points to the difficulties likely to be encountered in any wear study.

Griffith et al. (1978) continued to study socket wear in a series of 491 total hip arthroplasties examined after an average period of 8.3 years (range 7–9 years). This very detailed publication deals with many aspects of measurement of socket wear and answers various criticisms

Table 10.1. Correlation between depth of socket wear and the incidence of socket migration at 16.6-year follow-up

Wear (mm)	0	1	2	3	4	5	6	7
No. of cases	27	28	30	9	4	3	—	2
No. of sockets migrating	1	2	5	3	2	2	—	2
% of cases of socket migration	4	7	17	33	50	67	—	100

Table 10.2. Correlation between depth of socket wear and the incidence of socket migration. Patients were under the age of 40 years at the time of surgery with average follow-up 9.3 years

Wear (mm)	0	1	2	3	4	5	6
No. of cases	13	37	20	16	11	6	1
No. of sockets migrating	0	0	1	2	4	3	1
% of cases of socket migration	0	0	5	12.5	36	50	100

levelled at the method. The average rate of wear was 0.07 mm per year. Sockets implanted in males wore more than those in females. Although there was no significant difference between the ages of patients with low and with intermediate wear, deep penetration occurred in 12% of patients aged under 50 but only in 1.5% of patients over 60. There was no correlation between weight and the depth of socket wear or other joint involvement, but young and active patients predominated in the heavy wear groups.

In 1979 Charnley presented the results of a 12–15-year study. It became obvious that 25% of sockets may have to be revised eventually because of loosening. It is this finding probably more than any other that has led to the sudden upsurge of the uncemented arthroplasty. By 1979 loosening of the stem had already been accepted as the main long-term problem in vast majority of other series. Not so in Charnley's.

In 1984 the author reviewed the longest follow-up of the Charnley low-friction arthroplasty available at that stage. Ninety-three patients with 116 low-friction arthroplasties between them were studied. Their average age at low-friction arthroplasty was 53 years (range 20–71 years). The average follow-up was 16.6 years (range 15–21 years). The incidence of radiological socket migration was found to be 22.5%. Despite that the clinical results were excellent. The depth of socket wear was found to be 0.096 mm per year. What was interesting was the correlation between the depth of socket penetration and the incidence of socket migration. (Table 10.1). If there was a correlation between the depth of socket wear and the incidence of socket migration then this should be reflected in other studies.

In 1985 the author reviewed a group of 107 patients who were under the age of 40 at the time of the low-friction arthroplasty. The average

follow-up was 9.3 years (range 4–17 years). The patients with rheumatoid arthritis were almost completely excluded. (It was considered that multiple joint involvement would interfere with the index of function and thus of the socket wear.) The results from this series are shown in Table 10.2. The rate of socket wear was estimated at 0.2 mm per year.

From the two completely separate studies it became apparent that wear and loosening were closely related (Fig. 10.4). Every effort had to be made to study the problem of wear in detail. It must be pointed out that the study referred to in Wroblewski (1985b) was carried out before the Wroblewski (1984b) study but the correlation between socket wear and migration was not appreciated until after the latter study was completed. The dates refer to the time of publication only.

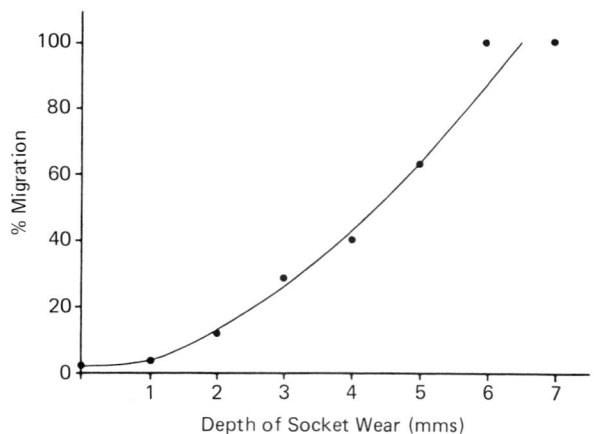

Fig. 10.4. The correlation between the depth of socket wear and the incidence of socket migration. Diagrammatic presentation of the results shown in Tables 10.1 and 10.2 combined.

a

b

c

Fig. 10.5.a Worn (and loose) socket at 9½ years. **b** Acrylic cast of the worn socket. **c** Shadowgraph showing the depth of wear (4.8 mm) and the direction of the penetration (coronal plane). Note the erosion of the socket bore rim.

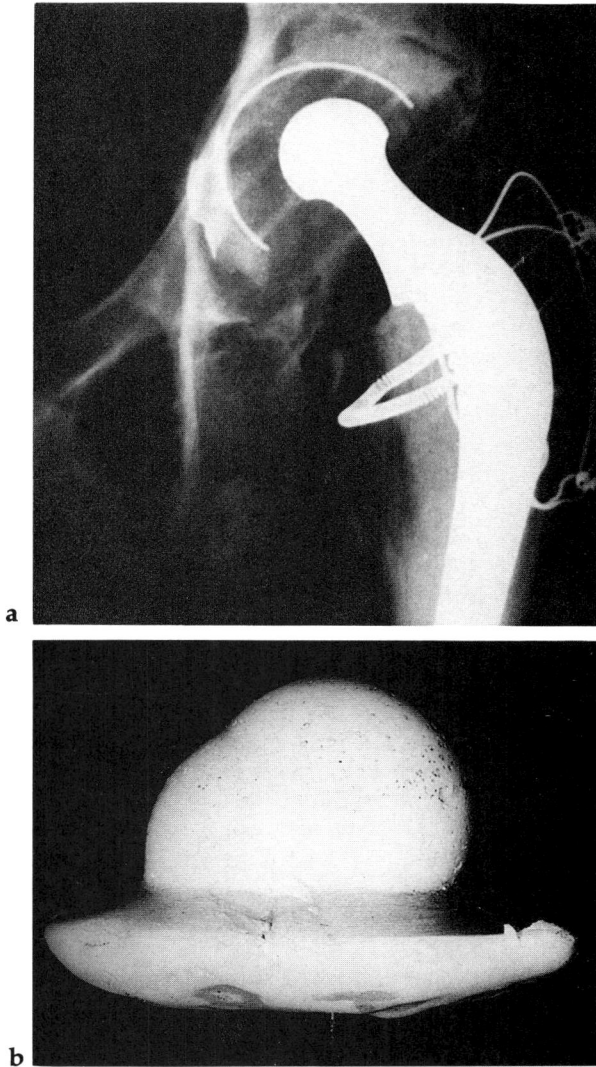

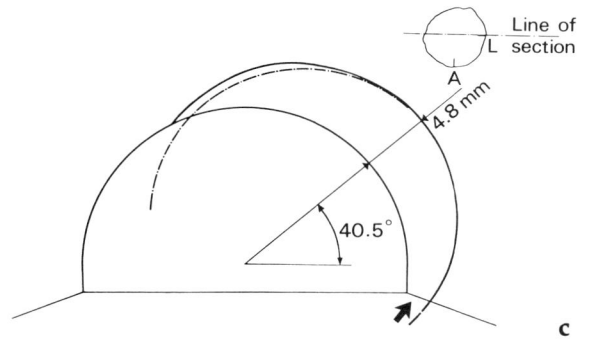

for further examination. Acrylic casts were made (Fig. 10.5.) incorporating the orientation marks made on the face of the socket. Using the shadowgraph technique the depth and the direction of wear of each socket were studied.

Correlation Between Real and Radiographic Wear Measurements

The findings confirmed a very close correlation between the real and the radiographic methods of measurement of socket wear (Fig. 10.6). Radiographic measurement tended to overestimate when real wear was below 2 mm and to underestimate when the real wear was more than 2 mm. On the whole the correlation was close enough to be of practical value in clinical situations with a better significance than 0.001.

Wear Measurement of Explanted Sockets

The study of 22 sockets removed at revision surgery was undertaken by Wroblewski (1985b). Sockets found loose at revision surgery (excluding revisions for deep sepsis) were marked for orientation while still in situ and then removed

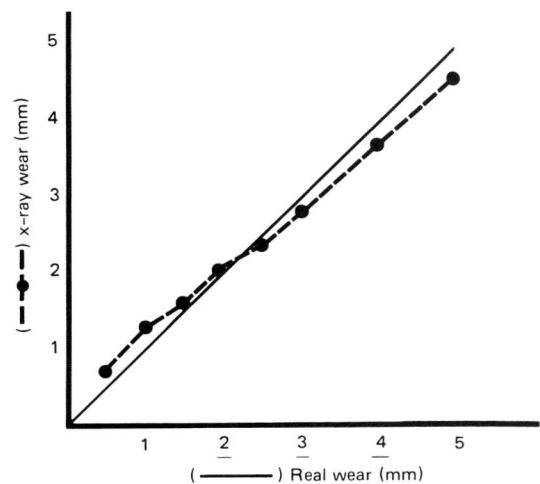

Fig. 10.6. The correlation between the real and the radiographic measurement of the depth of socket wear.

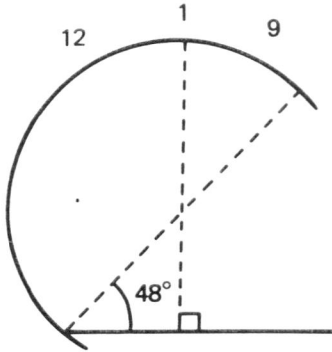

Fig. 10.7. Direction of socket wear. Diagrammatic representation of the direction of socket wear in the explanted sockets. Angle open laterally taken into consideration.

Direction of Wear

The sockets wear in a roughly cylindrical fashion as has already been pointed out by Charnley et al. (1969). The wear track was not always medial to the line drawn vertically upwards from the centre of the socket. Some sockets did wear on the very edge of the bore, well lateral to the vertical line (Fig. 10.7). This may have a bearing on the direction of load, possibly on the turning moment on the socket and on the likelihood of impingement as the depth of penetration increases with time.

Impingement

In some cases there was obvious evidence of impingement of the neck of the stem on the rim of the bore of the socket as shown by the enlargement of the socket bore margin in one direction, usually in the direction of wear. It was estimated that with the standard Charnley components the impingement probably started once the socket had worn somewhere between 0.4 and 0.56 mm. This statement was made on the following evidence: in the 14 cases with impingement the lowest depth of wear was 0.56 mm. In six cases without impingement the highest penetration was 0.4 mm. The rate of socket wear in this group of patients was 0.19 mm per year which correlated very closely with the findings for the under 40s group.

Atkinson et al. (1985a,b) and Isaac et al. (1986) studied sockets retrieved at revision surgery. The work was carried out at the University of Leeds with the full backing of the Institute of Tribology, the Department of Mechanical Engi-

neering and the Department of Metallurgy. The study was supported by the Department of Health and Social Security. The findings can be summarized as follows:

1. Worn HDP sockets showed three distinct regions: (a) a high-wear smooth area in the superior half of the socket; (b) a much rougher low-wear area where machining marks were still visible; and (c) a ridge separating the two areas (Fig. 10.8).

2. In the heavily worn sockets, rim wear due to impingement was observed.

3. All sockets showed pitting in both the low- and the high-wear areas. This was due to cement ingress occurring either at surgery or at some later stage (Fig. 10.8).

4. There was evidence of adhesive wear in the high-wear region, together with some abrasive wear (Fig. 10.9).

5. The ridge area showed two types of cracks, one type possibly due to poor sintering and the other type possibly due to cold flow of the material away from the heavily loaded area (Fig. 10.10).

6. The average rate of socket penetration was 0.19 mm per year, twice that of unrevised sockets (Griffith et al. 1978).

7. There was a very large range of individual penetration rates ranging from 0.005 to 0.623 mm per year.

8. Better agreement was obtained between radiographic and laboratory wear results, although laboratory results still underestimated in vivo penetration rates.

9. Scratches detected on the femoral heads (Fig. 10.11) were probably caused by particles of acrylic cement and may have increased the penetration rates.

10. Cement ingress had to be avoided. Results improved with better cementing techniques and with the introduction of flanged (ogee-flanged) sockets.

11. Three major factors were thought to affect the socket wear: (a) the level of patient activity; (b) the effective roughness of the femoral head; and (c) inherent variations in the wear factors of the polymeric materials.

--→

Fig. 10.9. Adhesive and abrasive wear of the socket. **a** Adhesive wear; the heaping up of HDP in the high-wear area. **b** Abrasive wear; grooves in the HDP not caused by the machining of the socket but occurring some time later.

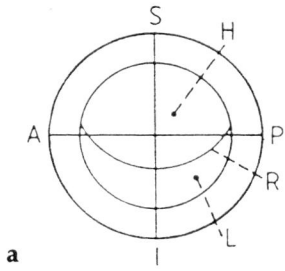

Fig. 10.8 Wear of the HDP socket: characteristic areas. **a** Diagrammatic representation of a typical appearance of a worn socket. *A*, anterior; *P*, posterior; *S*, superior; *I*, inferior (parts of the socket in relation to their position within the hip). *H*, high-wear area; *L*, low-wear area; *R*, ridge separating the low- and high-wear areas. **b** Low-power view of the inside of the socket. *H*, high-wear area; *L*, low-wear area; *R*, ridge. **c** Photograph of sectioned socket to show the characteristic appearance. **d** High-power magnification. Note the smooth high-wear area with pits due to cement ingress and the machining marks visible in the low-wear area. **e** Damage caused by cement ingress.

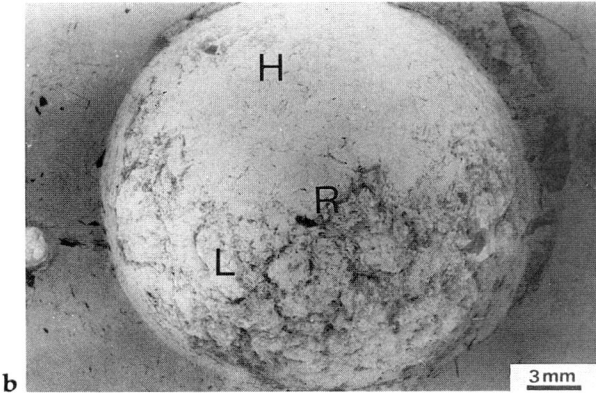

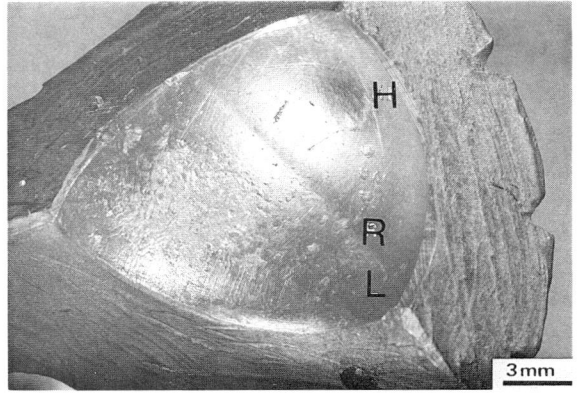

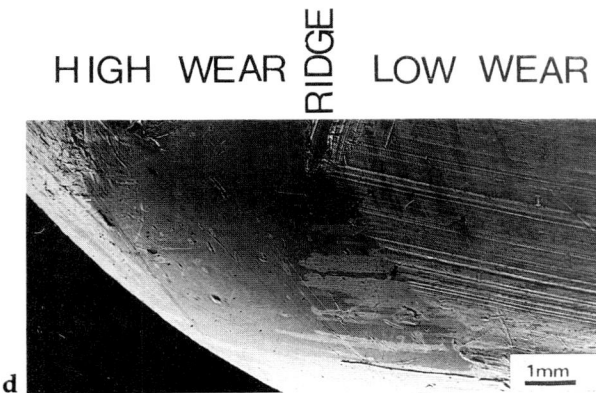

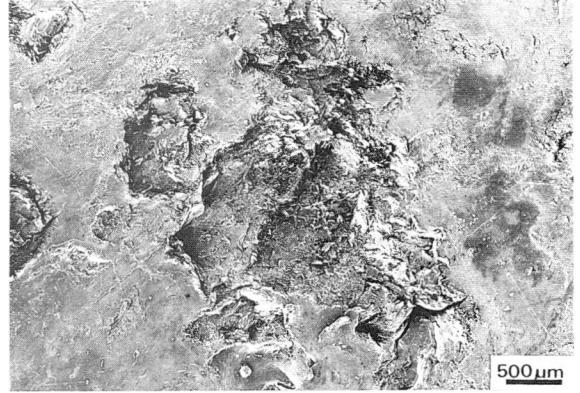

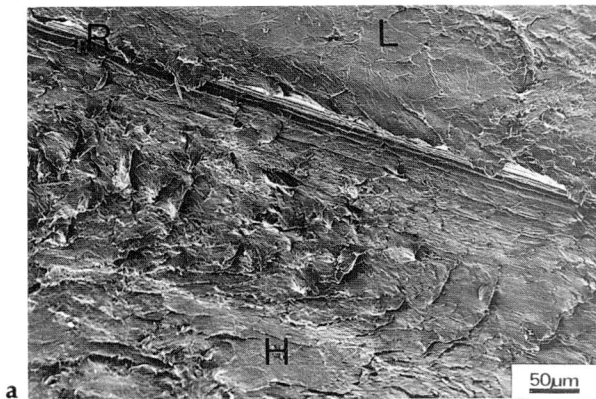

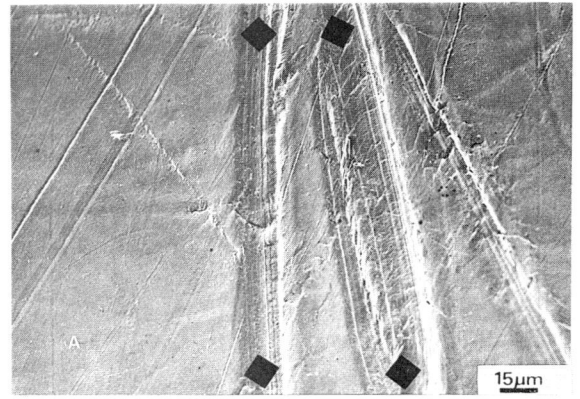

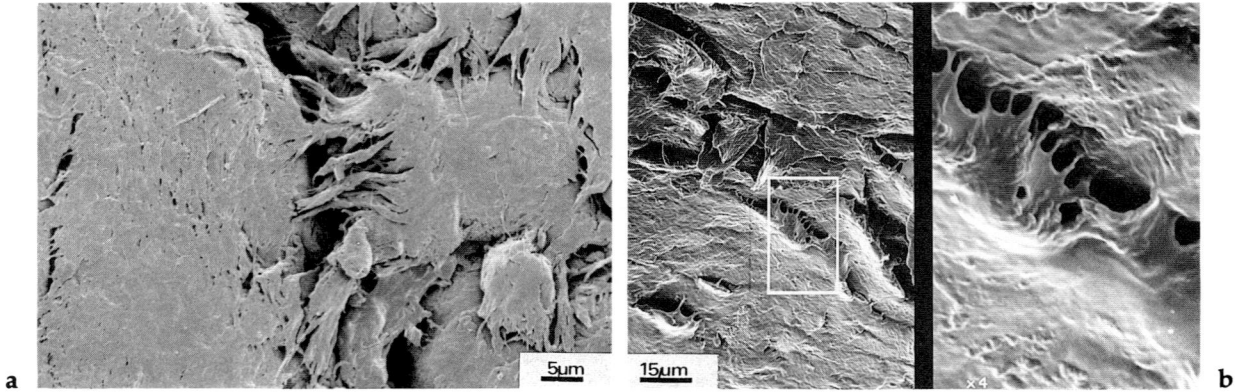

Fig. 10.10. Cracks within the HDP. **a** Could this be due to incomplete sintering? **b** Does this picture show cold flow of the HDP?

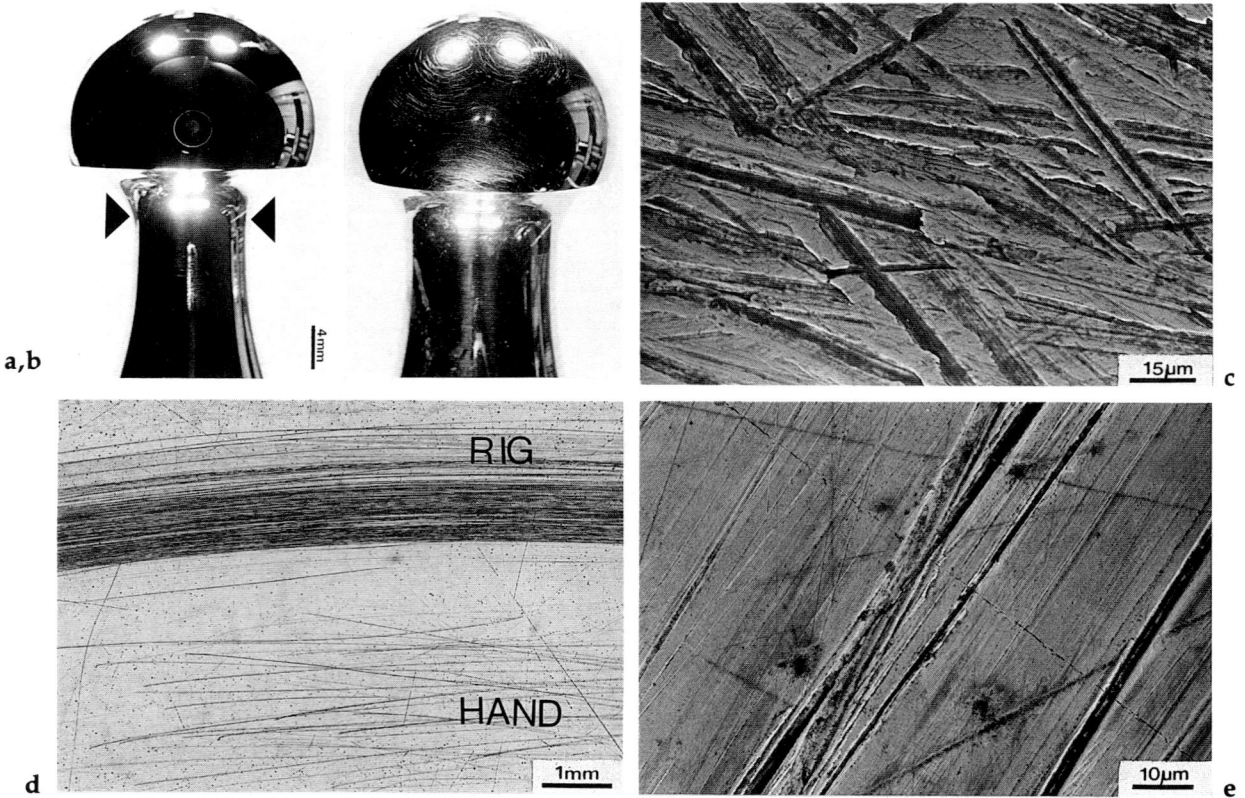

Fig. 10.11. Damage to the head of the femoral component. **a** Appearance as delivered by the manufacturer. (Note the reduced diameter neck.) **b** Appearance at revision some 8 years later. **c** SEM; damaged surface magnified. The grooves and the heaped-up ridges that cause the damage to the HDP socket. **d** The damage reproduced by using the acrylic cement in the test rig and by a hand-held specimen. **e** Magnified view of a part of **d**. Note the uniformity of direction as compared with **c**.

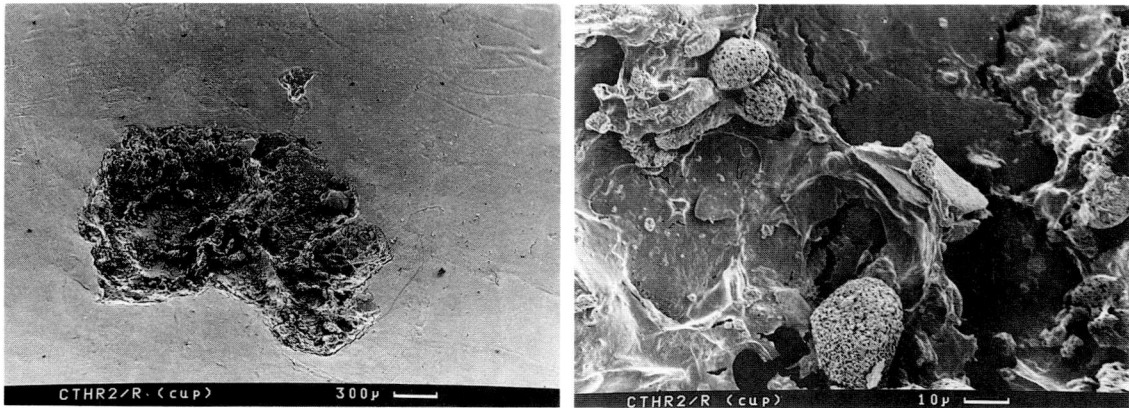

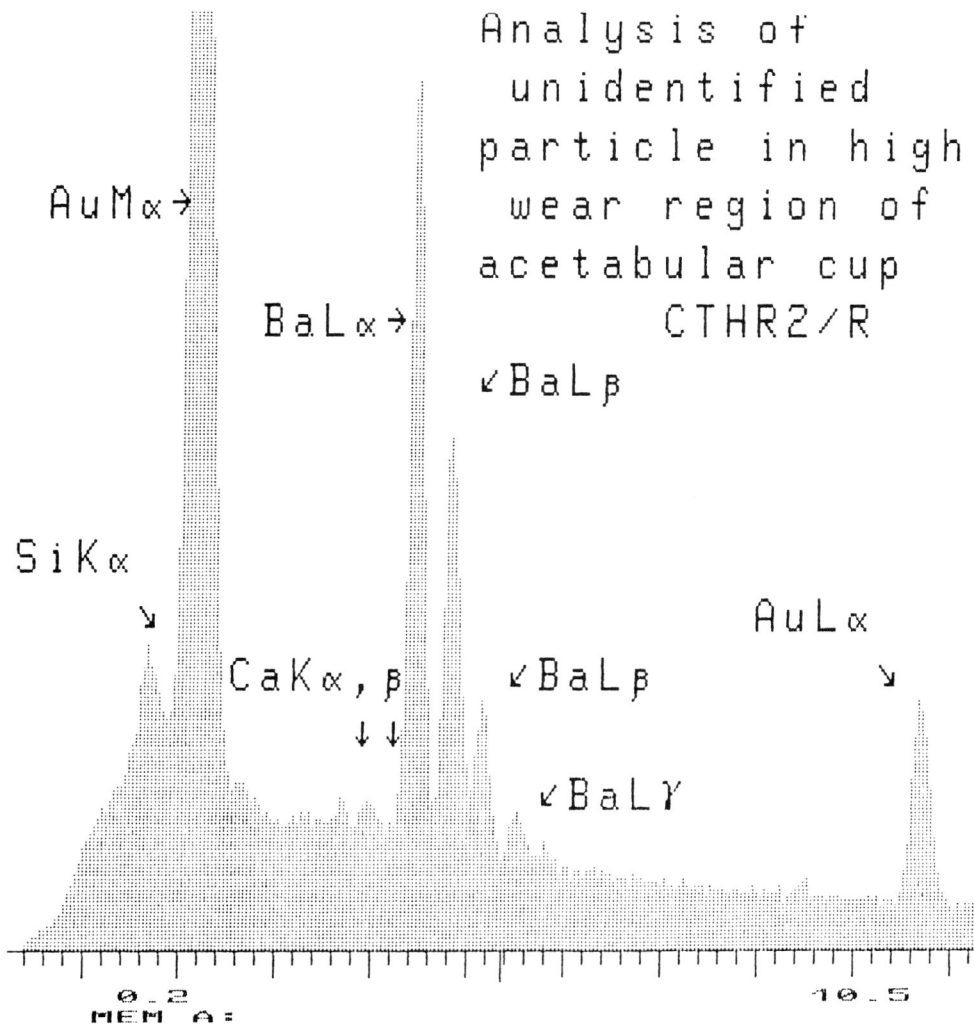

Fig. 10.12. Cement ingress into the articulation. *A*, a crater in the HDP caused by acrylic cement; *B*, pumice-like clumps of barium sulphate; *C*, analysis of the 'clumps' identifies them as barium. (The high peak for gold (Au) is due to the preparation of the specimen to avoid damage when analysed with the SEM; Si probably indicates presence of glove powder.) Photographs by courtesy of the Departments of Tribology and Mechanical Engineering, The University of Leeds.

The Effect of Cement Ingress into the Socket

The role the cement played in roughening the head of the femoral component was then examined in detail (Isaac et al. 1986). A total of 59 cups and 38 stems from Charnley low-friction arthroplasties were studied. The scanning electron microscope technique was used. Ingress of cement was confirmed (Fig. 10.12). Not only did it cause the pitting of the articulating surface of the cups but the barium sulphate (used to make the cement radio-opaque) contained as clumps within the cement damaged the surface of the heads of the femoral components, increasing its roughness from less than

0.02 µm Ra to 0.07 µm Ra, i.e. more than a threefold increase in roughness. The increase of in vivo roughness increased the penetration rates and reduced the life of the prosthesis. Wear and impingement leading to loosening is one possible cause of failure. Increase in the friction due to femoral head damage obviously also played its part as did the decreasing thickness of the socket wall.

Reduced Diameter Neck Stem

The advantage of reducing the diameter of the neck of the femoral prosthesis from the standard

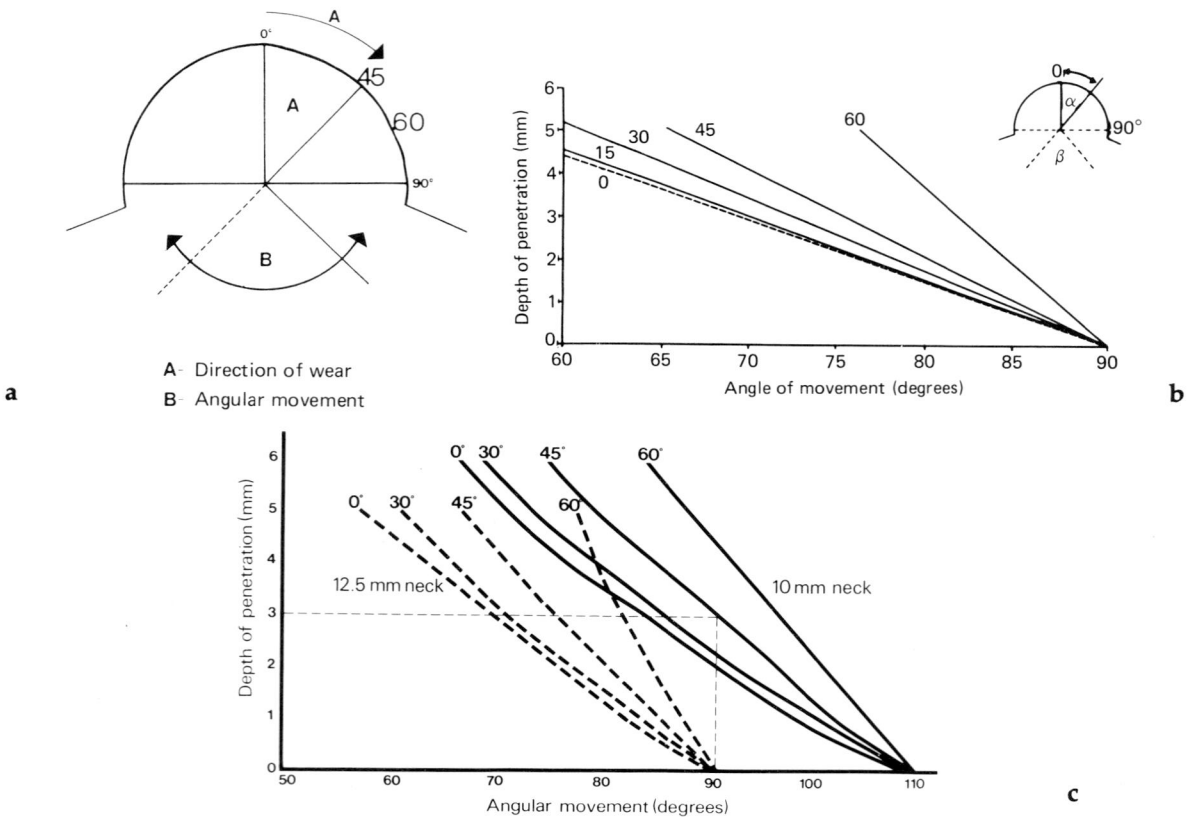

Fig. 10.13. Angular movements in relation to the depth of socket wear. a Schematic diagram of the socket: A, direction of wear 0°–90°; B, angular movements. b Restriction of angular movements (from the available 90°) according to the direction of socket wear (12.5-mm diameter neck); from 0° central wear to 60° peripheral wear. c Improvement in the angular range of movement with reduced (10 mm) diameter neck. The range of movements increased from 90° to 108°. In order to restrict the movement to 90° (as with the standard 12.5-mm diameter neck) at 45° wear path, the depth of penetration must be 3 mm.

12.5 mm to 10 mm was first suggested by Charnley to reduce impingement and dislocation. This design was made possible by the introduction of high nitrogen content stainless steel and the cold forming process used in the manufacture of the stem (Ortron 90, Chas. F. Thackray Ltd.). The advantages of the changed design are even more profound in the context of socket loosening. Using an experimental model it was demonstrated that for a 45° wear path (i.e. the wear path is directly upwards) the depth of penetration would have to be 3 mm before the 108° range of movements possible with the reduced-diameter neck design was reduced to 90°, i.e. that available with the old design (Fig. 10.13). In practical terms, a 3-mm depth of penetration would on average be expected to have taken place in 15 years in the under 40s group (0.2 mm wear per year) or 30 years in the 15–21-year follow-up group (0.089 mm wear per year). These are very optimistic figures. Long-term follow-up is awaited. The prospective study using the reduced neck stem design has been in progress since November 1983. No doubt the design will be copied by others.

Mechanical Testing of the Reduced Neck Stem

Before its introduction into clinical practice the reduced neck stem was extensively tested mechanically. The strength of the 10-mm neck in Ortron 90 was found to be identical to the strength of the 12.5-mm neck in 316L stainless steel, a design which has never failed in clinical practice in over 25 years. Tests have shown that the reduction of the neck diameter was not possible in 316L stainless steel. When tested, the

neck failed by bending. Using a similar design in chrome cobalt the neck failed by fracture.

Summary

Having at long last established the correlation between the radiological and the real wear measurements and having achieved very good correlation between the clinical and the experimental wear rates, the study of socket wear can be undertaken with greater confidence. Experimental findings can be extrapolated into clinical practice and radiographic measurements of socket wear can be carried out routinely and meaningfully as a part of long-term studies.

The lessons learned from the study of socket wear are as follows:

1. In the long term, socket loosening is related to wear and the resulting impingement of the neck of the stem on the socket rim.
2. Reduced neck diameters designed to delay the moment of impingement should be of long-term benefit.
3. Surgical technique must be directed towards avoiding the possibility of acrylic cement particles being drawn into the articulation.
4. Study of patients' function in relation to socket wear is essential.
5. A search must be made for materials which will further reduce friction and wear.
6. The study of friction and wear may prove to be more rewarding than the study of alternative methods of socket fixation.

11 Tissue Reaction to High-Density Polyethylene Wear Particles

Introduction

The study of tissue reaction to implant materials in general, and to wear products in particular, is within the domain of a specialist histologist. Unfortunately he may be unaware of the full history when examinng the specimen.

It is unlikely that the human body will respond specifically to a particular implant material, provided its chemical state, immunological response or mutation potential has not been affected. It is probably unrealistic to imagine that tissue would respond specifically to the range of materials already in use or likely to be used in the future. Such a state would imply unlimited possibilities of response to the vast ingenuity of the inventor and designer. It is more likely that the body responds to certain basic physical factors, e.g. the mere presence of the implant, its size, surface and function, any alterations in load transmission or changes in volume and pressure of the cavity housing the implant. Any wear products are likely to induce a response similar to that stimulated by the implant itself, provided their properties have not changed and provided they are not a by-product of a mechanical change affecting function of the implant.

Teflon

The earliest clinical experience with plastics in the context of total hip arthroplasty is that of Charnley using Teflon (polytetrafluorethylene, PTFE). Certain lessons have been learned, but caution and knowledge of the clinical methods used are essential for their interpretation. In the earliest stages of both design and the surgical technique, Teflon was used directly in contact with bone. First it was in the form of uncemented interposition shells then as an uncemented Teflon cup against a cemented metal stem. The immediate contact between the bone and Teflon resulted in wear of the plastic in contact with bone, as well as of Teflon in contact with Teflon. The failures occurred early and were associated with bone destruction by Teflon granuloma.

The wear of Teflon at the metal–plastic interface continued. The full thickness of the socket was worn in several years. From more recent studies it has become clear that the Teflon socket, even if cemented, must have become loose within a very short period of time. What was being observed was not only the tissue reaction to Teflon but also the result of socket loosening because of Teflon wear. The extensive destruction of the acetabulum was primarily due to loosening of the socket and this left the "joint cavity", with its contents of bursal fluid and wear particles, extending to the bone–cement junction.

The loss of the medial femoral neck (Fig. 10.1) was almost certainly mechanical in origin, the changes in volume and pressure at the bone–cement junction resulting from deflection and deformation of the implant under load. What is even more interesting than the appearance of

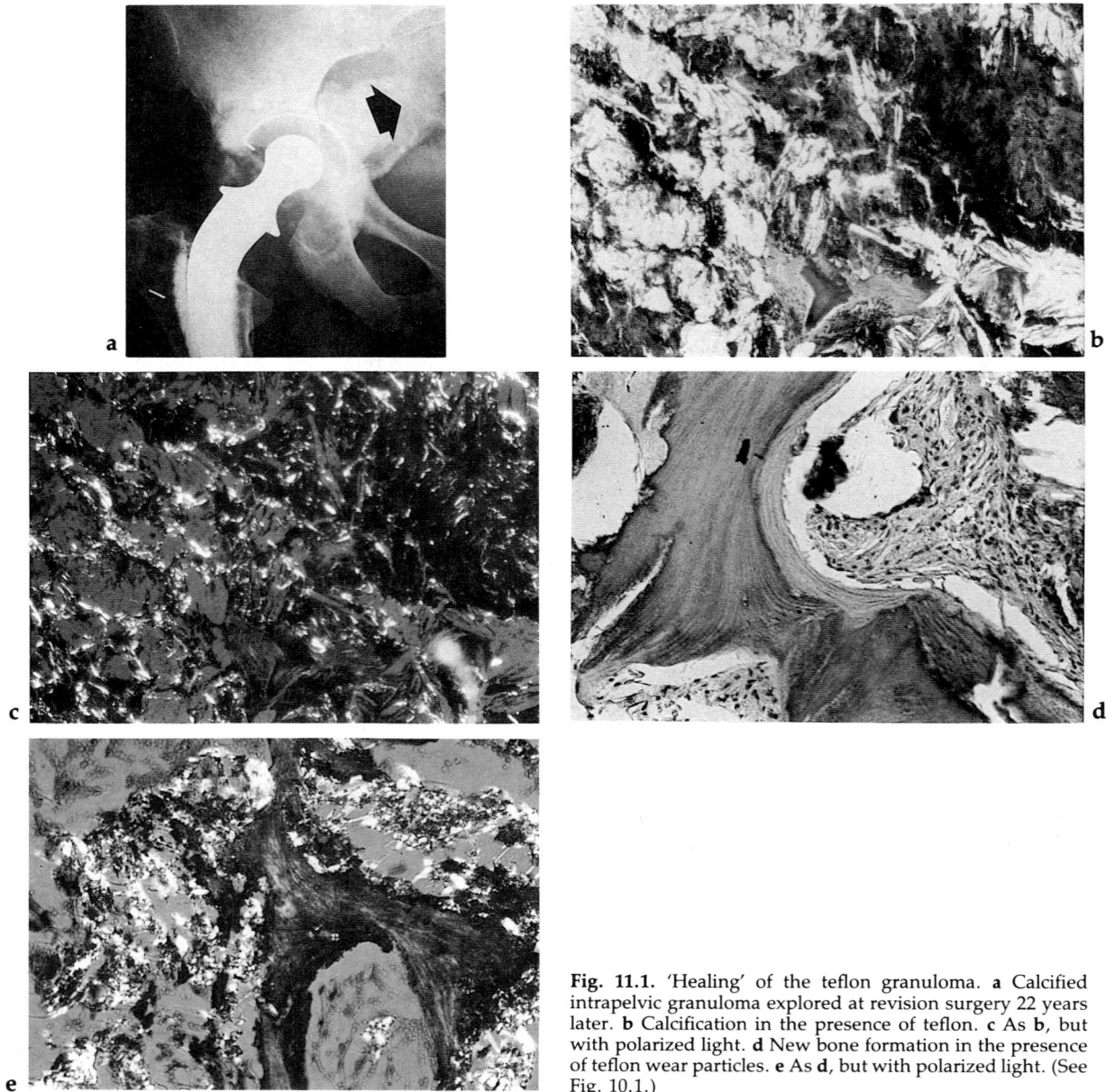

Fig. 11.1. 'Healing' of the teflon granuloma. a Calcified intrapelvic granuloma explored at revision surgery 22 years later. b Calcification in the presence of teflon. c As b, but with polarized light. d New bone formation in the presence of teflon wear particles. e As d, but with polarized light. (See Fig. 10.1.)

calcification is the even new bone formation within the granuloma (Fig. 11.1). The appearances of calcification and ossification are interpreted as evidence of the healing process, as with other granulomatous lesions, e.g. tuberculosis. This further supports the explanation that the tissue reaction is secondary to the mechanical failure and as such is reversible at least in part

and over a period of time. Thus for the typical changes of the plastic granuloma to appear, two factors are essential: wear particles from the plastic plus the hydrostatic changes within the joint cavity, the cavity now extending to the bone–cement junction. Once the movement has ceased, as it would do following revision, the granuloma would calcify. Thus the tissue response to Teflon wear particles was a foreign body reaction in general and not a specific response to the particular plastic.

High-Density Polyethylene

Because of its high-wear resistance the HDP cemented socket delays the onset of loosening and thus the changes associated with it. Despite well-documented evidence indicating its inappropriateness several further attempts have been made to articulate plastics directly against bone with predictable consequences (Fig. 11.2).

The unsuitability of HDP as a replacement for the femoral head has been pointed out (Wroblewski 1979). More recently the problem of the uncemented plastic socket has become apparent. The problem of HDP particles migrating down the medullary canal in an uncemented arthroplasty has yet to occur but no doubt it will, with time. In closing off the medullary canal, HDP cement restrictors were advised against to prevent any possible adverse tissue reaction (Wroblewski and van der Rijt 1984). The caution has been justified; sporadic cases of endosteal cavitation at the level of the HDP cement restrictors are now coming to light (Fig. 11.3).

The information from various studies suggests that, in the context of socket loosening, and possibly even on the femoral side, the mechanical effects of socket wear are more important than the biological response to the products of tissue wear. The evidence to support this is as follows:

1. The correlation between the depth of socket wear and the incidence of socket migration shows a consistent trend in the groups studied; As the depth of socket penetration increased so did the incidence of socket migration.
2. The demarcation of the bone–cement junction of the socket is closely correlated to findings of socket loosening as determined at surgery. The findings show quite clearly that the socket is loose far more commonly than hitherto suspected.
3. External wear, present in some 30% of revised sockets, shows that the source of the HDP wear particles may be other than purely at the articulation. For external wear to occur the socket must be loose, and is often found to be so (see (2) above).
4. When the turning moment on the socket is considered, together with thinning and deformation of the HDP socket shell as well as possibly an increase in friction due to the damaged head of the femoral component there is little doubt that the mechanical problems likely to lead to socket loosening are so obvious that there is little need to invoke the "tissue response" as the cause.

This is in contrast to the work of Willert and Semlitsch (1976) and Vernon-Roberts and Freeman (1977) and very much against what Rose and his colleagues (1980) have suggested: " . . . the chief clinical question is that of biological effects of the debris and not of mechanical problems due to dimensional changes."

The information on the subject of HDP wear and its effect on bone and the bone–cement interface suggests certain conclusions:

1. HDP wear particles by themselves are probably harmless.
2. The volume of HDP particles is only important because it is an index of mechanical changes within the socket, the implant–bone interface being affected secondarily.
3. The size of the individual particles may be more relevant; the larger the particles the more severe the changes.
4. Hydrostatic changes within the "joint cavity" in the presence of HDP particles will lead to bone destruction.
5. Any design employing a plastic in its articulation and allowing ingress of wear particles at the bone–implant interface may result in failure.
6. The changes are more likely to occur on the femoral side where a loose-cemented or uncemented stem acts as a non-return valve.
7. It is likely that other materials used for the articulation and resulting in wear may lead to similar changes under similar circumstances.

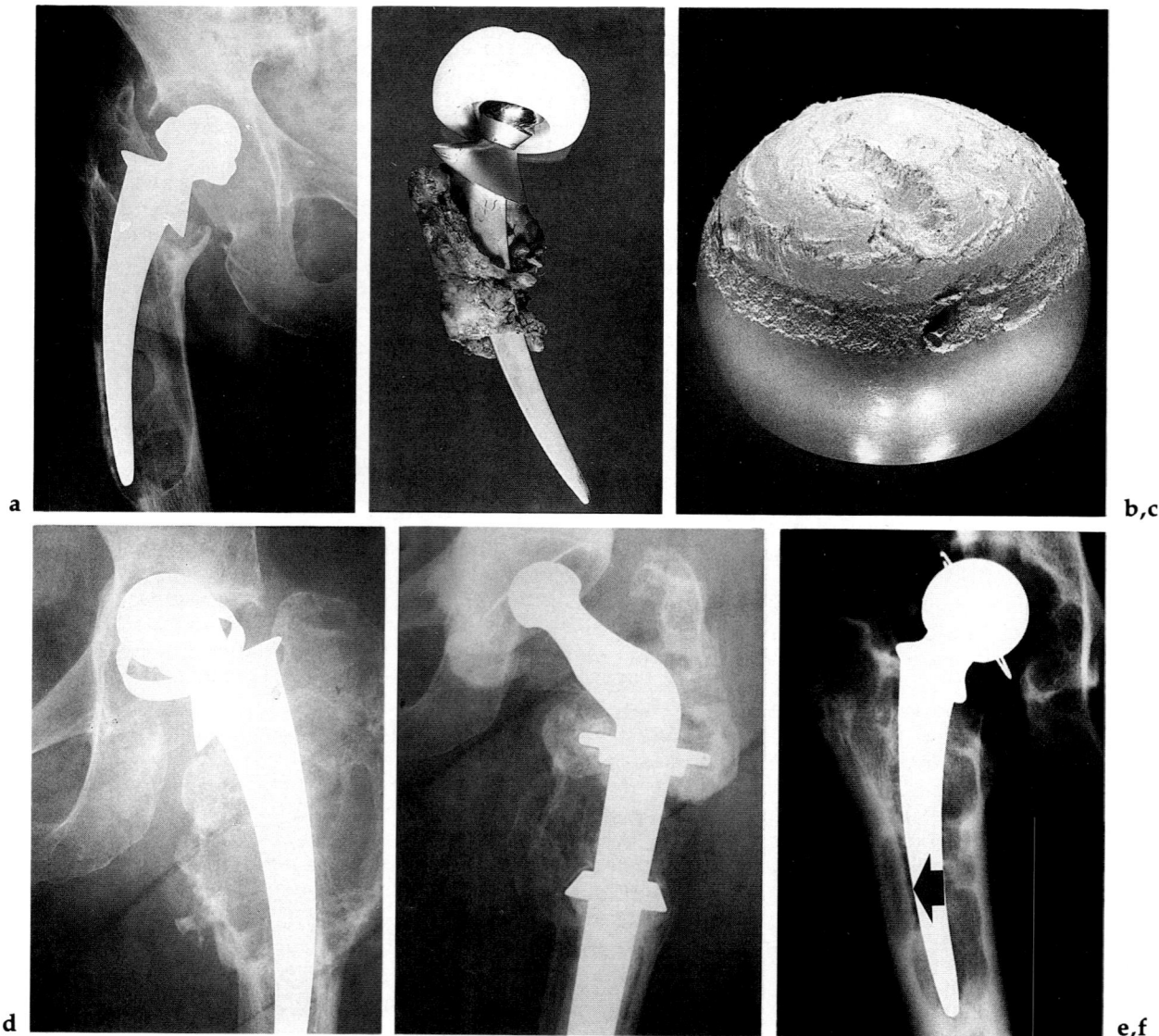

Fig. 11.2. High-density polyethylene articulating with the acetabular bone. **a** Uncemented stem and HDP head articulating with an acetabulum. A method used in the treatment of fracture of the femoral neck. Note the massive cavitation at the femur. **b** Specimen removed at revision. Granulation tissue round the proximal stem and the worn HDP head. **c** Close-up view of the HDP surface. **d,e** A further example of HDP wearing against bone. Note Nature's attempt to "heal" the lesion after proximal femoral replacement. **f** Endosteal cavitation from HDP granuloma in a loose cemented stem. **g** Post-revision radiograph clearly reveals the defect, neither packed with cement nor bone grafted. **h** Four years after revision. A healing process?

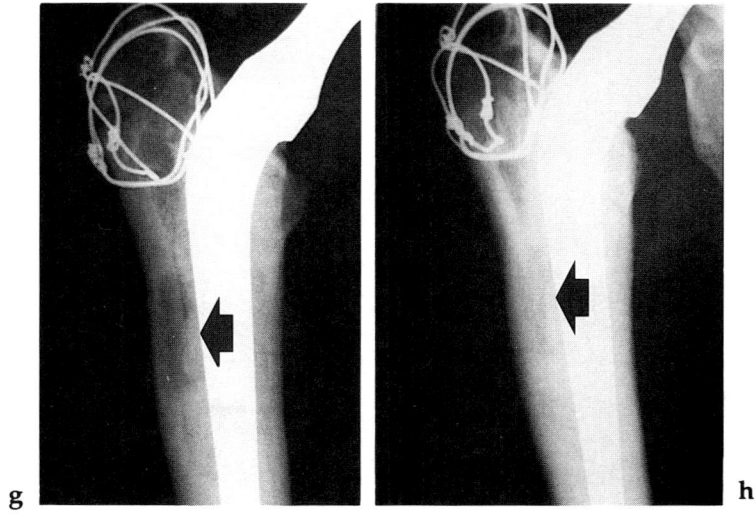

Fig 11.2. (*continued*)

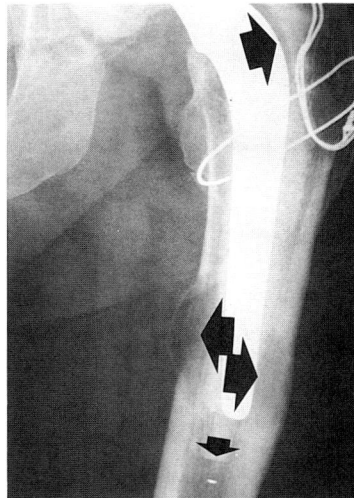

Fig. 11.3. Gross endosteal cavitation at the level of an HDP restrictor with a subsided stem.

12 Metal Backing of the Socket

It must be pointed out that Charnley was the first to use metal backing for the HDP socket, albeit an uncemented socket of the press-fit variety (Fig. 12.1). A total of 336 such "press-fit" sockets were used in clinical practice between November 1962 and December 1965. By December 1983 some 68 had been changed because of tilting or migration (Fig. 12.2). However, at that stage 16 remained in situ and functioned normally. A handful are still attending clinics (Fig. 12.3). It was because of an inability to maintain the press-fit socket in the correct position that its use was abandoned in favour of the cemented HDP socket.

With the Teflon experience fresh in the minds of surgeons, their uppermost thought was still the wear of the plastic. Any attempts to use metal backing at that stage would have obscured the possibility of HDP wear measurements. Such a situation was unacceptable. Furthermore, the small-diameter head allowed the use of a thick socket giving the advantages of relative rigidity, low-frictional torque and reasonable thickness of plastic to accommodate depth of penetration, three advantages in one scientifically worked out design.

The work of Harris and White (1982) came next. They recommended the use of metal-backed acetabular components. Their evidence was based on a comparison of 34 of their own cases using metal-backed cups with 43 cases of Dorr and Takei (1981) without metal backing. In both groups the patients were 45 years old or younger. The average follow-up in both groups was 6.5 years, with a minimum of 5 years and maximum of 9 years. They concluded that "in

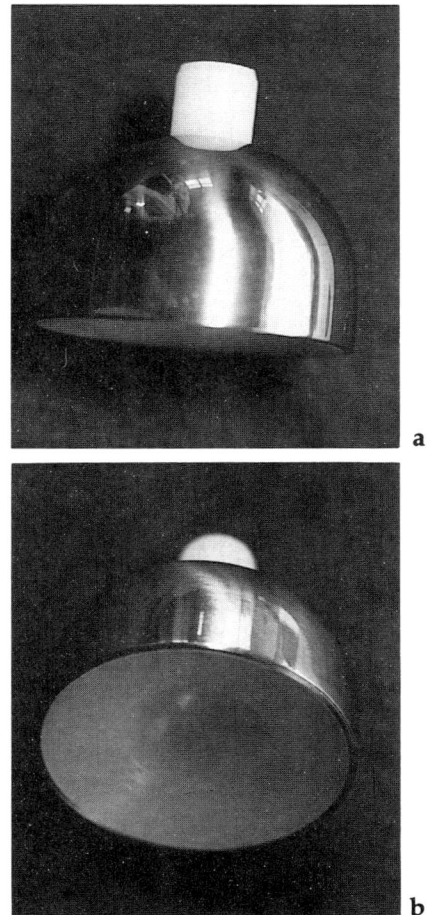

Fig. 12.1a,b. The Charnley press-fit socket, a cemented metal-backed HDP socket. The central HDP spigot was made to engage into the pilot hole of the acetabulum.

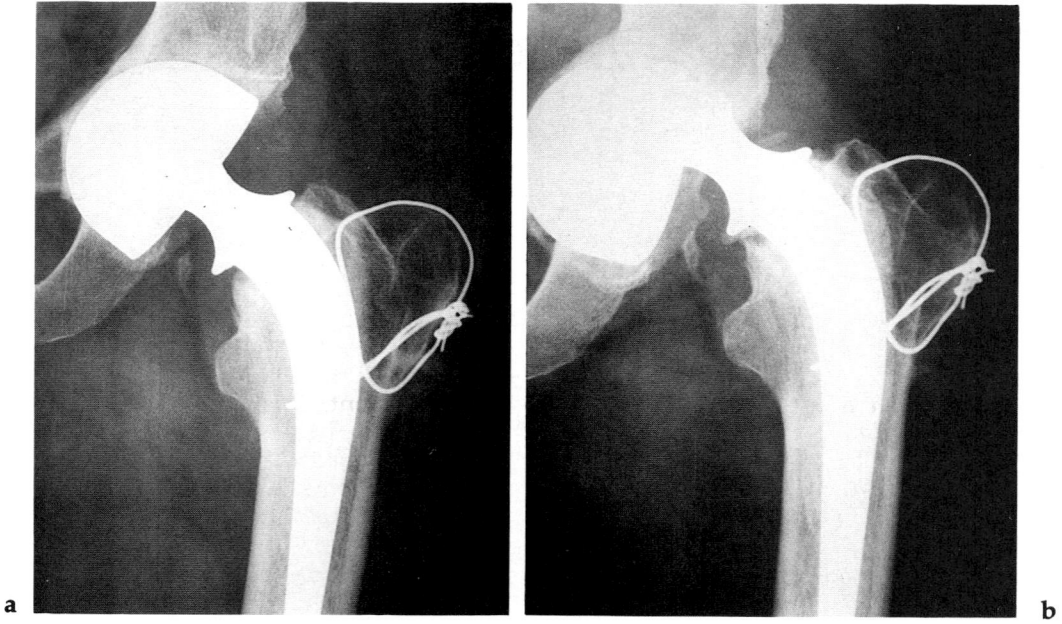

Fig. 12.2. Press-fit socket in clinical use. **a** Post-operative appearance. **b** Tilting and migration resulting in dislocation after 10 years of trouble-free service.

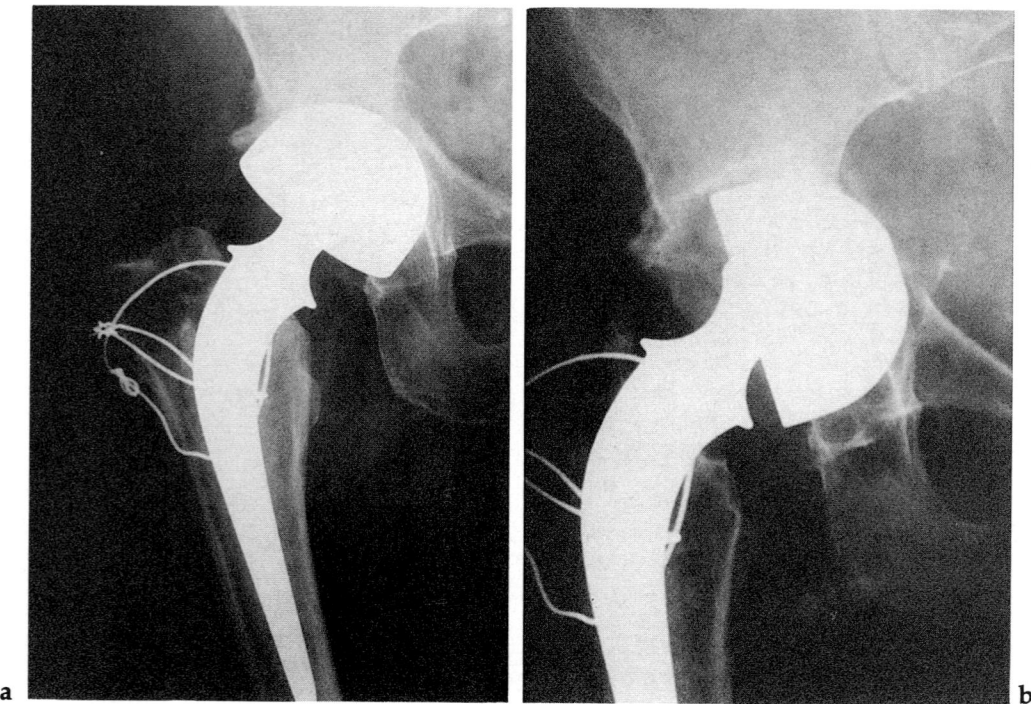

Fig. 12.3.a,b Long-term clinical success of the press-fit socket. Over 20 years' clinically excellent result despite the change in position of the press-fit socket.

view of these clinical data . . . we now recommend the use of metal-backed acetabular components for all total hip replacements". Although the difference between the results of the two groups was statistically significant, the authors did not make some of their statements entirely clear. Some of the statements need closer examination, e.g. "All hips except two had some radiolucent zone or zones at the cement–bone interface"; "A total of eighteen hips had radiolucent zones that were two millimetres thick at some point, but were not characteristic of impending failure." The first statement presumably refers to the two series of patients. If so then it could be rephrased as follows: "In only two hips was there no demarcation of the bone–cement interface." Stated thus it becomes obvious that in the rest the appearances of the bone–cement junction were other than perfect. The second statement is probably describing cases of socket loosening, presumably for the whole series, i.e. 18 out of 77 cases (23.4% at 6.5 years!). If on the other hand the 18 cases are from their own series of 34 then the failure rate at 6.5 years was 52.9%. If the 18 cases were from Dorr and Takei's series then the failure rate in that group was 41.9%. Whichever way the results are interpreted there is little room for optimism and none for recommending the routine use of a metal-backed socket.

It can be confidently stated that a zone of demarcation of 2 mm indicates loosening (Hodgkinson et al. 1989a) unless localized to the outer one-third of the bone–cement junction, though it doesn't necessarily indicate a clinical failure or the need for a revision. The fact that metal backing of the socket was recommended on rather inadequate evidence becomes obvious when the results of the "metal-backed" group were reviewed with follow-up of 11.3 years (range 10–13.5 years). At that stage "21 per cent have already required removal of the original acetabular component and 21 per cent more are definitely loose or have impending failure". Thus 41% have evidence of failure of fixation of the component. Furthermore "90 per cent of the acetabulae in patients who were below thirty years of age became loose" (Harris and Penenberg, personal communication 1986). It must be conceded that a number of cases in the Harris and White series were other than primary procedures, yet their original recommendation was unambiguously clear.

There is no denying that finite-element studies are more convincing than clinical results. It must also be accepted that metal backing may obscure some of the bone–cement changes and will make socket wear measurements difficult or even impossible. It is obvious that metal backing is not the answer to socket loosening and the results give no support to the original statement. The answer to socket loosening must lie elsewhere.

13 Loosening of the Stem

Introduction

Charnley, although not the first to use acrylic cement for stem fixation was the first to use it in the correct manner, i.e. as a grout, pushing it boldly down the medullary canal in quantity.

In Charnley's description of the surgical technique of the then new low-friction arthroplasty each stage was accurately detailed including the "two-thumb" method of inserting the cement down the medullary canal. Even in a later description (1971), the detail remained: "Ramming should be unhurried, allowing one second pause for viscous cement to move forward. 30 rams at one ram per second should be adequate" (Internal publication, 2nd revision, February 1971). In retrospect, this emphasis on the detail of the technique, although essential for any would-be users, can now be seen to be misplaced – the emphasis should perhaps have been more on the aim of the method. In order to gain a better understanding of the point under discussion it may be worthwhile analysing this aspect in some detail.

When preparing the medullary canal to accept a cemented stem the surgeon faces three variables: the size of the medullary canal, the amount of cement available and the size of the stem to be used. Initially two stems were available, the standard 45-mm offset "flat back" and a straight thick stem (STS) (a "flat back" with 3.75-mm offset) (Fig. 13.1) used in cases of conversions of previous intertrochanteric osteotomies, of which some 80–90 were being carried out each year. (For a period of time a straight narrow stem (SNS) was also used.) Thus the choice of stems was limited.

The amount of cement introduced down the medullary canal was largely determined by the detail of the technique and the availability of the standard 40-g pack of cement. The most important variable is obviously the size of the medullary canal and this is largely determined by the weight of the patient. It is this variable that should determine the size of the stem used and the amount of cement needed, assuming, of course, that medullary canal preparation etc. is good. In the early years of the technique this was not so. Very often the technique was virtually identical irrespective of the stem size and the size of the medullary canal. Thus in a large medullary canal, stem fixation was invariably better in the more distal, narrow portion and this led to fracture of the stem (Fig. 13.2). When the medullary canal was very wide the amount of cement was, by comparison, inadequate and stem loosening resulted (Fig. 13.3). Patients with narrow medullary canals fared well, a long plug of cement down the shaft of the femur functioning, purely incidentally, as a block, improving cement injection and stem fixation (Fig. 13.4).

With time, and with a better understanding of the problem, the preparation of the medullary canal became more deliberate, especially in the proximal portion. A flanged stem design was introduced to prevent the escape of cement through the open neck of the femur, thus improving cement injection and engaging the whole column of cement in load transmission. With the flanged stem design a selection of sizes became available.

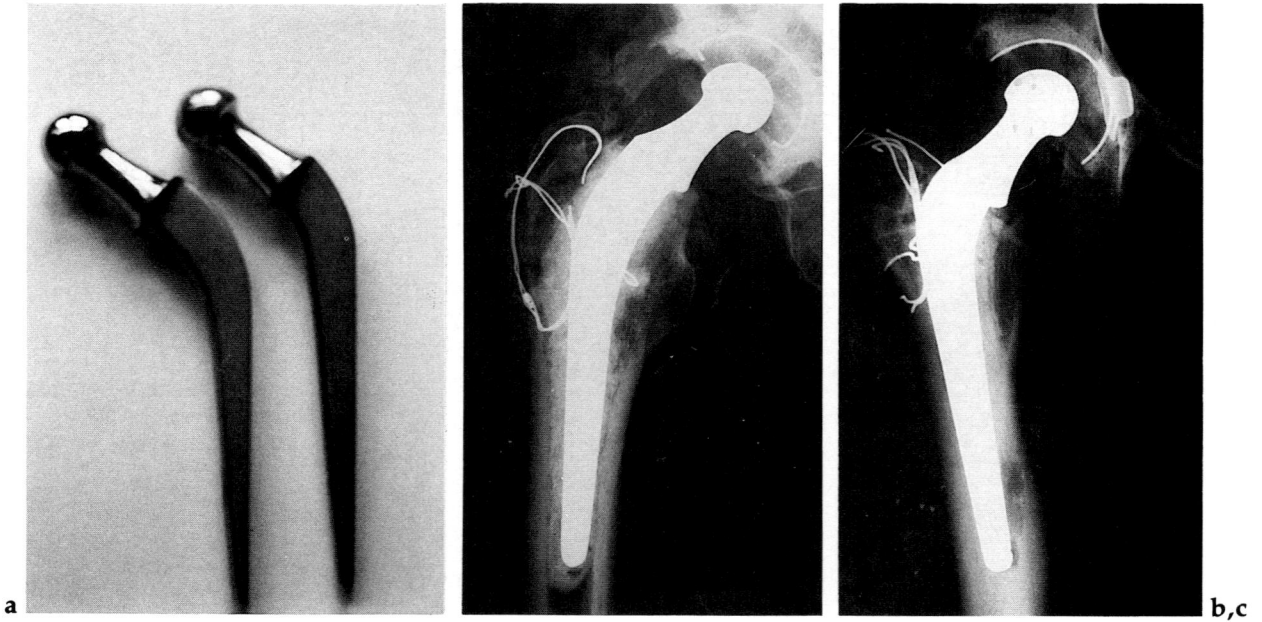

Fig. 13.1.a The initial choice of stems. **b** Standard, "flat back" 45-mm offset, as shown in clinical practice. **c** Straight, thick stem (STS) 37.5-mm offset, as shown in clinical practice.

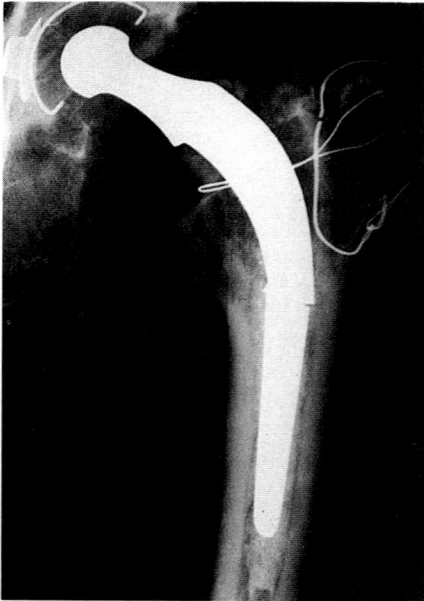

Fig. 13.2. Fractured stem. Note good distal fixation with lack of proximal stem support.

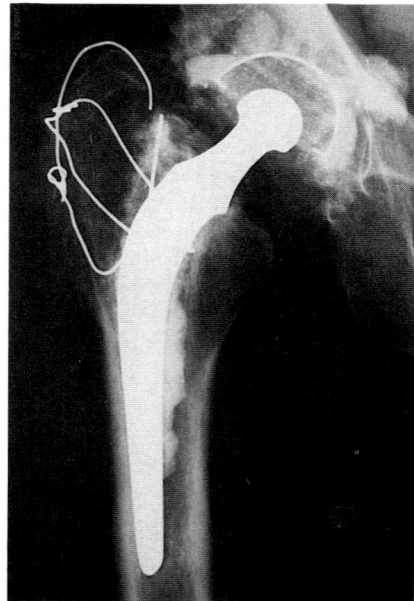

Fig. 13.3. Loose stem. Note large medullary canal, sparse cement for stem fixation and stem subsidence down to the lesser trochanter.

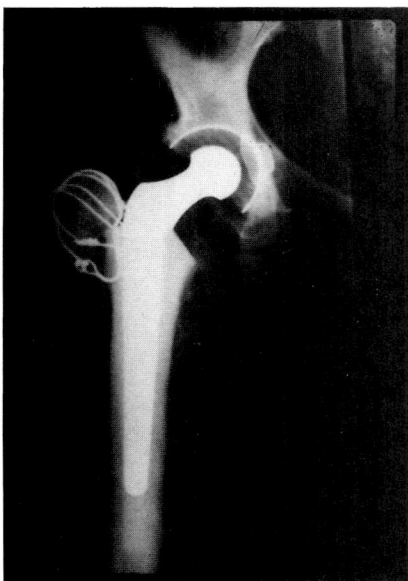

Fig. 13.4. Long-term success. Note narrow medullary canal, comparatively large amount of cement and stem filling the medullary canal.

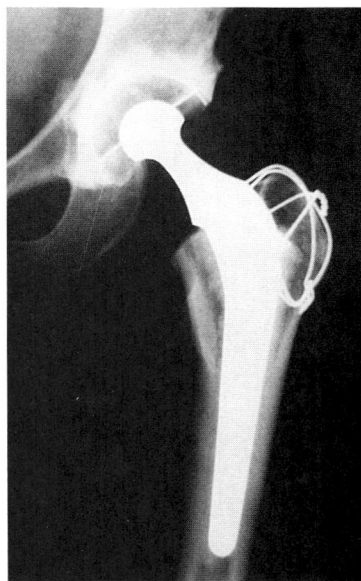

Fig. 13.5. Intramedullary cancellous bone block. The medullary canal is closed off with the cancellous bone block just distal to the tip of the stem. The stem is in a neutral position because of its size, the method of exposure and preparation of the medullary canal.

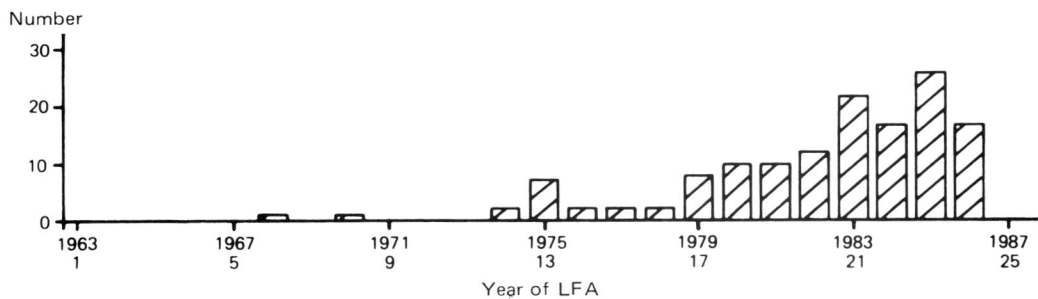

a

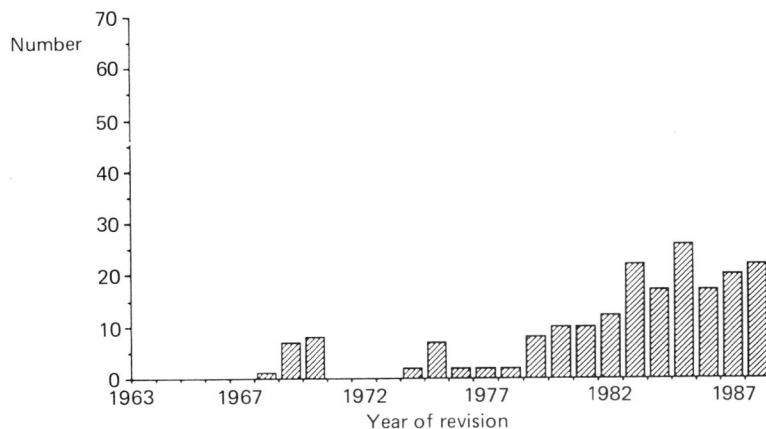

b

Fig. 13.6.a Declining incidence of revisions for stem loosening. Will the trend continue? **b** Apparently not! See text for possible explanation.

Table 13.1. Radiographic appearances of stems revised for loosening compared with the 15–21-year results (after Pacheco et al. 1988)

x-ray appearances	No. (%) revised for stem loosening (total 72 cases)		No. (%) at 15–21-year follow-up (total 116 cases)		Statistical significance
Unchanged at 1 year	12	(16.7)	70	(60.3)	$P < 0.002$
Separation of back of stem from cement	19	(26.4)	31	(26.7)	Not significant
Demarcation of tip of cement	43	(59.7)	21	(18.1)	$P < 0.001$
Fracture of tip of cement	12	(16.7)	4	(3.4)	$P < 0.001$
Endosteal cavitation	1	(1.4)	0	(0)	Insufficient data for analysis
Stem position					
Varus	7	(9.7)	16	(13.8)	Not significant
Valgus	42	(58.3)	19	(16.4)	$P < 0.001$
Neutral	23	(31.9)	81	(69.8)	$P < 0.002$
Previous surgery	22	(30.6)	5	(4.3)	$P < 0.001$
Weight (kg)	69		66		Not significant

Intramedullary Bone Block

In September 1977 the technique of intramedullary cancellous bone block was introduced (Wroblewski and van der Rijt 1984) to close off the medullary canal near the tip of the stem (Fig. 13.5). From then on the closed-off proximal part of the medullary canal could be fully packed with acrylic cement in the knowledge that the cement would be contained. The bulkiest stem which could then be introduced easily was used. Then washing and brushing of the closed-off medullary canal became the routine practice. It is apparent that the emphasis changed from the detail of the technique, i.e. how to carry out this part of the operation, to the aim of the procedure, i.e. sound fixation of the stem. This has obviously been reflected in the results; not only has the radiological finding of loosening of the stem been reduced to 0.3% (Wroblewski and van der Rijt 1984) but the incidence of revisions for stem loosening has also declined (Fig. 13.6).

The Pacheco Study

Dr. Victorino Pacheco (with others 1988), while working on a voluntary basis as a Research Assistant, has examined the problem of mechanical loosening of the stem in the Charnley low-friction arthroplasty. In a review of 19 161 LFAs carried out between November 1962 and December 1984 it is seen that a total of 1085 LFAs were revised for various reasons. In that group there were 72 stems revised for mechanical loosening. The object of the study was not so much to look at the incidence of stem loosening but to draw attention to certain radiological and clinical features which identified this group of patients as being at risk for stem loosening. The results of the study are summarized in Table 13.1 and must be examined in some detail. Comparison with the 15–21-year results (Wroblewski 1986a) sheds further light on the problem.

Unchanged Radiographic Appearances

In 17% of patients in the study the radiograph taken at 1 year was unchanged compared with that taken at the time of discharge. Thus a normal and unchanging radiographic appearance in a patient with good function is an encouraging finding; it indicates the likelihood of a successful long-term clinical result. (The comparison with the 15–21-year results confirms this; 60.3% had an unchanged radiograph at 1 year.) In the remaining 83% of patients there was a change of appearance within 1 year of surgery. This period of time was selected purely for convenience; it is at 1 year that the patients are most likely to be discharged from further follow-up and the time at which identification of cases "at risk" would be of practical advantage.

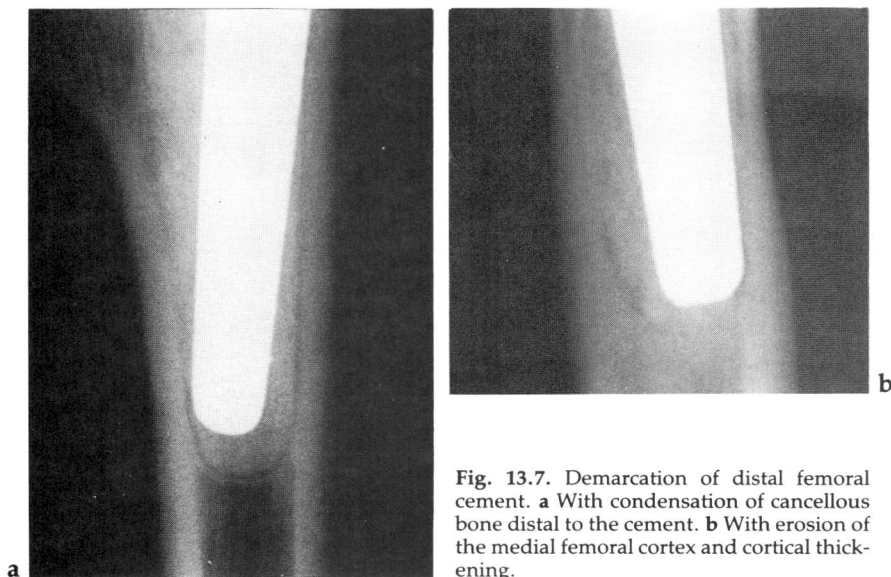

Fig. 13.7. Demarcation of distal femoral cement. **a** With condensation of cancellous bone distal to the cement. **b** With erosion of the medial femoral cortex and cortical thickening.

Demarcation of Distal Femoral Cement (Fig. 13.7)

This was present in 59.7% of patients in the Pacheco Study as compared with 18.1% in the 15–21-year follow-up group. The incidence of this finding did not seem to increase with time and if anything it probably declined. It was present in 52.8% of patients by the time of revision. Its early appearance is probably the result of condensation of the cancellous bone at the distal end of the stem–cement complex due to stress concentration caused by the slip of the stem or the stem–cement complex within the medullary canal. As such it is a radiological indicator of an early failure of stem fixation but not necessarily an indicator of long-term clinical failure.

Separation of the Stem from Cement (Fig. 13.8)

This is an indicator of a slip or tilt of the stem within the cement mantle. It was present in 26.4% of patients in the Pacheco Study and 26.7% of patients in the 15–21-year study. By itself it is probably of little clinical importance. However, it may often be associated with fracture of the proximal cement, endosteal cavitation, tilting of the stem, gross loss of bone stock and clinical failure. This is supported by

the incidence of this finding increasing to 45.8% by the time of revision.

Fracture of the Femoral Cement at the Tip of the Stem (Fig. 13.9)

This indicates a slip of the stem within the cement mantle, end-weight bearing of the prosthesis and fracture of the cement column under load. This may result either in tightening of the stem within the cement mantle, or in destruction of the proximal–medial cement. If progressive it will lead to distal migration and tilting or to a fracture of the stem. It usually presents within 1 year of surgery (16.7%) but the incidence did increase to 30.6% by the time of revision.

Endosteal Cavitation of the Femoral Cortex (Fig. 13.10)

Endosteal cavitation of the femoral cortex is almost certainly due to changes in volume and pressure caused by the micromovement of the stem–cement complex within the medullary canal. It presumably takes time to develop (unlike stem separation or cement fracture) and then additional time to lead to sufficient loss of the femoral cortex to be obvious on radiographs. Thus it is not an early sign of failure of stem fixation (1.4%) but is certainly an indication of loosening of some standing – its incidence had increased to 34.7% by the time of revision.

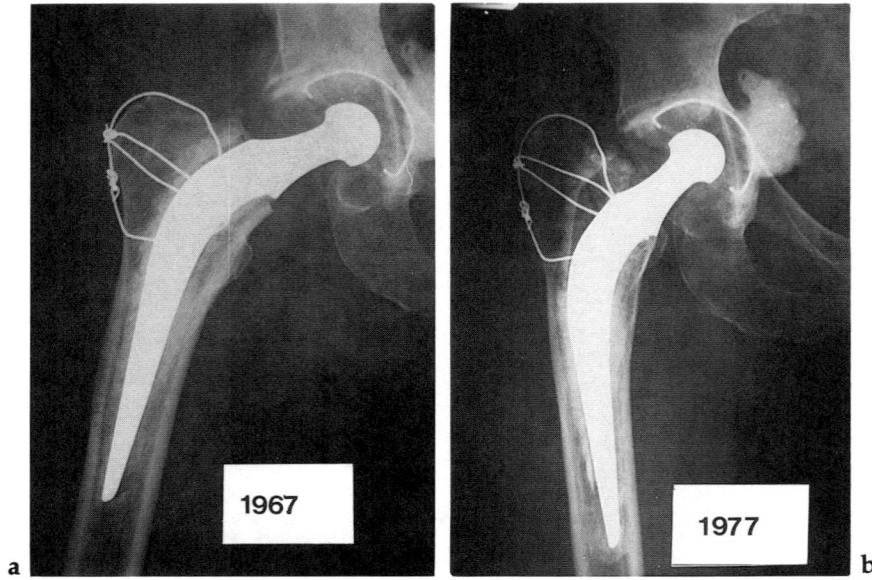

Fig. 13.8 Progressive separation of the lateral side of the stem from cement. **a** Early post-operative appearance. **b** Appearance 10 years later. The stem has subsided down to the lesser trochanter.

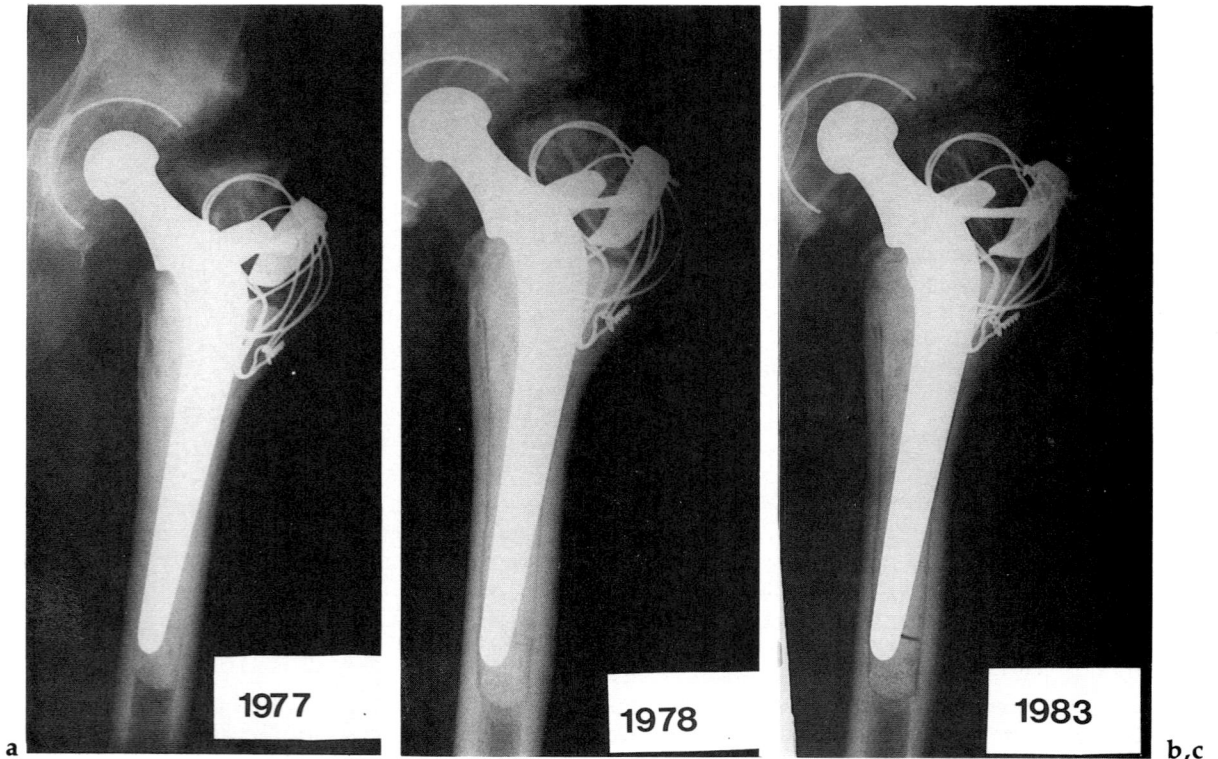

Fig. 13.9.a–c Fracture of the femoral cement at the tip of the stem. Progressive changes from after the operation in 1977 through to 1983.

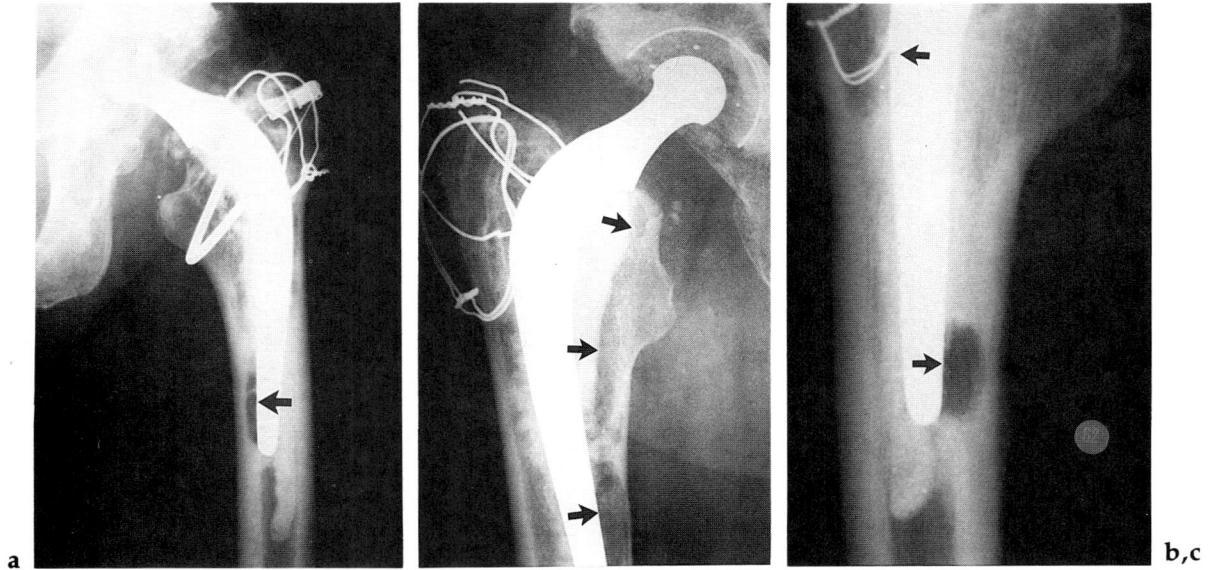

Fig. 13.10.a–c Endosteal cavitation of the femoral cortex. Examples of cavitation at various levels. Note the fracture of the stem.

Position of the Stem Within the Medullary Canal

Position of the stem within the medullary canal has, somehow, become synonymous with the quality of stem fixation. It has often been suggested that valgus is the desirable position whereas varus is indicative of failure. This is probably due to misinterpretation of some publications (see Chap. 14) and the fact that a description of a radiographic appearance strikes a cord more readily than does a detailed description of a surgical technique aimed at sound stem fixation.

In 58.3% of patients in the Pacheco Study the stems that were revised for loosening were placed in a valgus position. This may come as a surprise to those who believe that a valgus position for the stem is *sine qua non* for good fixation. This is not so. "Valgus" is a descriptive term of the radiological appearance of the position of the stem within the medullary canal. The valgus position reduces the "functional offset" of the stem and may even reduce the incidence of the stem fracture but it appears to be doing so at the expense of stem loosening, the emphasis being on position of the stem rather than its fixation. There was no difference between the two groups as far as "varus"

position was concerned, but stems placed in a neutral position, i.e. centrally down the medullary canal, gave the best results.

Previous Hip Surgery

The Pacheco Study has also highlighted the effect of previous operation on the eventual outcome of the LFA. Almost a third of the patients (30.6%) had had previous hip surgery (Table 13.2). This finding must be appreciated by surgeons who undertake uncemented total hip arthroplasties assuming that revision surgery will be easy. It may well be, but will the long-term results be successful?

Table 13.2. Previous hip surgery in patients whose LFA failed because of stem loosening (after Pacheco et al. 1988)

Operation	No.
Intertrochanteric osteotomy	11
Fracture fixation	3
Total hip arthroplasty	3
Femoral head replacement	3
Cup arthroplasty	1
Fusion	1
Total	22

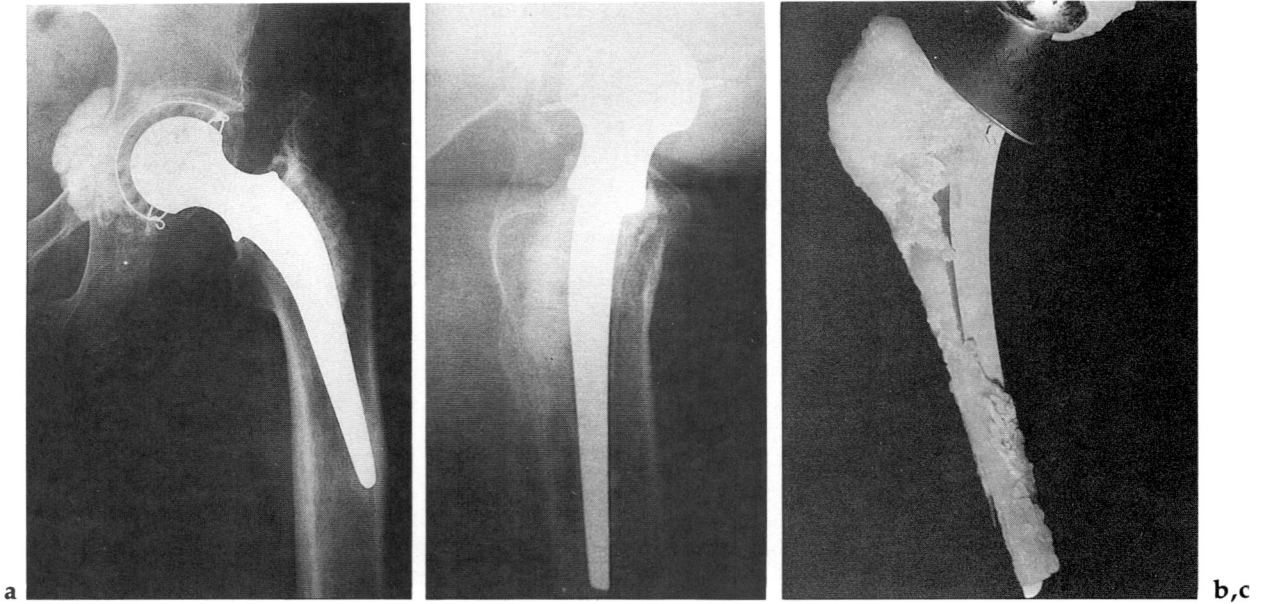

a   b,c

Fig. 13.11.a,b The problem of a limited exposure. The stem is "with cement" rather than "cemented". **c** Typical example of cement distribution due to limited exposure.

Primary to Revision Surgery

The problem of stem loosening can further be analysed in two distinct ways: first as a complication arising some time after surgery and thus related to the length of the follow-up; alternatively as a yearly problem seen in the light of the evolution of the operation from the earliest cases to the most recent ones. The first method of analysis is likely to give a pattern of revisions for stem loosening based on the length of the follow-up (and the number of patients still attending) while the second will be a better measure of numbers being revised each year as well as a reflection of any improvements in the technique of the operation. This latter method of analysis would also indicate likely future trends, and these could be used to make planning more logical. Thus revision for stem loosening may have to be carried out, exceptionally, within the first year following the operation or more than 15 years later.

Inadequate fixation is still probably the most common problem to be overcome. Sometimes it is due to lack of understanding of the demand likely to be imposed on the arthroplasty, but more recently it has been due to the fashion for limited exposure (Fig. 13.11). The numbers of patients affected increases with time after the operation, to peaking in the ninth post-operative year, then declines gradually (Fig. 13.12).

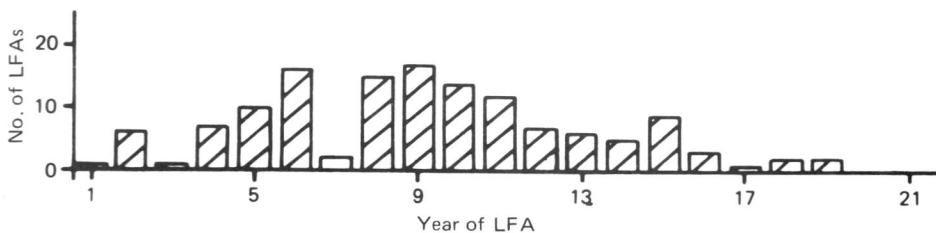

Fig. 13.12. Loose stem in the Charnley LFA. Time interval from primary to revision surgery.

The need for revision for stem loosening first presented in 1968, 6 years after the introduction of the LFA, and did not really become a regular problem until 1974, the twelfth year of the technique. Since 1979 (the seventeenth year of the Charnley LFA) the number of Charnley LFAs being revised has steadily increased and it was only in 1986 (the twenty-fourth year) that there was some indication of a reduction in numbers (Fig. 13.6). (The increase we are witnessing in the twenty-fifth year is probably due to the expected increase of secondary revisions.)

No simple explanation of this pattern of revisions for stem loosening can be offered. It is freely accepted that the first 6 years of the technique were not necessarily free from cases of stem loosening. It is unlikely, however, that any of the cases were revised in other units. The pioneering nature of the work was fully realized by Sir John Charnley and greatly respected by others. The components did not become freely available, on Sir John's insistence, until the second half of 1970, 8 years after the introduction of the technique into clinical practice. It is hard to imagine that with the strict control over the follow-up, the technique and the components, other surgeons would venture into revisions of an operation they were possibly not fully versed in. The 6-year period (1962–1968) of freedom from revisions for stem loosening and fracture as well as for socket loosening gives support to the explanation offered.

Today, however, revisions are invariably tackled earlier because of a better understanding of the problem and the need for preservation and improvement of the bone stock. Furthermore, with increasing follow-up time cases are now presenting for second or even third revisions. Thus their inclusion in any further analysis will obviously affect the overall result; such cases must be studied separately.

Two other factors makes continuation of such analysis less meaningful, and these are the non-uniform selection of the components and the non-standard operative technique. It is for those reasons that some cases from the Centre for Hip Surgery, Wrightington Hospital, will have to be excluded from further reviews. Although there will be fewer remaining cases, they will have the benefit of continuity of the concept of the Charnley LFA.

In cases with the longest follow-up, and where the technique of stem fixation has been correctly performed, the radiological appearances are most encouraging. With the better understanding of stem design and function the indications are that a perfect and a permanent stem fixation for the majority, if not for all, the cases is a real possibility.

Radiological Appearances of Failure of Stem Fixation

Gruen and colleagues (1979) published their classic description of "modes of failure", recognizing four mechanisms (pistoning, mid-stem pivot, calcar pivot and bending cantilever) as well as defining seven zones around the cemented stem. Although the mechanism of failure is easy to recognize in some cases it is by no means clear in all. Descriptive terminology such as "pistoning" implies an "up and down" movement which probably does not take place other than of the stem–cement complex within the femur. "Mid-stem pivot and calcar pivot" are probably a reflection of the technique just as much as they are of the mechanism of failure, while "bending cantilever" is part of the very nature of the concept and technique and does exist, by design, from the first moment of the stem insertion. However, it does not necessarily imply immediate or long-term failure.

Patterns of Failure of Stem Fixation

Several patterns of failure of stem fixation can be recognized radiologically. Their recognition is of interest not only for descriptive purposes but because their understanding has a bearing on the surgical technique, stem design, the likely clinical outcome and the indication for methods of management. It must be accepted that some overlap between the patterns of failure exists and the following simple description must not be looked upon as a rigid compartmentalization; it merely attempts to present a two-dimensional picture of a three-dimensional problem. The mechanisms of failure may be classified as follows:

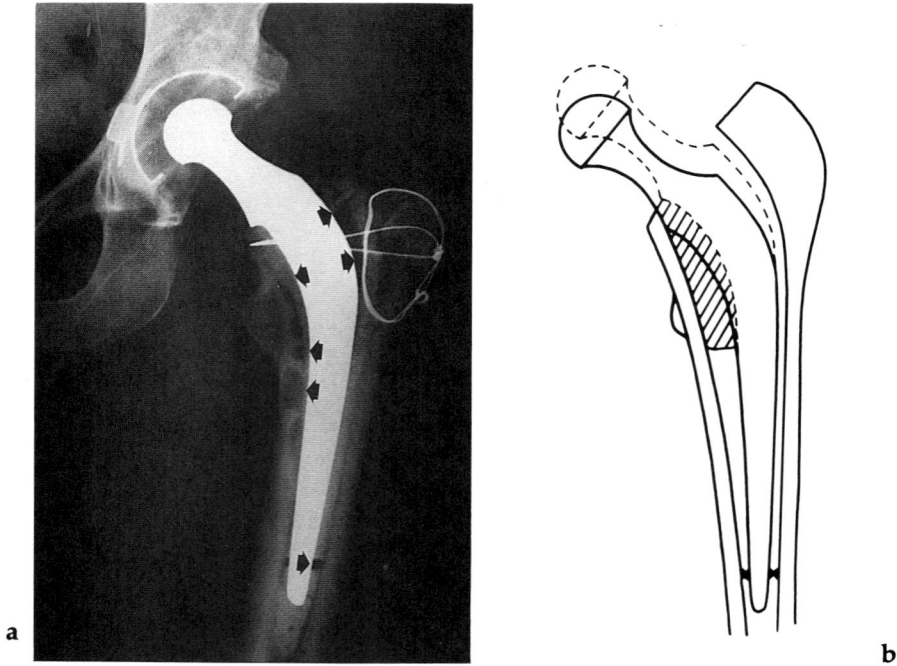

Fig. 13.13. Slip of the stem within the cement mantle. **a** The stem is end-weight bearing. Its slip within the cement mantle is shown by the fracture of the cement near the tip of the stem and separation of the lateral aspect of the stem from the acrylic cement. Note endosteal cavitation medially. **b** Diagrammatic representation of the changes that must take place in the proximal femur. These must be most marked medially because of the curved portion of the stem, its distal slip and deflection under load.

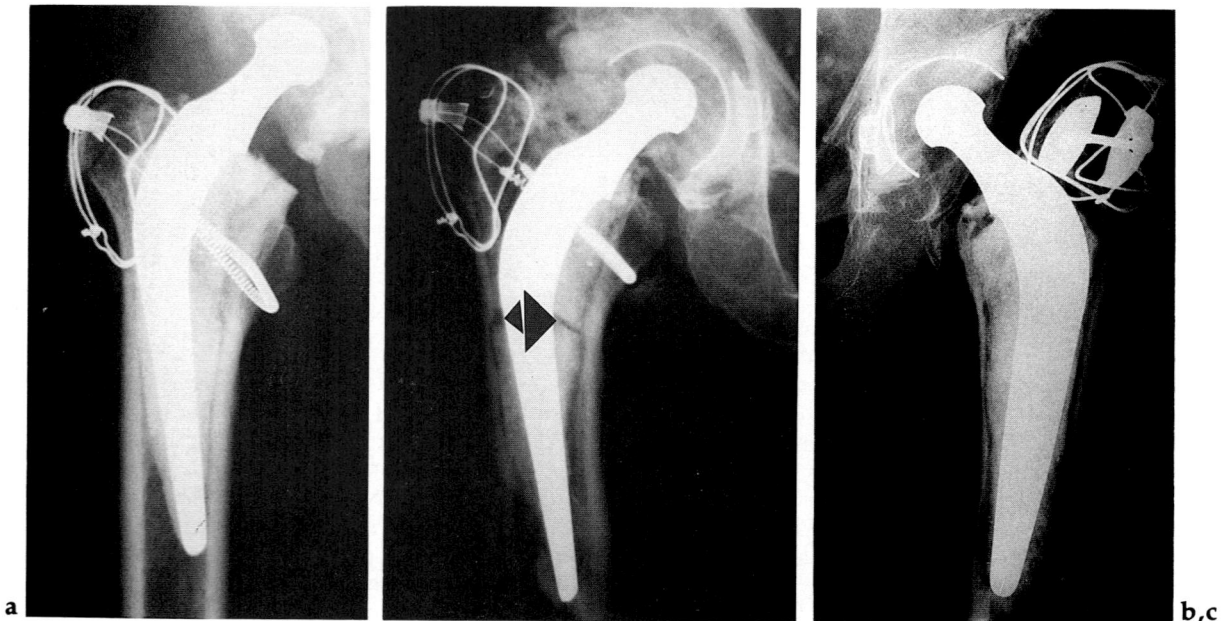

Fig. 13.14. Slip of the stem–cement complex within the medullary canal. **a** Post-operative appearance. **b** Fourteen-year follow-up. Stem–cement complex slipping "en masse" down the medullary canal. No gross stem tilting, no endosteal cavitation. Note the cement fracture at the level of the mid-stem. Occasional discomfort on activity. **c** Slip of the stem and intact cement. Some pain on activity.

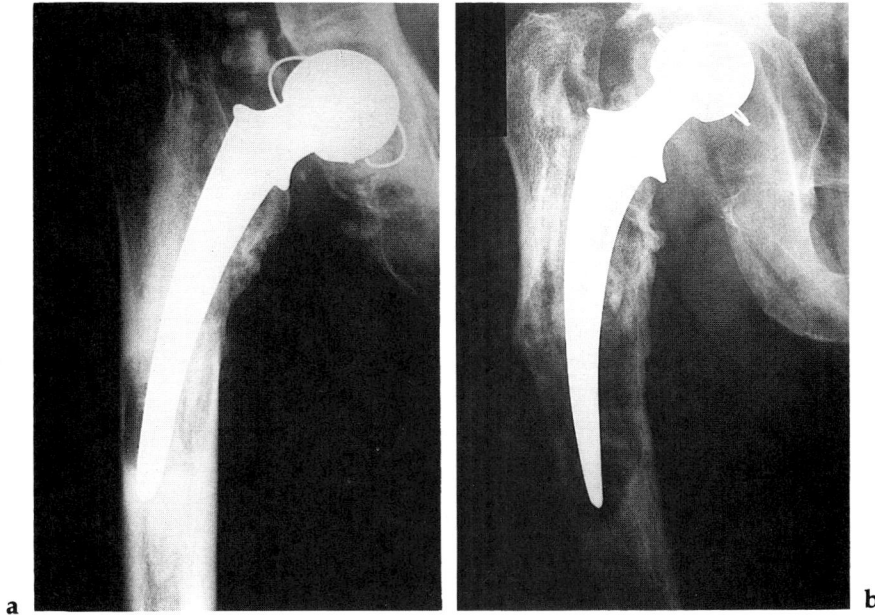

Fig. 13.15. Stem tilt. **a** Stem probably never fully supported medially. Progressive tilting into varus markedly destructive to the medial femoral cortex. Cavitation at the tip of the stem laterally. **b** Stem tilt with gross destruction of the femoral cortex and fracture of the femoral shaft.

1. Slip
   a. Stem within the cement mantle
   b. Stem–cement complex within the medullary canal
2. Tilt
   a. Stem
   b. Stem–cement complex
3. Pivot
   a. Cement
   b. Bone
   c. Stem–cement

Slip of the Stem Within the Cement Mantle

As already pointed out, this is probably the most common occurrence with any design which employs a taper which by the nature of its surface finish allows a certain degree of slip of the stem within the cement mantle. (It is an integral part of the Exeter stem both in the design and the surgical technique.) It can be readily recognized by the fracture tip of the cement and at times there is an obvious separation of the back of the stem from the cement. It is probably harmless in isolation unless it leads to fragmentation of the cement at the calcar, loss of proximal support (Fig. 13.13), fracture of the stem or progressive loosening.

In treating slip of the stem within the cement mantle the lack of proximal stem support must be appreciated and corrected for by meticulous clearing of the cement and fibrous tissue, as well as by excavation of the lesser trochanter which involves removal of the anatomical calcar for cement injection into its strong cancellous bone. This will offer support for the stem in the postero-medial aspect, proximally, and is an essential part of treatment. To fail to do this is to invite early failure of the bone–cement junction and fracture of the stem by the hinging mechanism (see Chap. 14).

Slip of the Stem–Cement Complex Within the Medullary Canal

For this mechanism to become apparent the whole of the stem–cement complex must subside within the medullary canal. It may or may not be associated with fracture of the cement mantle (Fig. 13.14). The slip is usually slow, may be accompanied by condensation of the cancellous bone round the cement and is not usually markedly symptomatic. In fact the patient may

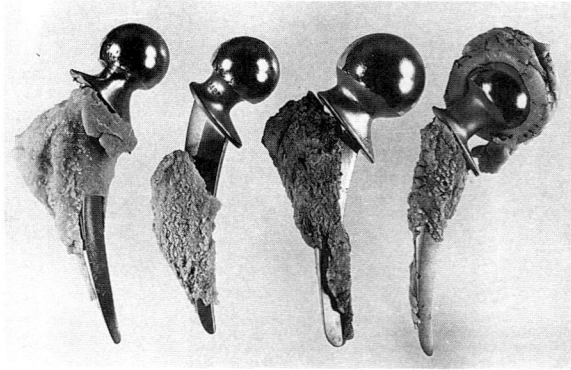

Fig. 13.16. Tilt of the stem–cement complex. Four examples of stem–cement complex removed at revision for deep sepsis. Note the amount of cement and its distribution.

revised late, no support at the lesser trochanteric level can be achieved and not only will an extended neck prosthesis have to be used, but also a longer stem becomes essential to by-pass the weakened lateral cortex. If neglected the mechanism is likely to lead to femoral fracture (Fig. 13.15).

Tilt of the Stem–Cement Complex

The whole implant comprising the stem and the cement tilts and migrates en masse, usually weakening the lateral, or at times the medial, cortex. It is common in cases of deep sepsis where well-injected cement fails at the bone–cement interface or in cases of previous revision where the femoral canal is no more than a smooth straight tube, its distal part having not been by-passed by the new stem and cement (Fig. 13.16). The symptoms are not necessarily severe and are usually restricted to the thigh when weight bearing. It is necessary to be aware of the possibility of femoral shaft fracture.

be remarkably free from symptoms apart from progressive limb shortening. However, revision should be undertaken if the slip reaches the proximal part of the lesser trochanter or if tilting or cavitation start to appear. Removal of the fibrous layer, careful exposure of the cancellous bone deep to the condensed cancellous layer and excavation of the lesser trochanter are essential. The new stem need not by-pass the previous level distally, provided no tilting or endosteal cavitation is present. If these features are present then the new stem should certainly be made to engage into the virgin canal distally, not particularly far but some 1–2 cm to prevent future stem tilting. If slip is excessive then the term "subsidence" is probably more apt.

Pivoting of the Implant Within the Cement

Pivoting of the implant within the femur can occur at several levels. The stem, with its surrounding mantle of cement which may or may not be intact, pivots on its tip which is supported by a column of well-injected cement (Fig. 13.17a,b). This type of pivoting is common in cases of deep sepsis or late mechanical failure. Apart from achieving proximal support, the new stem should be made to enter the medullary canal further distally, especially if a degree of tilting and cortical thinning or cavitation are present.

Tilt of the Stem

This is unfortunately a common problem. It is often a result of an inadequate exposure and inadequate fixation as judged by the position of the stem, the amount of cement as well as its distribution. The tilting is often slowly progressive initially and not severely symptomatic but it is markedly destructive to the femur. The endosteal cancellous bone, the lateral femoral cortex and the medial femoral neck are readily lost (Fig. 13.15). If revised early a result comparable with that of primary surgery may be achieved. If

Pivoting of the Implant Within the Bone

The stem–cement complex subsides and becomes supported on a layer of condensed cancellous bone which with time becomes obvious radiologically (Fig. 13.17c). This is no doubt a relection of some degree of load bearing distally. The proximal part of the stem–cement complex may become stabilized by wedging within the taper of the medullary canal. Distal migration, tilting or cavitation do not necessarily occur and are unusual in the early stages.

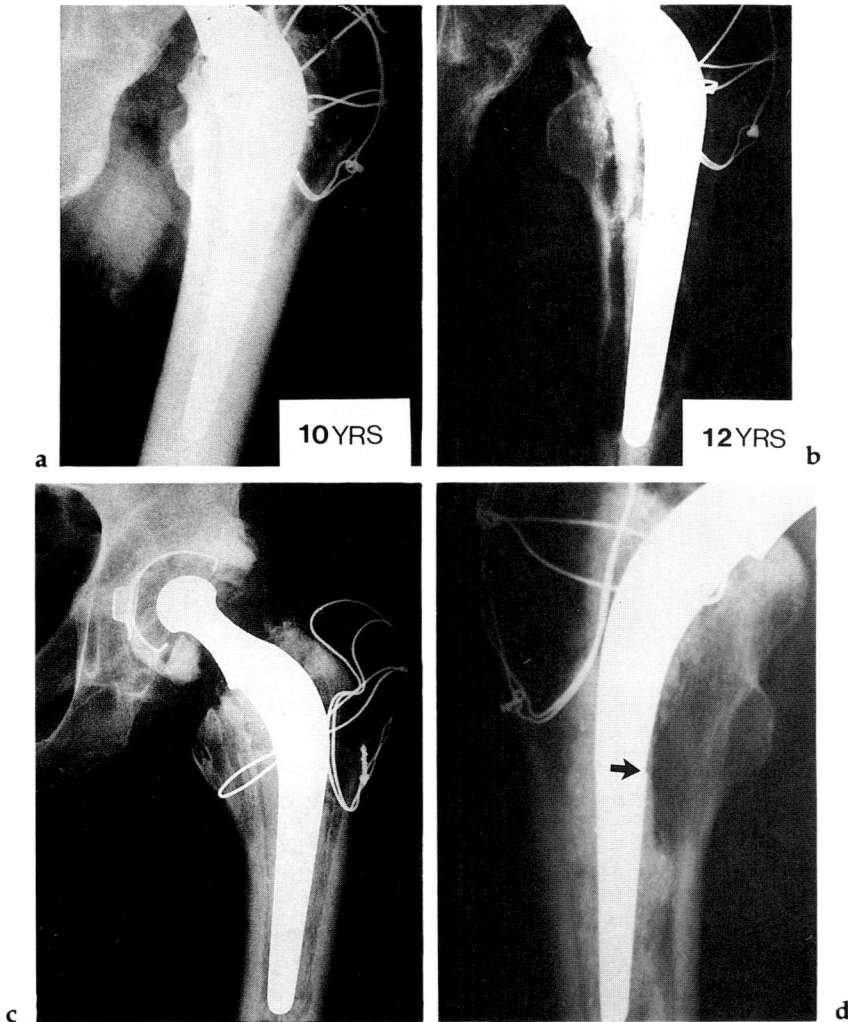

Fig. 13.17. Pivot. **a,b** Cement–stem pivots supported distally on a column of a well-injected cement. Gross cavitation of the shaft presenting between the 10th and 12th years of follow-up. Patient asymptomatic at all times. **c** Bone–stem pivoting on condensation of cancellous bone distal to the tip of the stem. Patient mildly symptomatic. **d** Stem–cement pivot: the proximal part of the stem pivots on its distal tip which is surrounded by well-injected cement. May lead to stem fracture.

Though not severely symptomatic this condition needs watching. Revision should be undertaken if the femoral cortex is in danger of being weakened by progressive thinning, or if tilting becomes imminent.

Pivoting of the Stem–Cement Complex

The distal part of the stem is embedded within a cement mantle. This mantle can be quite extensive (Fig. 13.17d) or no more than a token amount. The proximal part of the stem and some of the surrounding cement pivot within the medullary canal. Slip or subsidence is not marked and may not even be obvious. Endosteal cavitation can be very extensive and may present late. The most worrying aspect of this pattern of failure is its long-term effect, i.e. loss of proximal bone stock. It may be reflection of proximal stress shielding and distal load transfer. Revision must aim at proximal support of the stem and the by-passing of any weakened or cavitated cortex.

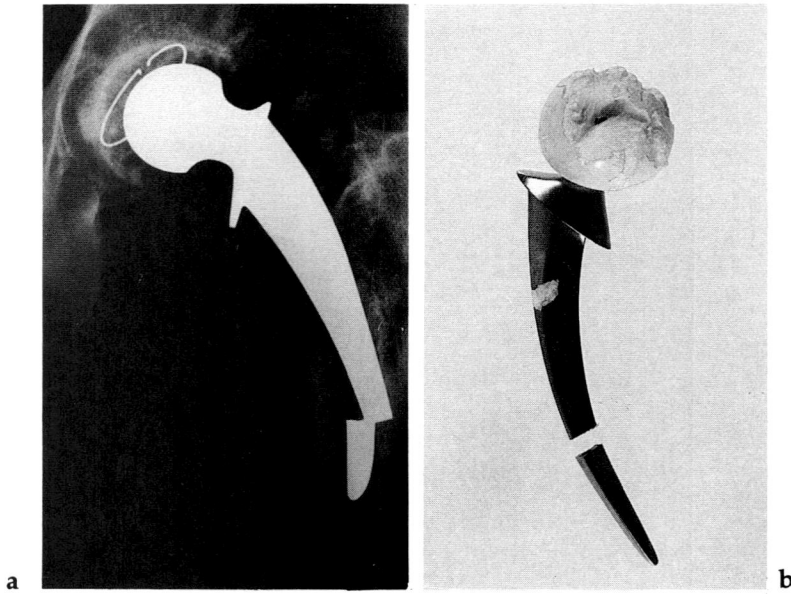

Fig. 13.18. Lack or loss of proximal support and stem fracture. **a** Fracture of the stem with a very short distal fragment. **b** Fracture of the stem of a femoral head replacement using HDP articulating within the acetabulum. Despite gross HDP wear and bone destruction, what little function was permitted was sufficient to fracture the stem.

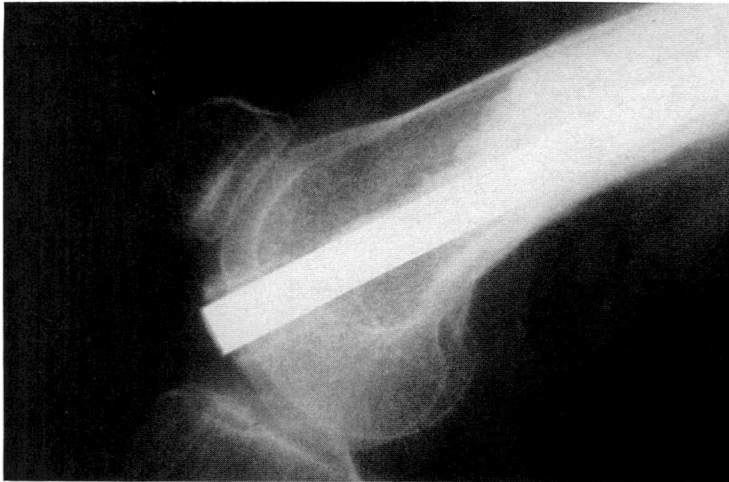

Fig. 13.19. Long stem in revision surgery. This stem is probably too long.

The Sequelae of Failure of Stem Fixation

Two further aspects of failure of stem fixation must be considered: the lack or loss of proximal support in the presence of good distal fixation, i.e. the cantilever mechanism of Gruen et al. (1979), and the cavitation of the endosteum caused by the changes in volume and pressure within the medullary canal.

Lack or Loss of Proximal Support in the Presence of Good Distal Fixation

This mechanical disadvantage often follows the slip of the stem within the cement mantle as described above. It may at times be the result of failure or lack of the proximal cement without an obvious distal stem slip. The sequence of events is probably as follows. The stem is well fixed distally. It may or may not be supported proximally. With time, and as a result of repeated deflection of the stem under load, the anatomical calcar becomes resorbed. The cement mantle fails, the stem loses its support then bends and fractures (Fig. 13.18). The new stem need not be made to extend past the previous level distally but its proximal support is essential.

Endosteal Cavitation

This indicates loosening and changes in volume and pressure of some standing (Figs. 13.10 and 13.13). In this context wear debris almost certainly play an undesirable part. If occurring early, especially near the tip of the stem, endosteal cavitation may indicate sepsis.

Although oversimplified this classification of modes of failure gives a better understanding of the problem and offers some practical hints as to the management. Revisions must not be equated with long stems (Fig. 13.19) but with the knowledge of the problem and the likely outcome. It is early recognition and treatment that offers the best results. Delays often necessitate more complex treatment and certainly lead to poorer results. Once fixation and support have failed a combination of mechanisms will be in operation governed by the direction and magnitude of the load and the strength or weakness of the femoral cortex.

Recognition of patterns of failure and their management may be exciting and rewarding but the skill lies in the prevention at primary surgery.

14 Fracture of the Stem

Introduction

Fracture of the stem has been the most dramatic complication of the Charnley low-friction arthroplasty. By virtue of its presentation and the wealth of material made available for study, it is comparable to the loose sockets retrieved at revisions some years after primary surgery. The failure of the stem being an event rather than a process (as with stem loosening) is likely to reflect the state of the arthroplasty, the role of the stem as well as the function of the hip joint in general. The two, the fractured stem and the worn socket, have really been the "flight recorders" of the arthroplasty.

Study of various aspects of the complication made it possible to identify patients and stem designs that were likely to be at risk and radiographic appearances that pointed to the likelihood of failure. The mechanism of the fracture was established from the examination of the fragments and subsequently confirmed experimentally. This finding has also given good insight into the pathology of other hip conditions.

Revision of these cases gave early opportunity to evolve various aspects of the revision technique and instrumentation. There was also a chance to look at other aspects of the operation.

The first case of fracture of the stem in the Charnley LFA (Fig. 14.1) presented in 1968, the sixth year of the Charnley technique. Retrospectively some undesirable features can be seen on examination of the radiographs of which the lack of proximal support of the stem is most obvious. It is this lack or loss of proximal support of the stem in the presence of good distal fixation that is the problem. Either as a result of the surgical technique or due to subsequent changes, the proximal support is absent or lost. This increases the lever arm and the bending moment. Although it is accepted that the distal part of the stem must be fixed, this quality of fixation is relative; it can involve most of the stem or the very tip only (Fig. 14.2). It is the disparity between the unsupported and the supported part of the stem that will lead to fracture.

It is probably correct to assume that any stem design or any method of stem fixation which must leave an unsupported extramedullary portion is potentially at risk for fracture because of the inherent cantilever beam arrangement.

Charnley reviewed a series of early fractured stems pointing out the salient features:

The mechanical situation which would favour fatigue fracture of a prosthesis is defective support by the layer of cement which is interposed between the bone of the calcar and the concave upper part of the stem of the prosthesis, when this is combined with firm bonding of the lower part of the stem of the prosthesis in the stiff tube of cortical bone composing the femur at this level. Bending stresses at each load-bearing step, caused by the offset of the head of the prosthesis from the axis of the stem, would be concentrated at the junction of the upper part, deflecting under load, with the rigidly supported lower part. (Charnley 1975 p. 115).

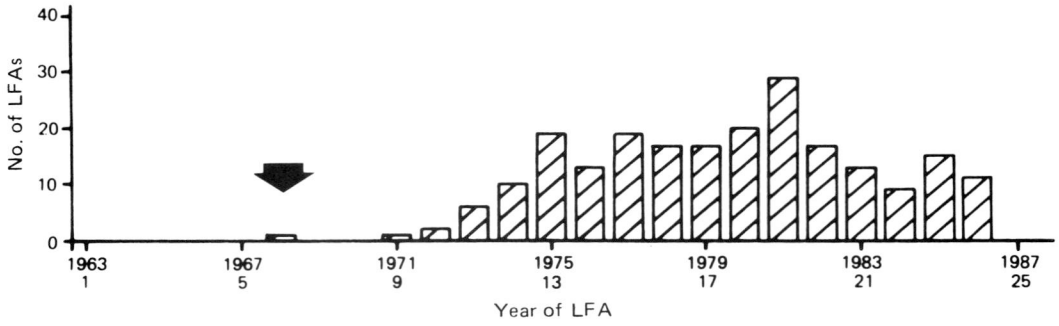

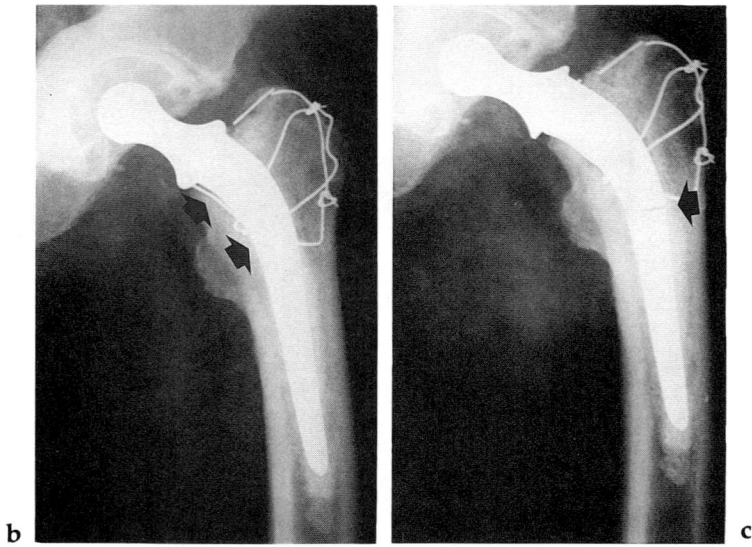

Fig. 14.1. Fracture of the first stem in the Charnley LFA, a 1968. Fractured stem presents as a complication. b,c The first fractured stem: note the lack of proximal stem support; retrospectively obvious on the immediate post-operative radiograph.

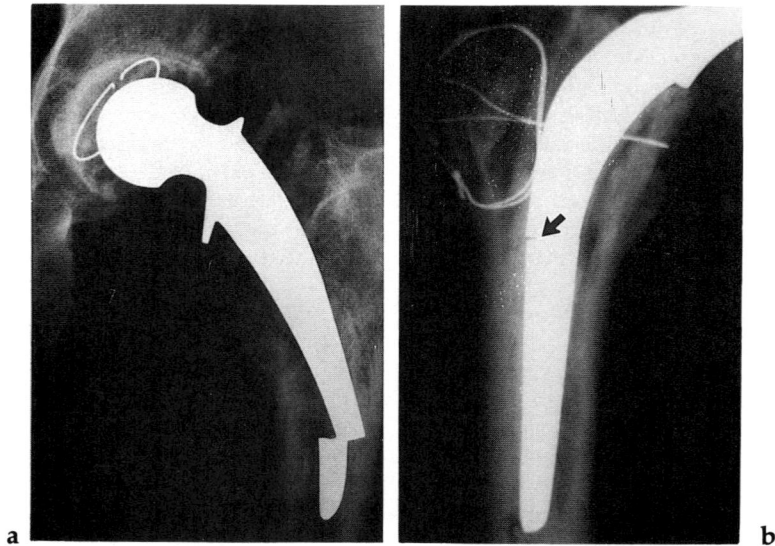

Fig. 14.2.a Very distal fracture of a curved stem. b A more typical level of fracture of the stem.

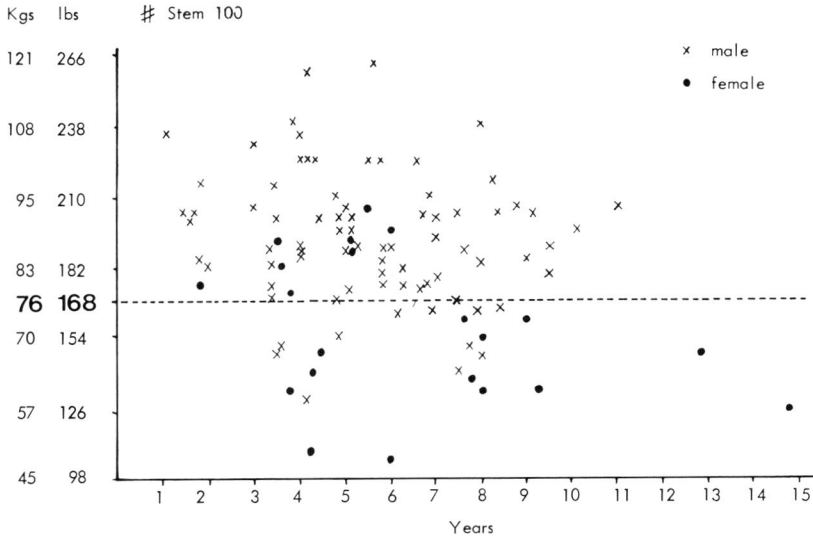

Fig. 14.3. Time to failure of the original Charnley "flat-back" stem. All except two out of 100 stems have failed within 11 years from the time of the operation. This pattern supported the suggestion of a "fatigue limit" for the stainless steel stem. (*Dotted line*, average weight of patients without a fractured stem.)

The author (Wroblewski 1982a) reviewed 120 cases, including the group previously reported by Charnley. All stems were of the original "flat-back" variety. The material was EN58J stainless steel. The incidence of fracture was established at about 1.15%. It must be accepted that because of the many parameters involved such as age, weight, sex, activity level and the length of follow-up, this figure is only an estimate, and now only of historical value. The incidence is based on an original group of 3983 hips which had at the time of the review passed the 11-year "at risk" period. This group produced 46 fractures, hence the incidence calculated as 1.15%.

When the graph of the "time to failure" is examined, it becomes apparent that a large proportion failed within the 11-year period from the time of surgery (Fig. 14.3). This part of the study recorded the time to failure and not the time to revision.

Although the majority of patients presented within days or weeks of fracture, in some cases the delay was much longer, on occasions as long as several years. The graph of "time to revision" (Fig. 14.4) shows a more extended period. The 11-year follow-up period in fact picked up 97.5% of the fractures. Although a handful of stems did fracture later, they were from the early Teflon days and their function could not be considered normal.

The relatively clear-cut at risk period for stem fracture suggests a "fatigue limit" phenomenon.

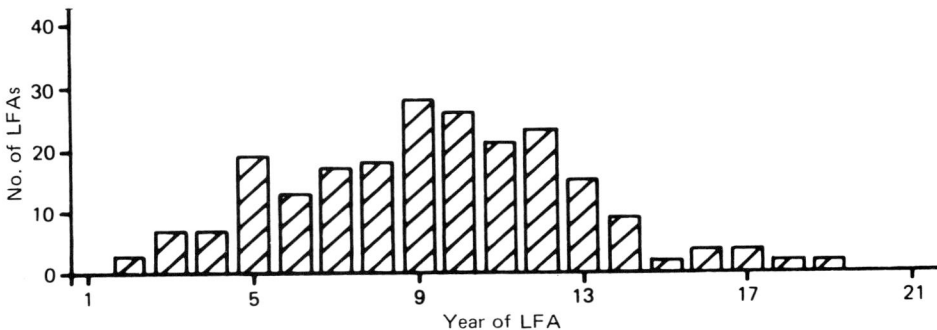

Fig. 14.4. Fractured stem: time to revision. The incidence increases gradually from the post-operative year to peak in the 9th year, followed by a gradual decline over the next 10 years.

Table 14.1. Condition of the contralateral hip as a measure of function in patients with a fractured stem (Wroblewski 1982a)

Hip contralateral to the fractured stem	No.	Per cent
Normal	47	40.9
LFA	54	47.0
Osteoarthritic	10	8.7
Fused hip	2	1.7
Infected LFA	1	0.9
Fractured stem	1	0.9

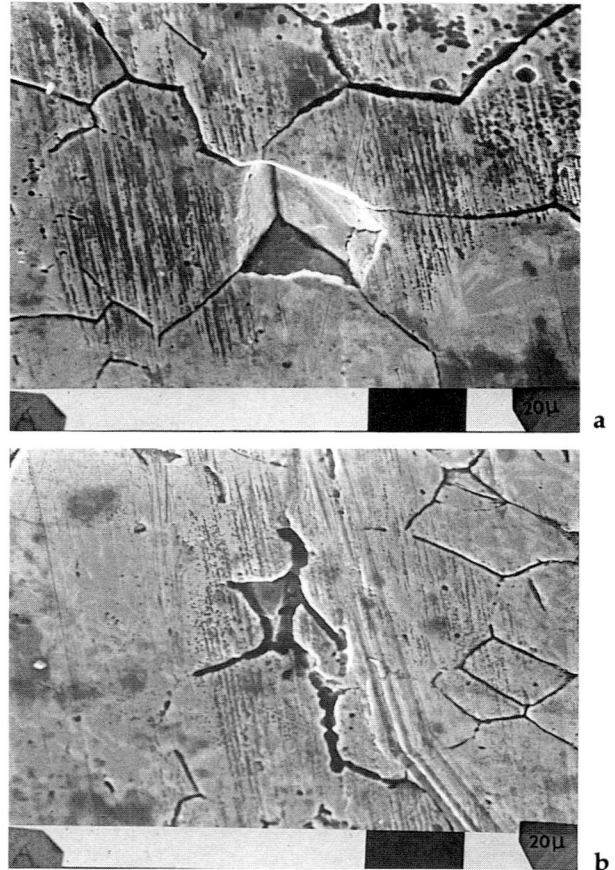

Fig. 14.5. Scanning electron microscope evidence of stem corrosion. **a** Defect in the crystal pattern. **b** Typical "running man" of corrosion. (Photograph courtesy of Salford University.)

(A stainless steel component stressed cyclically within its limit of strength will not fail provided that limit is not exceeded and provided the environment is non-corrosive.) If we accept the "fatigue limit" then we can assume that the environment is probably non-corrosive. If this is so, then there is much more to be gained from improving design and surgical technique than from the introduction of expensive "corrosion-resistant" materials. (Corrosion in the context of total hip arthroplasty is defined as "progressive destruction of metal by body fluids".) Since there is nothing progressive about the incidence of the fractured stem we can, once again, assume that the environment is unlikely to be corrosive to the extent suggested by the definition.

The evidence of corrosion can be seen on examination of the scanning electron microscope specimen (Fig. 14.5). Whether this corrosion is the cause of failure or the effect of fretting between the stem and the cement is within the realm of the corrosion expert, who cannot be expected to make a judgement based on limited evidence.

Patients' Function

It is probably correct to say that a fractured stem may be a reflection of the patient's function following the operation. If patients' function is to be judged by the state of the hip on the side contralateral to the fractured stem, then Table 14.1 shows quite clearly that in 87.9% this function could be considered normal. In the other 8.7% the contralateral osteoarthritic hip was not significantly symptomatic.

Patients' Weight and Time to Fracture

There was a linear relationship between patients' weight and time to fracture indicating quite clearly that heavy patients fractured the stem early (Fig. 14.6). The average weight for the 92 males with fractured stems was 88.3 kg (194.3 lb) and for the 28 females, 71.9 kg (158 lb).

It may be of interest to point out that 53 patients (46.1%) had gained weight (an average of 8.7 kg or 19.1 lb) between the LFA and the fracture of the stem. Thus it cannot be accepted that it is the patient's immobility *before* the operation that contributes to this weight gain. Although patients must be encouraged to maintain their correct weight we may have to accept that ageing brings with it the problem of weight gain.

Surgical Technique

The importance of the surgical technique can to some extent be estimated. All stems in the study were of a single design. Patients could be divided into two groups: those operated on in the unit and those referred from other centres. Even within the unit individual surgeons could be identified if required and their surgical techniques compared by analysing the radiographic appearances, the incidence and the time to failure of the stem.

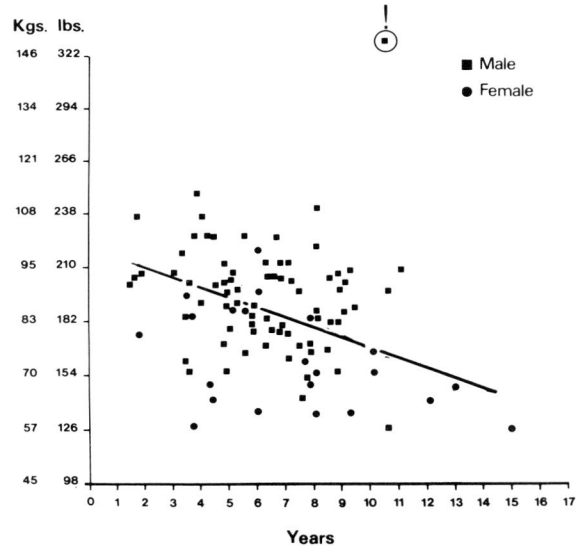

Fig. 14.6. Correlation between patients' weight and time to fracture. Heavy patients fractured the stem earlier than light patients. Note the lonely male weighing over 322 lb!

Radiographic Appearances

Fracture of the Femoral Cement

Of 113 cases where radio-opaque cement was used, fracture of the femoral cement at some level was present in 51.3% as seen on pre-revision radiographs. The most common site was near the tip of the stem (29.2%); in 15% of cases the fracture was at the medial femoral neck and in 7.1% at both those sites.

Endosteal Cavitation of the Femur

Endosteal cavitation of the femur was present in 24.8% of patients in the study and was observed at the calcar, often extending to the level of the lesser trochanter or beyond. In only three cases was the cavitation present near the tip of the stem. In 26 out of 28 cases the endosteal cavitation appeared after the first year following surgery. This would suggest that the changes of cavitation do not occur instantaneously but take time to develop. They then present radiologically when sufficient of the cortex has been excavated to "show through" on the radiographs. Occurring at the calcar, as it did, endosteal cavitation of the femur would have led to

bone resorption, loss of proximal stem support and stem failure.

This late appearance of endosteal cavitation has sinister long-term implications. It is almost certainly a result of the surgical technique which allows repeated pumping action of the bursal fluid and debris within the cavity. Sufficient evidence exists now to indicate that the cavitation is purely a result of mechanical changes in volume and pressure and not some direct "noxious" effect of the cement or HDP particles.

In situations where the movement ceases, the cavitation regresses and calcifies. Unfortunately the calcar is not the site where this is likely to occur.

Early Radiographic Signs of Failure of Stem Fixation

In 92 cases serial radiographs were available which allowed a more detailed study of stem subsidence or tilting. The radiographic criteria used to define the "stem at risk" were:

1. Separation of the back of the stem from the cement.
2. Fracture of the cement at the tip of the stem.
3. Fracture of the cement at the calcar.
4. Endosteal cavitation of the femur.

(Fracture of the cement at the calcar may be difficult to establish radiographically as the fracture occurs in compression and often without separation. Endosteal cavitation on the other hand is a *late* sign.)

Based on the four criteria, radiographic evidence for the "stem at risk" was present in 77.2% of patients (71 cases) within the first year following the operation. Using only the first three criteria 69 stems were shown to be at risk for a future fracture; two showed radiographic evidence at 2 weeks post-operatively, 26 at around 6 months and 41 around the first year. (Any surgical technique which avoids those early changes must be considered a step in the right direction.)

In a group of 21 cases the "at risk" signs were not present on the 1-year radiograph. The two groups are compared in Table 14.2. Comparison of the two groups readily shows the earlier failure of the stem in the "at risk" group. Although a normal 1-year radiograph is reassuring it does not guarantee that there will be no further complications.

Position of the Stem Within the Medullary Canal

The position of the stem within the medullary canal, as observed on the AP radiograph, has been the subject of much discussion, much of it, unfortunately, without clear appreciation of the problem. An assumption has usually been made, quite incorrectly, that the fixation of the stem has been correct and adequate, so that the only point for debate was the position (varus or valgus) of the stem. This is not at all surprising. Varus and valgus are terms readily assimilated, recognized and expressed. Stem fixation, on the other hand, is a technique that cannot be simply expressed, except possibly by reference to long-term results, and demands understanding of all aspects of the procedure. Thus position of the stem became equated, sadly, with the surgical technique.

It is clear that variations in the position of the stem within the medullary canal in the coronal plane are only possible if:

1. The medullary canal is wide.
2. The femoral stem is relatively narrow.
3. The position of the stem is not maintained at preparation, trial reduction or cementation.

Table 14.2. The outcome of the "at risk" stems compared with those considered not at risk from 1-year radiographs (Wroblewski 1982a)

Femoral stem	No.of cases	Weight		Time to stem fracture (month)
		kg	lb	
At risk	71	84.5	186	67.5
Not at risk	21	83.6	184	84.8

Thus a wide medullary canal closed off distally, the bulkiest stem that will be accepted, a well-prepared cancellous bed, adequate packing of the medullary cavity with cement and proper introduction of the stem in the line of the medullary canal are likely to give a neutral stem position. Thus the final position of the stem is the result of the technique. An analysis according to the varus/valgus stem position in 120 stem fractures has shown the following:

1. On average the patients with a "valgus" stem were significantly heavier than the patients with a "varus" stem.
2. On average the stems of the "valgus" patients probably did fracture significantly earlier than those of the "varus" patients.
3. If patients weighing 80 kg (176 lbs) or more are considered then the weights of the varus/valgus groups are comparable yet the stems of the valgus patients fractured significantly earlier (Table 14.3).

It is true that more fractured stems were in the varus position (67) than in the valgus position (23) but this is probably no more than a reflection of the proportion of cases overall at the stage of the evolution of the operation.

Varus/valgus terminology is of descriptive value only. Although it probably reflects the method of exposure and the technique of stem fixation, it must not be equated with the quality of the long-term result.

Table 14.3. Varus or Valgus position of the stem and time to fracture in patients weighing 80 kg or more (Wroblewski 1982a)

Stem position	No.	Average Weight		Average time of fracture (months)
		kg	lb	
Varus	38	94	206.9	72.8
Valgus	23	93	204.6	60.5

Table 14.4. Comparison by weight and time to fracture of patients from the Hip Centre and referred patients. The difference is statistically significant (Wroblewski 1982a)

Source	No. of cases	Average Weight		Time to stem fracture (months)
		kg	lb	
Referred	24	83.5	183.6	56.6
Hip Centre	96	85.0	187	77.7

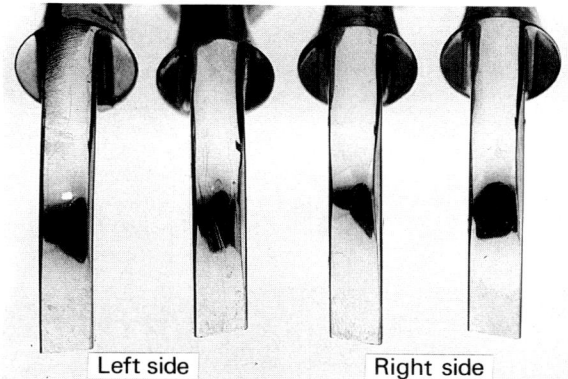

Left side   Right side

Fig. 14.7. Obliquity of the fracture. When viewed from the lateral side of the fractured stem (the "flat back") the obliquity of the fracture became apparent allowing the identification of the side of stem origin, i.e. left side or right side. The obliquity of the fracture also suggested that the mechanism was not that of simple bending – an element of torsion must have been present.

Comparison of Cases from Two Sources

The availability of patients from two sources, i.e. from the Hip Centre and referred from other units, made it possible to carry out a comparison by weight and time to failure. The results are obviously not intended to be a criticism, merely a statement of findings, and are shown in Table 14.4.

The Mechanism of Fracture of the Stem in Total Hip Arthroplasty

Fracture of the stem in the cemented total hip arthroplasty began to be seen at a time when the problem of wear of the Teflon socket had been overcome by the introduction of high-density polyethylene, and it was considered that the remaining problems, if any, would be resolved with time and improved technique. Further changes were considered to be "the gilding of the lily", to use Sir John Charnley's expression from 1968.

A number of explanations were offered at that stage: faulty metal, faulty manufacture or faulty design. In fact, as has already been pointed out, the main problem was in the surgical technique.

Attempts to reproduce fracture of the stem experimentally have so far failed, primarily because of the lack of understanding of the mechanism leading to that complication. In experiments the stem was invariably supported at the base of the neck, in a "valgus" position, while the load was applied in a vertical direction, in the same plane as the neck of the stem.

However, examination of 70 fractured stems has revealed a very consistent pattern, which if accepted could be used confidently to analyse any fractured stem and identify the mechanism of the fracture. This, in conjunction with the review of serial radiographs, could be used to predict such a complication, point to the salient desirable features of a total hip arthroplasty or be a measure of radiological success of a new technique. The features studied were as follows:

1. Obliquity of the fracture.
2. Bending of the proximal fragment.
3. Fracture wave.
4. Fracture lip.

Obliquity of the Fracture

Because of the geometry of the original Charnley stem the "flat back" (actually the lateral side) of the stem could be used as a convenient reference point. When viewed from the lateral side it was obvious that the fracture line was never exactly transverse; it was always oblique, i.e. at an angle to the long axis of the stem. This angle varied from 2° to 20° (Fig. 14.7) and in some cases it was difficult to measure, though such cases were

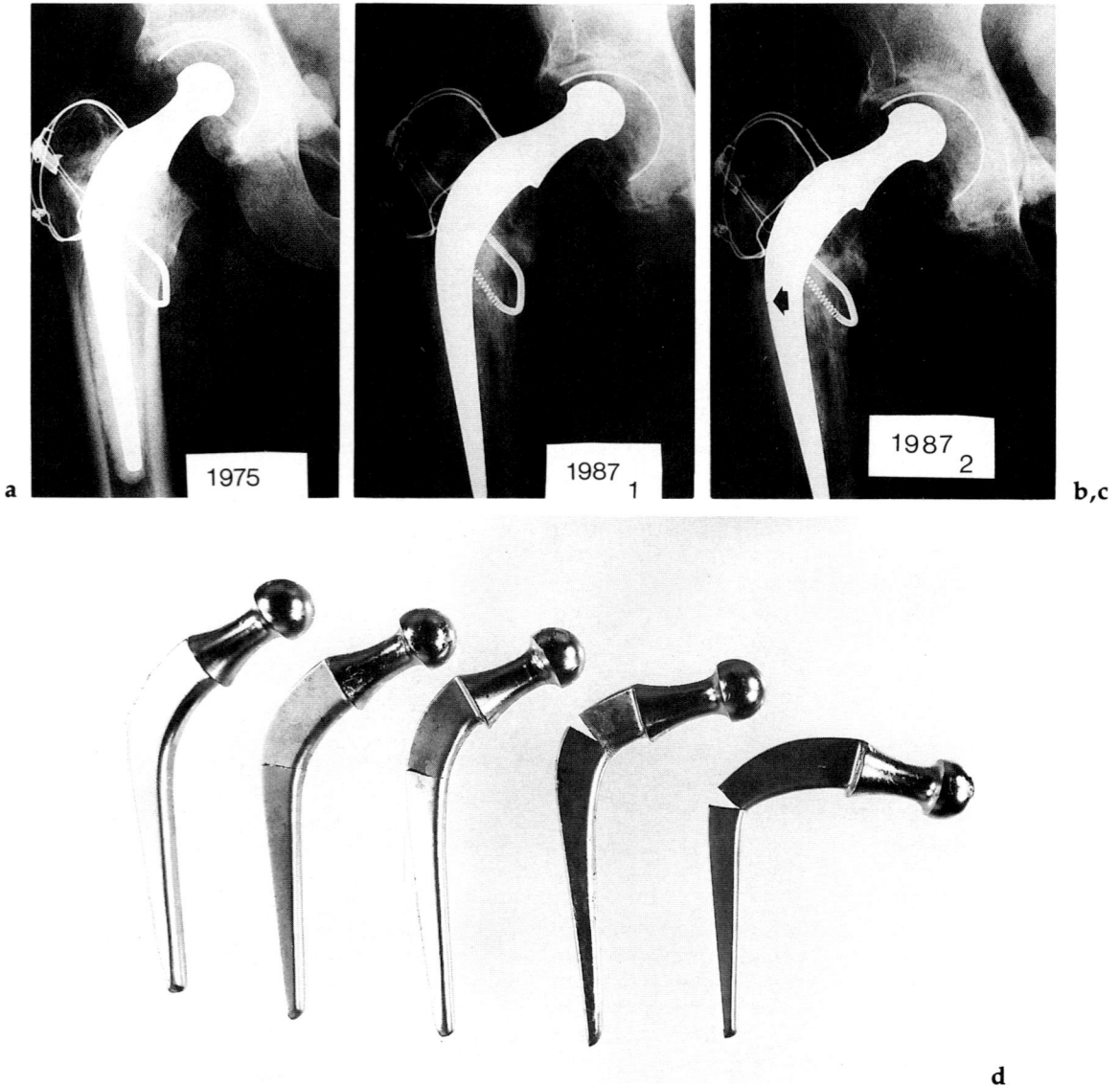

Fig. 14.8. Bending of the proximal part of the stem. **a** Post-operative appearance, 1975. **b** Bending stem and worn socket, 1987 (1). **c** Fractured stem, 1987 (2). **d** A more graphic picture of the stages of stem fracture. (Specimens removed at revision.)

extremely rare. The slope of the fracture could be used to identify the origin of the stem, i.e. right or left hip. Thus in the left hip the fracture sloped towards the left side and in the right hip towards the right side.

If the fracture line was not at right angles to the long axis of the stem then a mechanism other than pure bending must be responsible for causing the fracture. Obliquity implies torsion.

Assuming uniformity of stem implantation then the obliquity of the fracture line, as viewed from the lateral aspect, must be a reflection of the angle of the load in relation to the long axis of the stem. As such it probably mirrors the length of the stride of the patient and is probably proportional to it. This aspect has not been investigated so far, yet may add to our understanding of the problem.

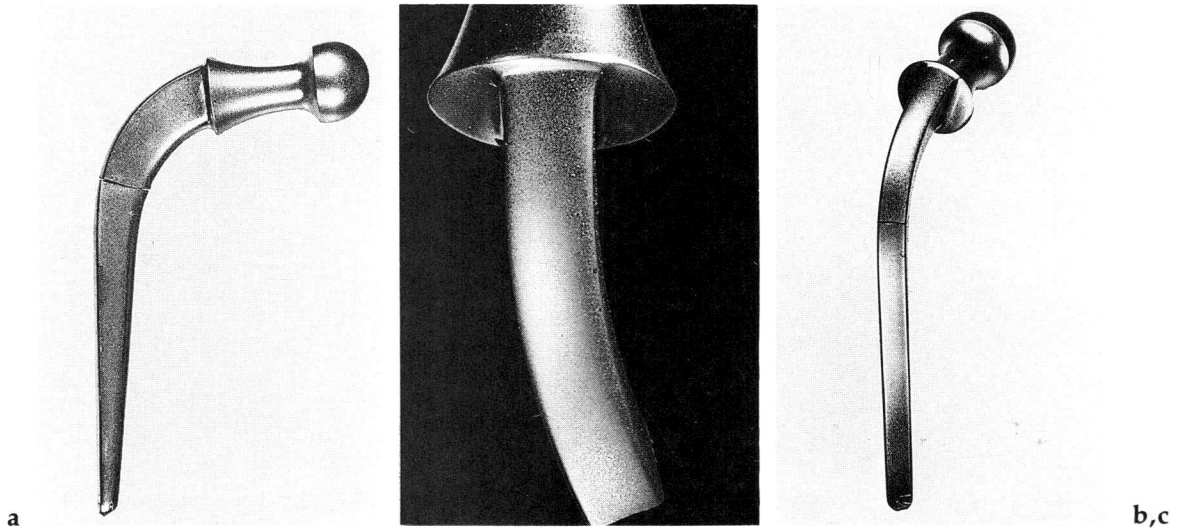

Fig. 14.9. Bending–torsion of the proximal fragment. **a** The bending element is obvious. **b,c** Torsion is more easily recognizable where the fragments are still in contact, i.e. before the fracture becomes complete.

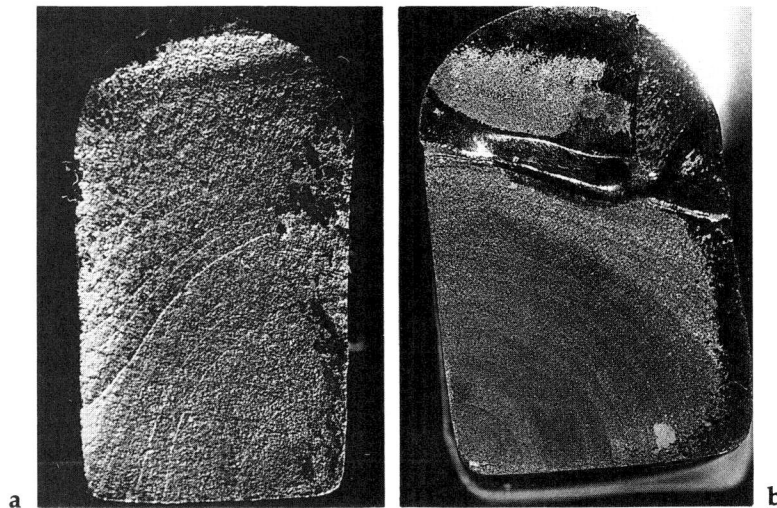

Fig. 14.10. a,b Fatigue fracture wave. Its origin is at or near the antero-lateral corner of the stem.

Bending of the Proximal Fragment

Bending of the proximal part of the stem into a varus position was at times very obvious on radiographs (Fig. 14.8) before the stem actually fractured. Thus bending preceded the fracture. (Any stem that appears bent on an AP radiograph is almost certainly bent. Deviation from the true AP by rotation of the stem around its long axis would make the stem appear straighter, provided foreshortening has not taken place.) When the fracture was examined it became obvious that it was not the result of a pure bending deformity but of a bending torsion of the proximal unsupported part of the stem in relation to the distal fixed part. Whether or not

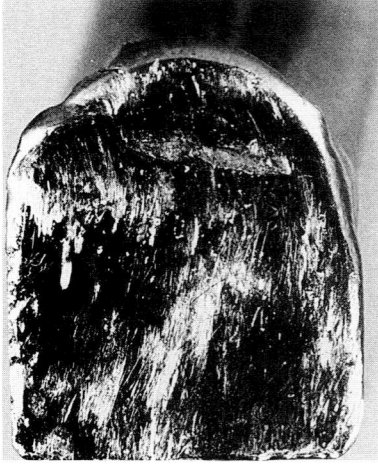

Fig. 14.11. Polished fracture surface caused by fracture surfaces rubbing together. Result of walking on a fractured stem.

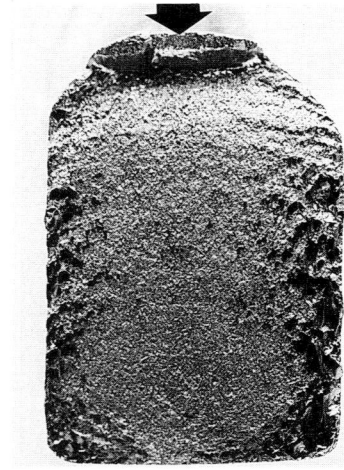

a

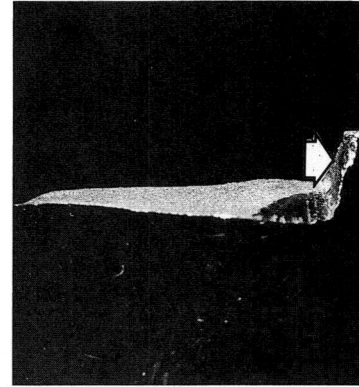

b

Fig. 14.12. a,b Fracture lip: the most medial part of the stem and the only part which fails suddenly.

this bending could be accurately assessed depended on the length of the proximal fragment; the longer and thinner the fragment the more readily was this pattern recognizable (Fig. 14.9). What is more, the proximal part was always rotated downwards and backwards, suggesting that the load was in fact from the antero-superior direction (or that the hip was predominantly loaded in flexion).

Fracture Wave

In cases where revision was carried out soon after the fracture had occurred, the fatigue fracture wave (tidal or beach mark) could be easily made out (Fig. 14.10). The origin of the wave was usually at, or close to, the antero-lateral square edge of the stem. From there the wave extended progressively towards the opposite part of the stem. In itself this is no more than the fatigue wave which is normally associated with failure of a metal component by the fatigue mechanism. What is of interest is the site of origin and the direction of propagation; both suggest once again that the mechanism is bending torsion. The antero-lateral aspect of the stem, being angular, acted as a stress riser. This fatigue wave was obviously not discernible if the

fracture ends had been polished as a result of walking after the fracture had occurred (Fig. 14.11).

Fracture Lip

The only part of the stem to fail suddenly was the fracture lip (Fig. 14.12). This is the most medial part of the stem, and its sudden failure often accounted for the rather dramatic clinical presentation of the complication. The sequence of events is as follows.

The proximal part of the stem lacks or loses its support while the distal part is well fixed. Repeated bending torsion of the proximal part leads to the typical sequence of events ending in

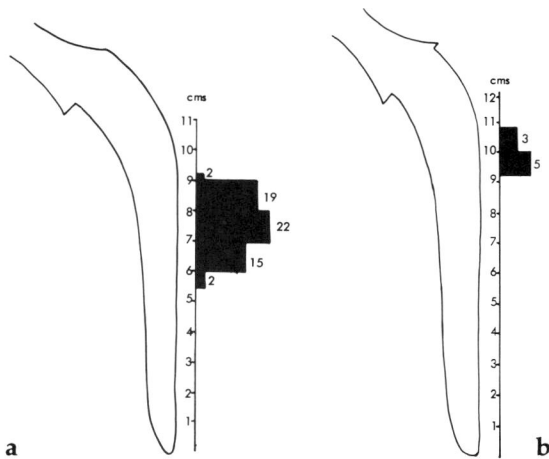

Fig. 14.13. The segment at risk: comparative level of fracture. **a** The standard 45-mm offset. **b** The straight stem 37.5-mm offset.

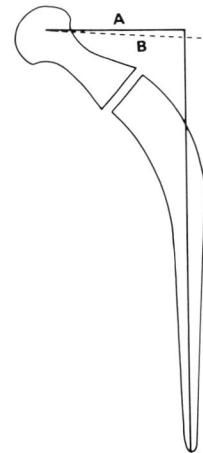

Fig. 14.14. Measuring the stem offset: *A*, as suggested by the accepted definition; *B*, as established from examination of fractured stems (probably more correct as it defines the functional offset.)

stem failure. The most likely load is that imparted during normal walking, the highest and most frequent load to which the hip joint is subjected other than occasionally.

At the "heel strike" the hip is loaded in flexion; at "toe off" the body is projected upwards and forwards, hence the load on the hip must be downwards and backwards. The load being out of line with the neck of the stem results in torsion rather than bending. It is not a "to and fro" bending of the stem but repeated bending torsion, the load being in the antero-superior direction. The recovery takes place during the non-load-bearing phase of the walking cycle so there is no reversal of the direction or magnitude of the load. Reversal would be against the two peak loads in the walking cycle and would indicate a "backward and forward" progression during walking, obviously a rather bizarre suggestion.

offset and the "straight stem" 3.75-mm offset, showed a definite "at risk" segment (Fig. 14.13). With a straighter stem the segment was somewhat higher than with the standard stem; it was also narrower in the straighter stem measuring some 2 cm as compared with 4 cm in the standard stem. This finding would suggest that the "functional" as opposed to the "design" offset is different and should probably be taken not from the centre but from the lateral edge of the stem (Fig. 14.14). After all, the fracture starts on the surface of the stem shaft and not within it. This would also explain why the curved "banana" stem should fracture rather low (Fig. 14.15). The offset of the stems as suggested by Charnley (1975) is probably more correctly interpreted thus (Fig. 14.16). This would probably go some way to explaining the reason for a lower fracture in a more curved stem.

The Level of Fracture of the Stem

Although no doubt it was a result of stem design as well as the "functional offset" of the stem within the skeleton, it is interesting to note that the two stems then in use, the standard 45-mm

Fracture of the Stem Following Revision Surgery

Fracture of the stem following revision for the same complication, although mentioned, has not been the subject of a detailed publication. However, examination of such cases gives an

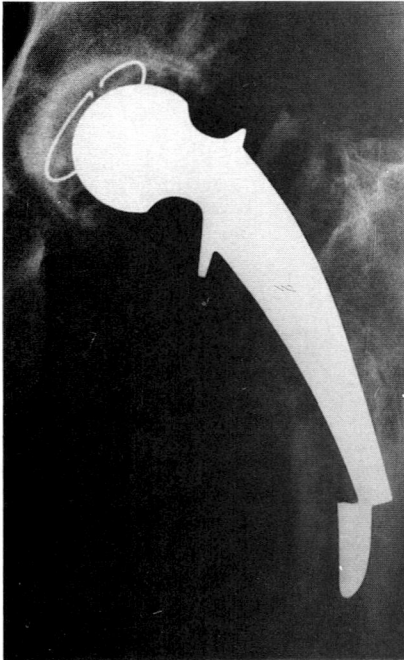

Fig. 14.15. Very low fracture of a curved stem.

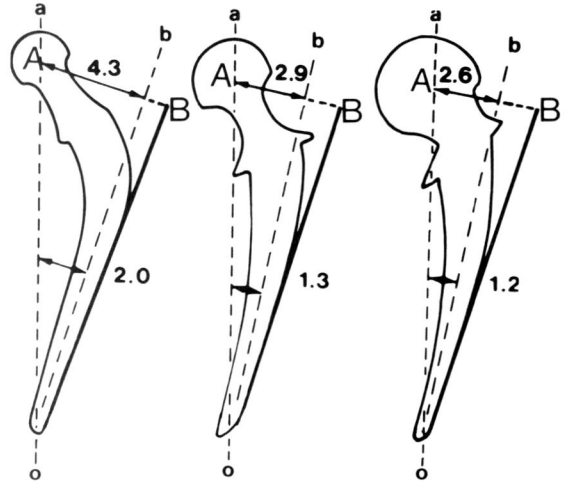

Fig. 14.16. An alternative interpretation of the "offset" of the stem. *a–b*, accepted definition (after Charnley 1975); *A–B*, definition suggested from examination of fractured stems. This would also go some way to explain why curved stems fractured more distally down the shaft of the stem.

interesting insight into the mechanism of fracture and thus into a detail of the surgical technique of both primary and revision surgery that was not fully appreciated until then.

The Pattern

Out of a total of 220 revisions for stem fracture, 15 have fractured again, an incidence of 6.8%. All were in very heavy patients weighing over 85 kg (187 lb). The only female in this group was over 180 cm in height and weighed 89 kg (196 lb). The time to failure followed closely the pattern already recorded from the whole series. The mechanism of failure was surmised from examination of the removed specimens and confirmed experimentally.

The Specimens

The most striking finding was the continuity between the proximal fragment of the stem and the proximal part of the cement, at revisions the stem and the cement readily coming out as a single unit (Fig. 14.17).

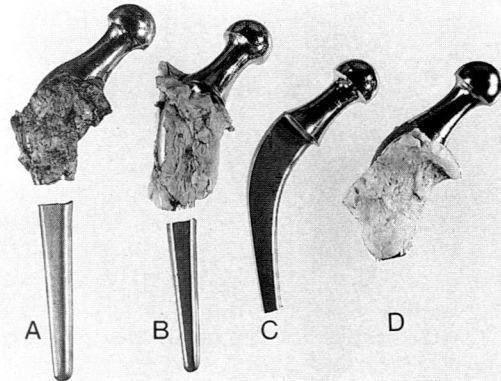

Fig. 14.17. A "hinging" mechanism of stem fracture. *A, B* and *D*, typical findings at revision: the proximal cement is bulky and is extracted with the proximal fragment of the stem; *C*, the more common mechanism of "counterlever beam"; the proximal stem fragment is devoid of cement.

Radiographs

The radiographs of the cases in question were examined. (Unfortunately photography does not reveal the details adequately.) What became apparent was the early failure at the junction of the old distal cement and the new proximal cement.

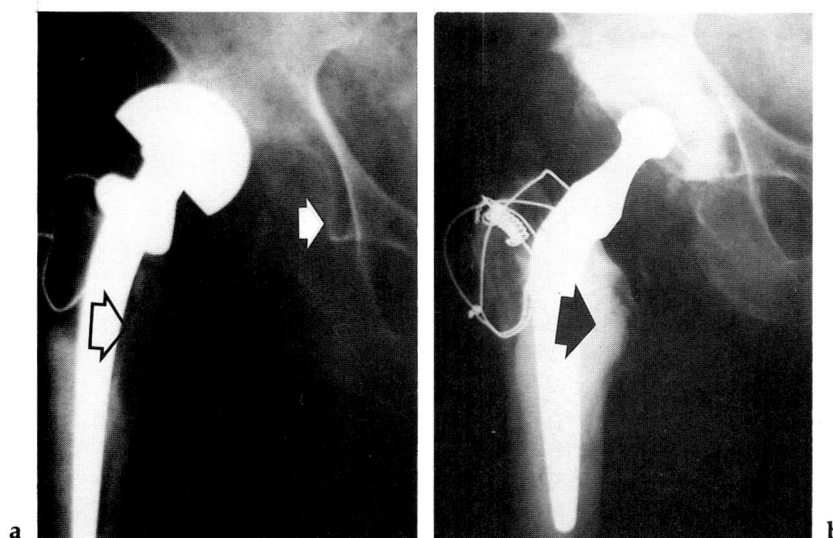

Fig. 14.18. The use of the lesser trochanter in revision surgery. The lesser trochanter is excavated and packed with cement to provide support for the stem in its proximal, postero-medial position. **a** Before revision. **b** After revision. (A case of migrating bipolar arthroplasty due to deep sepsis.) Note the tear drop.

Mechanism of Stem Fracture

The mechanism of stem failure is interpreted as follows. The proximal part of the femur is not adequately prepared at revision for a fractured stem. The fibrous layer at the bone–cement junction is probably not completely removed, the condensation of cancellous bone deep to it is not curetted and the strong cancellous bone of the cavity of the lesser trochanter is not exposed for the cement injection. The new stem, with fresh cement, is fixed in position. It becomes obvious that an excellent fixation is maintained distally while proximally the stem is merely surrounded by the cement. The stem subjected to the load deflects and the "end to end" junction of the old and new cement fails, readily allowing it to hinge on the distal cement column. The distal fragment may, at least theoretically, back fractionally out of the cement mantle then be literally torn apart by hinging. The mechanism is exactly the same as that involved in taking apart a fly-fishing rod, a trick readily appreciated by the angling fraternity.

Experimental Confirmation

If the hinging mechanism was in fact the mode of failure then it could be readily reproduced experimentally. This was in fact the case. The proximal portion of the stem was surrounded by a mass of cement while the distal part was embedded in the fixation medium, the distance between the two being only a fraction of a millimetre. The specimen was fatigue tested, the stem failing in the predicted manner.

Clinical Implications

It is obvious that both at primary and revision surgery support of the proximal part of the stem is essential. Attention to the detail of preparation of the medullary canal, exposure of the strong cancellous bone, correct cementing technique, closure of the distal medullary canal and stem positioning is most important. In this context the role of the calcar, both the anatomical and the surgical, must be appreciated. It must not be thought that new materials or stem designs can be a substitute for an adequate technique.

In practice, use should be made of the cavity of the lesser trochanter in revision surgery (Fig. 14.18). In primary surgery, if the anatomical calcar is poor, as it often is, especially in the elderly, it should be removed exposing the strong cancellous bone deep to it.

Reaming of the medullary canal to the cortex, however, is likely to lead to failures due to loosening at the bone–cement interface.

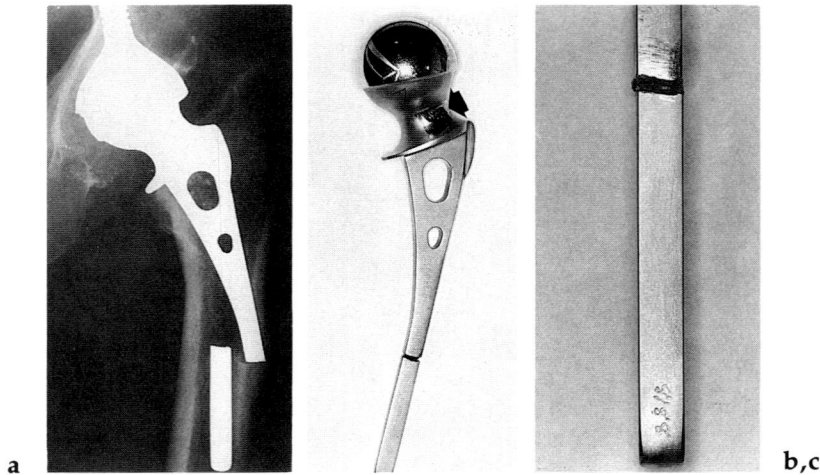

Fig. 14.19. Mechanism of fracture of the uncemented metal-to-metal Ring stem. **a** Fracture of the Ring stem, left side. **b** Gross notching and polishing of the neck of the stem resulting from impingement on the anterior socket rim. **c** Obliquity of the stem fracture to the right, the opposite side to that found with the cemented stem (see Fig. 14.7) suggests the mechanism postulated. (Photographs by courtesy of Mr. M. Lynch.)

Recent Developments

It will not be out of place to point out here that with the better understanding of the demand imposed on the arthroplasty, improved stem design and the introduction of high-nitrogen-content stainless steel (ORTRON 90, Chas. F. Thackray) there has not been a fracture of the Ortron stem reported. The slight increase in fractures seen over the 2 years 1975–1976 (Fig. 14.1a) was probably due to very late fractures in patients who after years of indifferent function had the LFA carried out on the contralateral side, thus improving their activity level.

It must be recalled that the 11-year "at risk" period refers to patients with normal function and not merely the time interval between the operation and the fracture.

Fracture of the Stem in the Uncemented Metal-to-Metal Arthroplasty

This apparently rare complication has not received detailed attention. Ring, the greatest exponent of the procedure, did not mention the problem when reviewing 1000 cases (Ring 1968). Jones (1979) mentioned four stem fractures in a series of 1219 metal-to-metal Ring arthroplasties, an incidence of 0.33%. Whether this reflects the quality of the components or the clinical result is a matter for debate. What is of interest is the probable mechanism of the fracture of the uncemented Ring stem, not reported hitherto, i.e. impingement of the neck of the stem on the anterior part of the socket. In flexion, the neck impinges on the socket rim thus fixing the proximal part of the uncemented, and therefore loose, stem. The femur, now free to move around the shaft of the stem strikes the distal part of the stem from behind leading to a fatigue fracture of the stem. The fixed part of the stem is now proximal and the unsupported and under load part distal. The obliquity of the fracture towards the right side, i.e. in the opposite direction to that seen with the cemented stem, confirms the mechanism of the fracture (Fig. 14.19).

A metal on plastic uncemented articulation may be protected by the possible shock-absorbing effect of the plastic socket, but the metal on metal or ceramic on ceramic hip is likely to be at risk for this complication. It need not present as a stem fracture but is more likely to reveal itself as damage to the components, initially at the site of the impingement, and loosening of the components eventually.

It may be of long-term interest to see if such a mechanism of failure will be observed with other uncemented designs.

15 Fracture of the Shaft of the Femur

Introduction

Individual surgeons' experiences with the problems posed by fracture of the femoral shaft in patients with total hip arthroplasty is not great, primarily because the complication is fortunately rather rare, and secondly, because it is an emergency, transfer of the patient in the acute stages is not advisable. Cases that are transferred are often those with failure of union after attempted conservative treatment.

The classification proposed by Khan and O'Driscoll (1977) offers a good "working scheme" and is to be commended. The problem to be tackled can usually be classified in one of three ways:

1. Fractures distal to the implant.
2. Fracture of the femur in the presence of a loose stem.
3. Fractures involving the stem–cement complex.

1. Fractures distal to the implant can be treated conservatively and will unite (Fig. 15.1) as pointed out by Charnley (1966). Care must be taken not to miss the loosening of the stem.

2. Fractures distal to or involving the distal part of the stem–cement complex and associated with stem loosening can present a technically difficult problem, in fact two problems in one: that of a fractured femur and that of a loose stem. Attempts to treat such a fracture by cementing a long stem may be misconceived (Fig. 15.2) and

are no more appropriate than attempts to treat femoral fractures by the same method. Attempts to hold the fracture using a plate may also be doomed to failure (Fig. 15.3). The problems must be identified and treated deliberately. In this sphere the work of Sven Olerud (Olerud and Karlstrom 1984) is to be commended. (Khan and O'Driscoll also reported one such case in 1977.) Olerud manages the two problems by a single method, using a cemented femoral stem slotted down the intramedullary nail. This allows the distal femoral fragment to "ride up" and unite while controlled by the intramedullary nail and avoids the problems associated with keeping the fragments separated. This has been the author's method of choice in the handful of cases that have presented themselves for treatment (Fig. 15.4).

A selection of modified Charnley stems have been made available together with a choice of Kuntscher nails (Fig. 15.5). Alternatively the proximal part of the femur may have to be replaced (Fig. 15.6) and this is a really major undertaking.

A word of warning: to use a combinaton of a stem and a Kuntscher nail, even if fixed with acrylic cement, is to invite the possible problem of fretting and failure of the system. The most likely outcome would be fracture of the nail. This must be made clear to the patient. The operation is used as a salvage procedure, to ensure fracture healing. Further surgery may have to be undertaken. Meanwhile the use of support for ambulation is indicated.

It is in order to avoid problems of this nature that timely intervention for stem loosening is

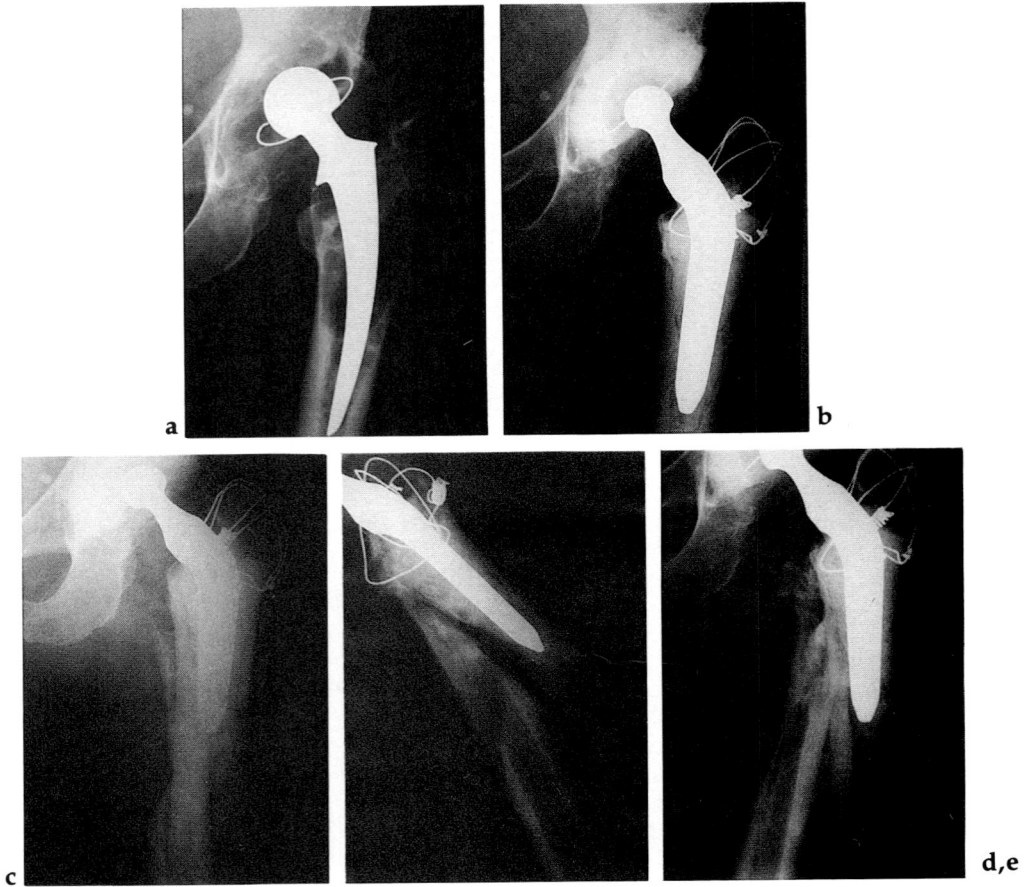

Fig. 15.1. Fracture of the shaft of the femur managed conservatively. **a** Pre-revision radiograph. The problem was deep infection with loosening of the components. **b** Post-revision appearance: a shorter stem was used. **c,d** Fracture of the femoral shaft following a very severe fall. **e** Union achieved with conservative treatment, 3-year follow-up. (What is the next step if loosening of the stem occurs?)

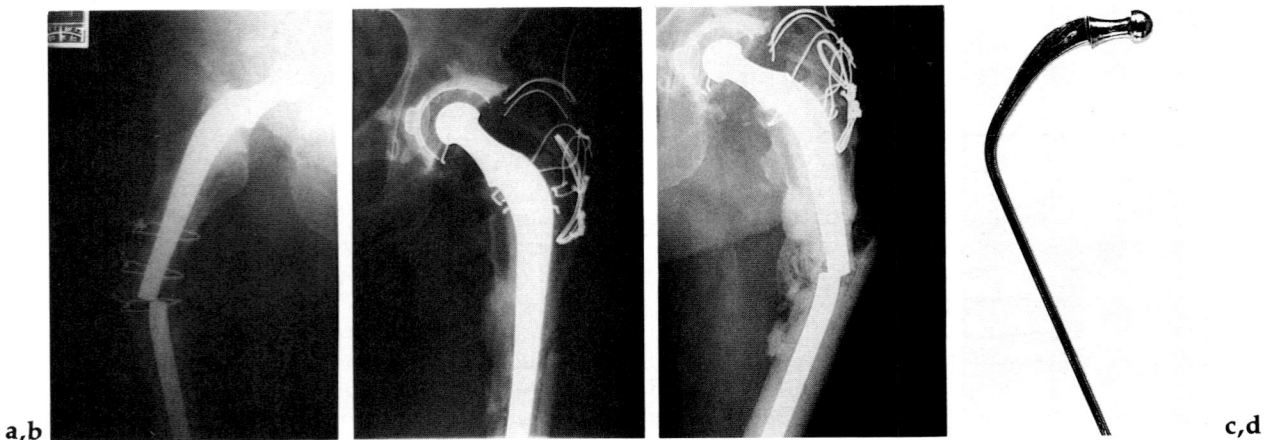

Fig. 15.2. A long stem used in an attempt to secure fixation of the fracture of the femoral shaft distal to the tip of the stem. **a** The result of keeping the fracture fragments apart. **b** Revision using a long stem. **c** Non-union and fractured stem. **d** Bent stem removed at revision. The clinical history of the specimen is not known.

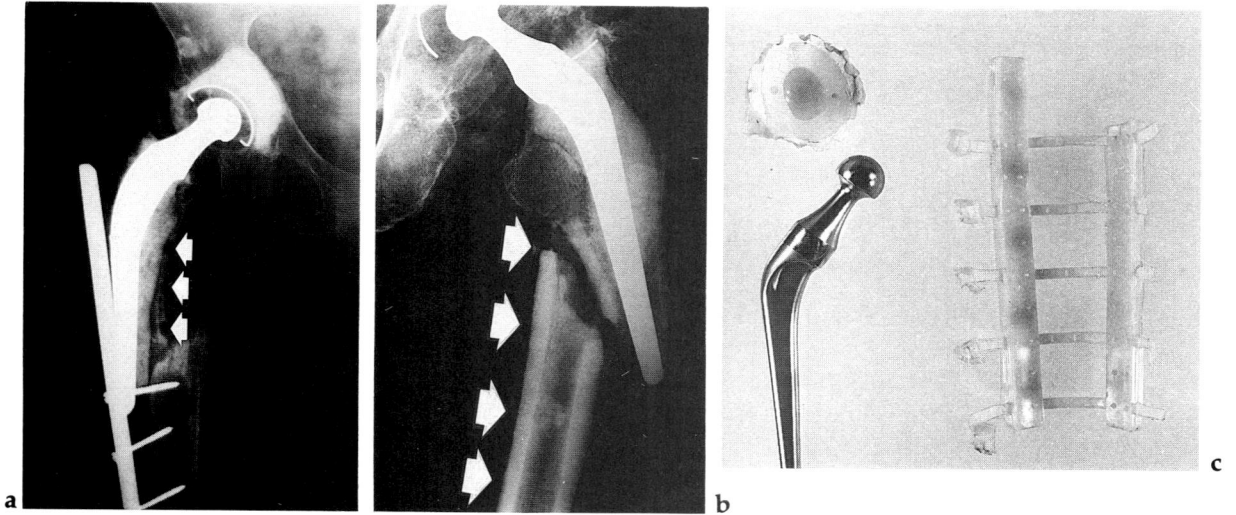

Fig. 15.3. Attempts at fracture fixation in the presence of a loose stem. **a** Plate, screws and HDP straps. **b** HDP plate and straps. **c** Specimen removed at revision.

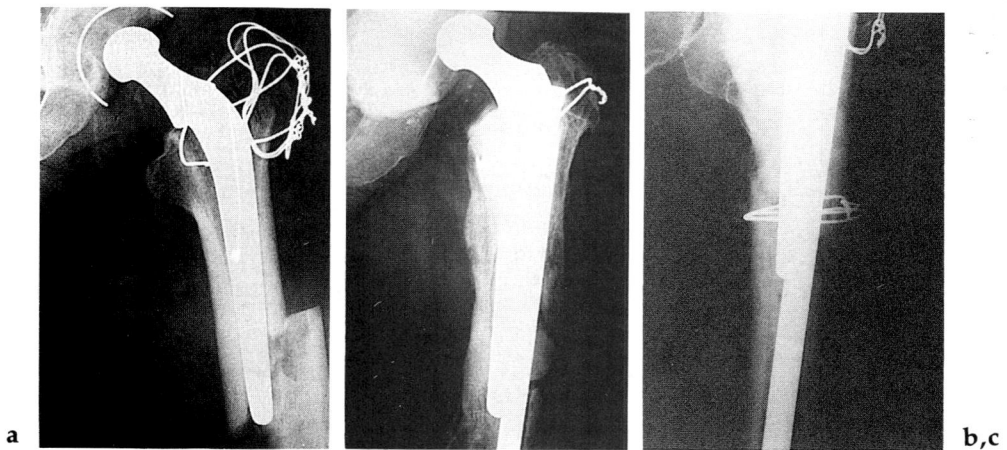

Fig. 15.4. Kuntscher nail and a modified Charnley stem. A combination used with success. **a** After several attempts, including revision complicated by deep infection with a sinus, the patient was referred for further surgery. **b** Seven years after revision using a Kuntscher nail and stem combination. **c** Case shown in Fig. 15.3b. Bony union achieved 18 months later.

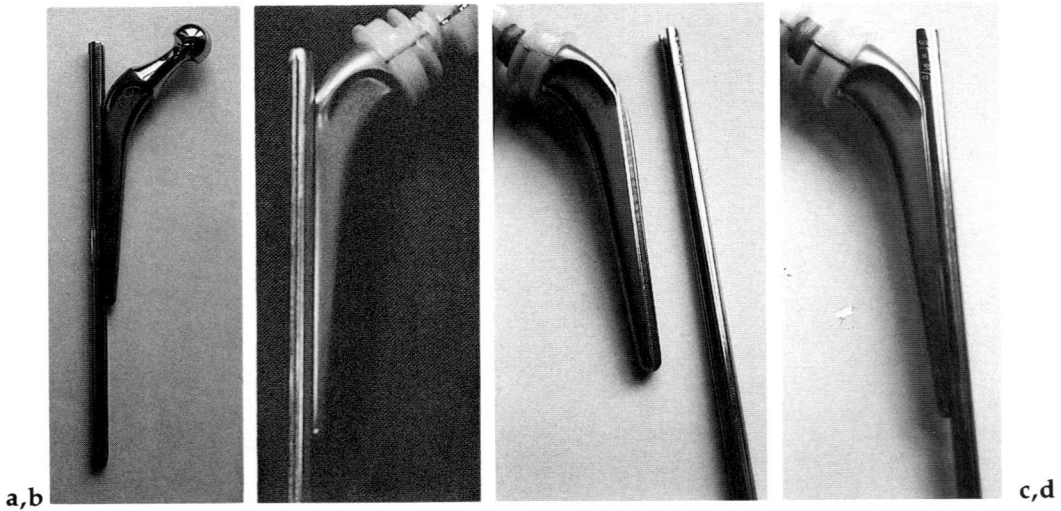

a,b   **c,d**

Fig. 15.5. a,b Kuntscher nail and modified Charnley stem. **c** Before assembly. **d** After assembly.

indicated even if it means operating solely on the basis of radiographic changes. A loose stem acts as a stress riser and predisposes to femoral fractures.

Two things must be watched out for:

a. The flail proximal fragment and a loose stem within it.
b. Mobile fracture of the femur which easily angulates during manipulation.

The first is overcome by retaining the east–west Charnley retractor resting on the pin retractor and the proximal femur while the cement is removed from the proximal (and at times the distal) fragment. At the same time the excessive angulation of the femur is avoided by the "leg holder".

The second can be dealt with by formally exploring the fracture site (removing the acrylic cement from the distal fragment at this stage), reducing it and securing the hold with the Charnley bone-holding forceps. The long Charnley curette serves very well as an intramedullary rod during manipulation once the cement has been removed.

The fracture having been fixed with the Kuntscher nail the stem is introduced and the arthroplasty tested for stability. (No attempt need be made to get a tight fit of the nail into the distal femoral fragment; the object is to allow the distal fragment to "ride up" against the proximal part of the shaft, allowing compression and hopefully union.)

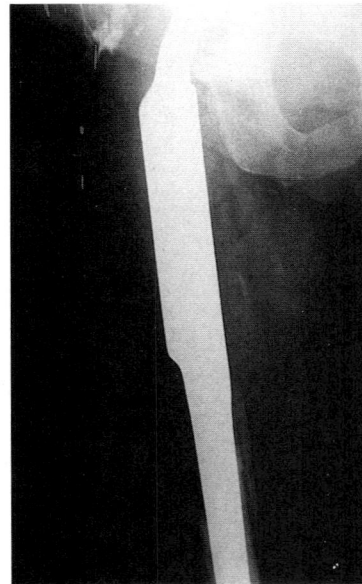

Fig. 15.6. Failure to save the proximal femoral fragment. Delay in revision, gross loss of bone stock and inability to save the proximal femoral fragment demands proximal femoral replacement. (This decision may have to be taken at the time of the revision and must be considered *before* surgery.)

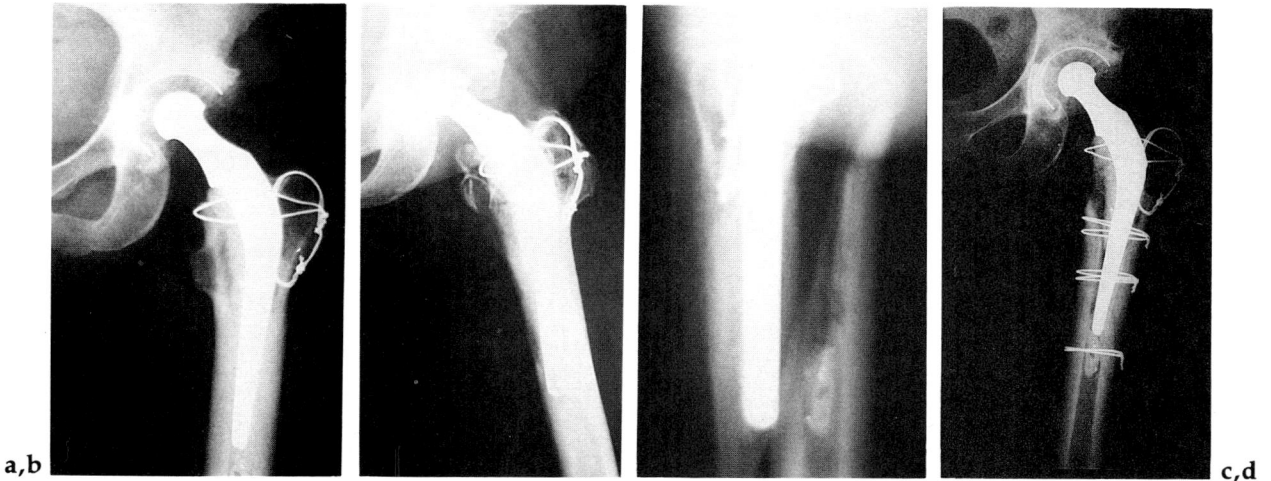

Fig. 15.7. a Fracture of the shaft of the femur involving the stem–cement complex. **b** Appearance at 12 years. Normal function. **c** A severe fall resulted in a spiral fracture of the proximal femur. The lateral radiograph gives a better indication of the problem. **d** Appearance after open reduction and fixation with circlage wires. (Note the comminution at the level of the medial femoral neck.)

After inserting the trochanteric wires the position of the Kuntscher nail is checked to ensure that the slot is placed medially to accept the stem in a neutral orientation. Some 2 cm of the nail is left protruding proximally. This will avoid the nail being pushed "out of sight" when the stem is introduced. The medullary canal and the cavity of the nail are packed with cement and the stem is inserted down the slot of the nail. Once the stem is fully in place the Kuntscher nail is tapped fully home until it is out of the way of the trochanteric bed. When the cement has set the hip is reduced and the trochanter reattached in the routine fashion.

The post-operative routine is 3 weeks' bed rest. No traction or splintage, apart from the abduction pillow, is used. An anti-rotation tibial pin, retained during the period of bed rest, is of help in controlling external rotation of the limb but need only be used if indicated. If the patient's general health permits 6 weeks' non-weight-bearing and 6 weeks' partial weight-bearing are recommended. The method has been remarkably helpful in the management of what otherwise can be a difficult problem.

3. Fractures involving the stem–cement complex are probably best explored, formally reduced and secured in place with circlage wires (Fig. 15.7). Even if stem loosening becomes obvious eventually some type of revision can be performed with what can now be a relatively anatomical proximal femur.

It must be emphasised once more that a loose stem acts as a stress riser and may lead to femoral shaft fracture. If only for that reason revision must not be delayed.

16 Heterotopic Ossification

Introduction

The study of the aetiology and treatment of cases of heterotopic ossification is a complex subject. Some of the complexity is no doubt due to the lack of an agreed definition, some to the variable interpretations of radiographic appearances. Thus various descriptive terms have been used: significant and insignificant by Taylor et al. (1976); faint, moderate and marked by Wilson et al. (1972). In an attempt to define the extent of the ossification Ritter and Vaughan (1977) recognized three grades, while Brooker and others (1973) described four grades.

At the Hip Centre at Wrightington Hospital only two well-documented cases are on record (other than the trimming of a prominent greater trochanter at the time of removal of trochanteric wires) where exploration has been carried out specifically for the excision of ectopic bone. However, in a very comprehensive study DeLee and others (1976) recognized 10 potential groups, but excluded, by definition, those patients with ectopic areas smaller than 5 mm in the greatest dimension.

The condition did not become a subject of discussion until the advent of total hip arthroplasty. It is, therefore, probably correct to assume that the operative procedure has a role to play and either contributes to it or actually causes it.

Muscle ischaemia from retraction has been suggested as a possible cause (Hamblen et al. 1971) though it is difficult to imagine why ischaemia should contribute to new bone formation and yet at the same time be a cause of non-union, which is apparently due to a lack of "new bone". Wilson and others (1972) have found that in some 30% of the cases deep sepsis was suspected. Previous hip surgery has also been implicated (Patterson and Brown 1972). This was supported by Brooker and his co-workers (1973) but not confirmed by DeLee et al. (1976) except in cases where previous surgery did produce new bone. Prolonged operative time and excessive blood loss were considered to be important (Bisla et al. 1976; Reigler and Harris 1976). Trochanteric osteotomy was not thought to be a contributory factor (DeLee et al. 1976).

As a method of prevention careful removal of bone dust was suggested (Bonnin 1972) although with routine wound irrigation the incidence was still 30% (Ritter and Vaughan 1977). Diphosphonate was found to be of help in reducing the incidence (Finerman 1977), while in established cases excision and radiotherapy were employed. More recently indomethacin was found to be effective. It would certainly assist further studies if some agreed parameters were adopted for the purpose of the definition and assessment of the extent of the heterotopic ossification.

Proposed Definition

Post-operative heterotopic ossification is accepted to be present when soft-tissue calcification/ossification between the pelvis proximally

Table 16.1. Details of patients studied

Osteoarthritis	
Primary	55
Secondary	
Congenital dysplasia	25
Trauma – femoral neck fracture	2
– fracture dislocation	2
Slipped femoral epiphysis	1
Paget's disease	1
Quadrantic head necrosis	1
Synovial osteochondromatosis	1
Rheumatoid arthritis	7
Primary protrusio acetabuli	4
Ankylosing spondylitis	3

Table 16.2. Results of the prospective study

	No. of patients	No. of LFAs	Average age	(range)
Men	36	38	57.7	(21–80)
Women	64	72	60.0	(32–80)
Total	100	110	59.2	(21–80)

and the greater trochanter, the femoral neck and the lesser trochanter distally, which was not seen on the immediate post-operative radiograph, appeared on subsequent examinations, the follow-up being not less than 1 year.

This definition would exclude all the cases where "shadows" are obvious on the post-operative radiographs. These "mature" with time to form obvious areas of ossification. Whether such cases should be included or not has not been clearly stated. It can be argued that since the ossification is present on the immediate post-operative radiograph there is nothing *new* about it, heterotopic though it may be. Provided a clear distinction is made between *new* ossification and *that which is present immediately post-operatively but matures with time*, and the time limit is specified, this aspect of the subject need not be controversial.

Definition of the extent of the ossification may demand greater attention to detail. The classification of Brooker et al. (1973) has become the one most widely quoted because of its relative clarity, yet it has significant drawbacks. Group I is probably clear although the extent of ossification within other groups may obviously vary tremendously and will, to an extent, depend on the distance between the pelvis and the proximal femur. This distance will in turn depend on the position of the socket and the effective length of the neck. Thus a deep or a high socket and a short neck of the femoral component (or a subsided stem) may transfer the case from group II to group III or from group III to group IV, without the extent of the ossification actually increasing. This aspect is in fact clearly seen in Brooker et al.'s original paper (1973). The figure illustrating group IV shows high placement of the socket and low section of the femoral neck,

both of which bring the greater trochanter closer to the pelvis and increase the apparent extent of ossification.

Ideally one would like to estimate the mass and volume of the heterotopic bone. Such methods may be difficult because of the interference of the metal stem or tedious because of the extensive investigations required, and being such would not find favour with the majority of surgeons other than for research purposes.

The Incidence

In order to establish the incidence of heterotopic ossification in the Charnley LFA according to the proposed definition, a prospective study was carried out in 100 patients who between them had 110 LFAs. A trochanteric approach was used in all cases and careful attention was paid to the removal of femoral and acetabular reamings. No irrigation was used. The assessment was made by comparing post-operative and 1-year radiographs and making a tracing of the areas of the ectopic ossification. This allowed an easy review and comparison without repeated referral to the radiographs. The details and results are shown in Tables 16.1 and 16.2.

In this prospective study the incidence of heterotopic ossification was 20.9%. In men the incidence was 26.3% while in the females it was 18.1%. In 20 hips (18%), the area of heterotopic ossification was directly above the tip of the greater trochanter. In 18 of them it remained as an isolated island while in five it became continuous with the greater trochanter by the second year. The size varied from 3 to 38 mm in the greatest dimension. In 14 cases it measured less than 20 mm. In three of the hips ectopic bone was also present at the level of the medial femoral neck and measured 3, 4 and 28 mm.

There were also four other cases where soft-tissue calcification was seen on the immediate post-operative radiograph and increased in

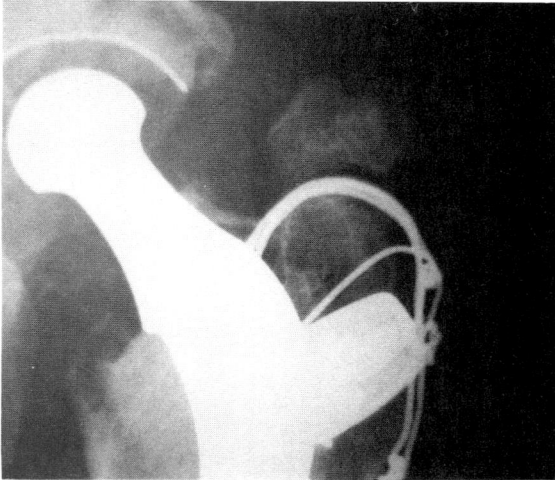

Fig. 16.1. A typical example of heterotopic ossification over the tip of the greater trochanter. In this case associated with deep infection.

density during the follow-up period. In two cases the calcification was above the greater trochanter and in two it was at the medial femoral neck. There were no cases of heterotopic ossification on the pelvic side. According to Brooker's classification 16.4% were group I and 4.5% group II.

Two points of interest must be highlighted, i.e. the site and the extent of the ossification.

The Site

Penosteal stripping regularly occurs at the tip of the greater trochanter during introduction of cholecystectomy forceps; retraction of the capsule takes place as the Gigli saw is introduced, then again as the trochanteric wires are inserted. At the medial femoral neck it occurs as the capsule and fibrous tissue are stripped during dislocation of the hip and femoral neck section (Fig. 16.1).

The Extent

The areas of heterotopic ossification identified in the prospective study were never as extensive as

groups III or IV described by Brooker, and were usually restricted to isolated areas, mainly near the tip of the greater trochanter. This site featured in 20 out of 23 cases (87%). This surely must have something to do with the periosteal elevation at various stages of the procedure.

There remains one question to be answered: What is the cause of heterotopic ossification in total hip arthroplasty? If the cause is inclusion of bone marrow and cancellous bone in the operative site then avoiding this "contamination" should reduce the incidence. Furthermore, inclusion of cancellous bone and bone marrow should increase the incidence. If on the other hand the periosteal stripping is the cause then it should not be difficult to reproduce it clinically.

Inclusion of Cancellous Bone in the Operative Site

Eleven hips were studied. In nine a piece of cancellous bone measuring not less than 10×5 mm was inserted into the tissue plane between the capsule and the abductor mass before re-attachment of the trochanter. In one it was placed within the capsule, lateral to the neck of the femoral stem. In one other patient, a female of 20 with avascular necrosis due to femoral neck fracture, cancellous bone from the femoral head was placed round the neck of the prosthesis in a deliberate attempt to stimulate heterotopic ossification and thus avoid an excessive range of movements and a possible subluxation of the LFA.

When the cancellous bone was inserted near the tip of the greater trochanter, seven out of nine hips produced heterotopic ossification. In only one case could it be shown radiologically that the ossification "progressed" from the inserted bone to the tip of the greater trochanter. In the other six the ossification appeared to start at the tip of the greater trochanter. Whether or not the cancellous bone inserted became involved or contributed to the extent of ossification was not possible to determine. The radiological appearances were no different from those observed in the first part of the study and none of the patients had clinical symptoms or restriction of movement.

Of the two cases where cancellous bone was placed within the capsule one remained unchanged by 7 months, while in the second

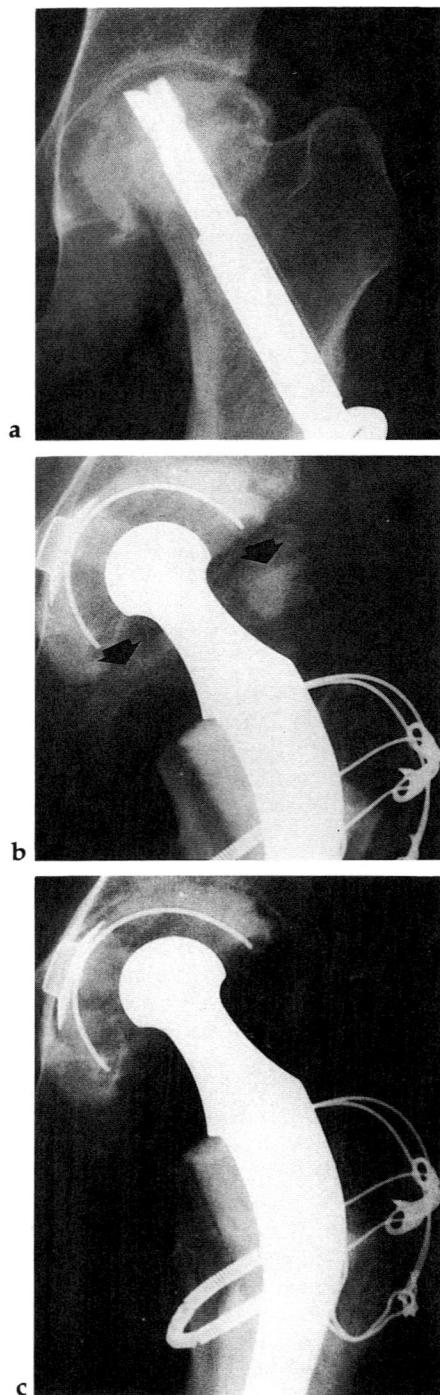

most of the cancellous insert was resorbed (Fig. 16.2) and the object of reducing the range of movements was not achieved; 37 months and one pregnancy later the patient had an excessive range of movements and had had two episodes of subluxation.

Periosteal Stripping

This is something that can be produced readily, accidentally or deliberately, at the time of the exposure of the hip joint. The areas most commonly involved are the tip of the greater trochanter, the medial femoral neck and the vastus lateralis ridge, where stripping of the periosteum may be readily seen if the trochanteric osteotomy is attempted before complete division of the soft tissues or if the vastus lateralis is stripped deliberately as it usually is when the greater trochanter is placed in position 2 or 1 as seen in Fig. 16.3.

It would also be expected that any "limited" exposure which demands forcible retraction would result in the same problem. This has been repeatedly demonstrated in cases of double cup arthroplasty; the exposure demands preservation of the blood supply to the femoral head, therefore limited exposure and retraction with periosteal stripping is not unusual with the resulting high incidence of heterotopic ossification. Stripping of the psoas tendon of the lesser trochanter produces heterotopic ossification in almost one-quarter of cases (Fig. 16.3c) (Dominguez et al. 1989b).

Excision

Since heterotopic ossification has not been found to be of significant clinical importance there have been no opportunities to study the results of treatment of this condition in the Charnley LFA.

In an attempt to find out whether excision resulted in recurrence, and if so, to what extent, Fahmy and the author (1982) used a planimetric method. Twenty-three sets of radiographs were reviewed from 21 patients where following the LFA a "significant" amount of new bone had

Fig. 16.2. The fate of intracapsular inclusion of cancellous bone. **a** Fractured neck of femur, internal fixation and avascular necrosis. **b** Post-operative radiograph showing the cancellous bone placed within the capsule. **c** Appearances 6 years later. Cancellous bone completely resorbed.

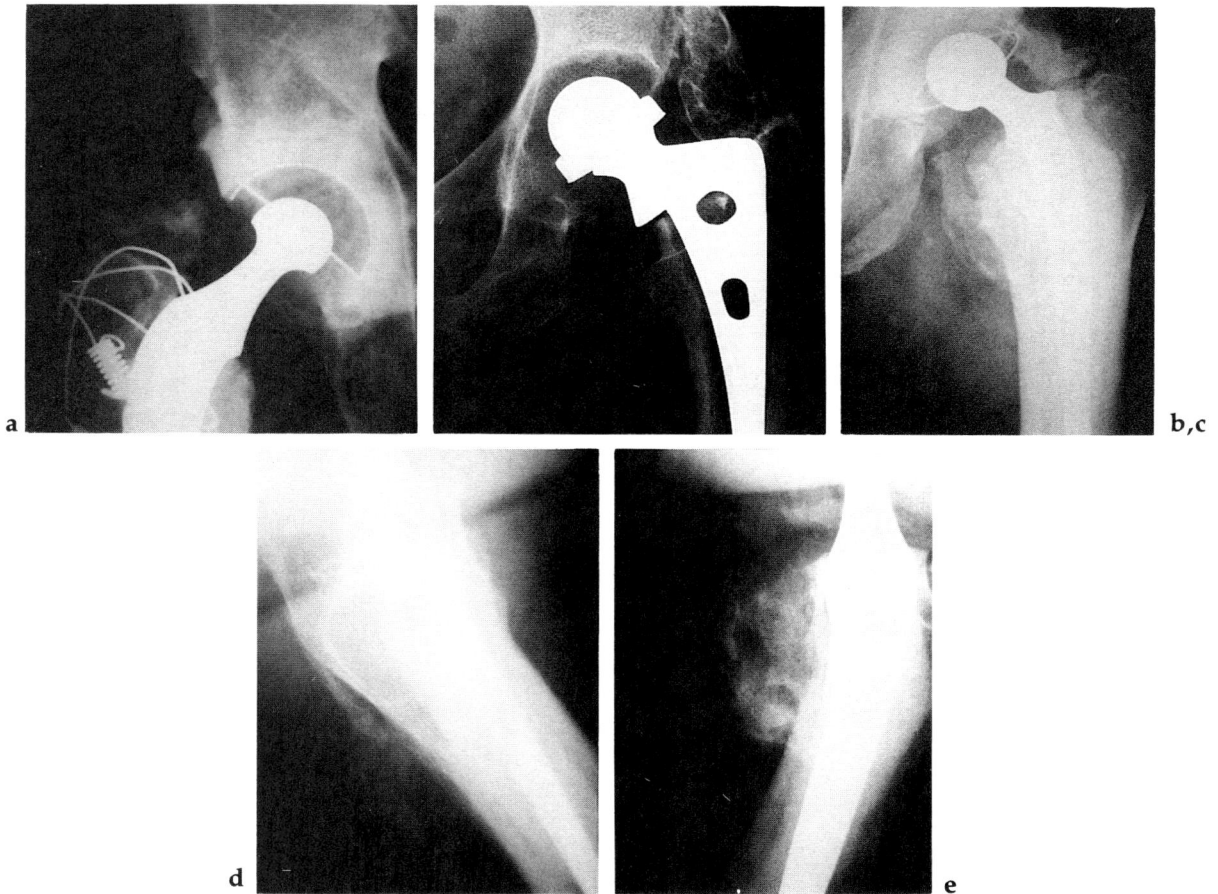

Fig. 16.3. Heterotopic ossification and its relation to exposure. **a** Transtrochanteric approach. **b** Liverpool approach with partical elevation of the abductors. **c,d** Posterior approach with stripping of the psoas, abductors and gluteus maximus. **e** Direct lateral approach.

formed which had to be excised at revision surgery. Standard radiographs allowed a direct comparison for each case and for the results of the whole group. For each case four tracings were made and the results expressed in cm^2 (Fig. 16.4). The tracings were made of the following areas:

1. Area following the LFA.
2. Area before the revision.
3. Area following the revision.
4. Area at final reviews.

Thus subtraction of the first area from the second area gave the extent of the ossification following the LFA. The difference between the second and the third areas was equivalent to the area of the bone excised, while the difference between the third and the fourth areas was the area of ectopic bone recurring following the excision.

One of the 23 cases studied was revised for a loose stem; all the others were revised for a fracture of the stem. All except one of the patients were males. Twenty had osteoarthritis while three had rheumatoid arthritis. Five had had previous hip surgery; two had had an

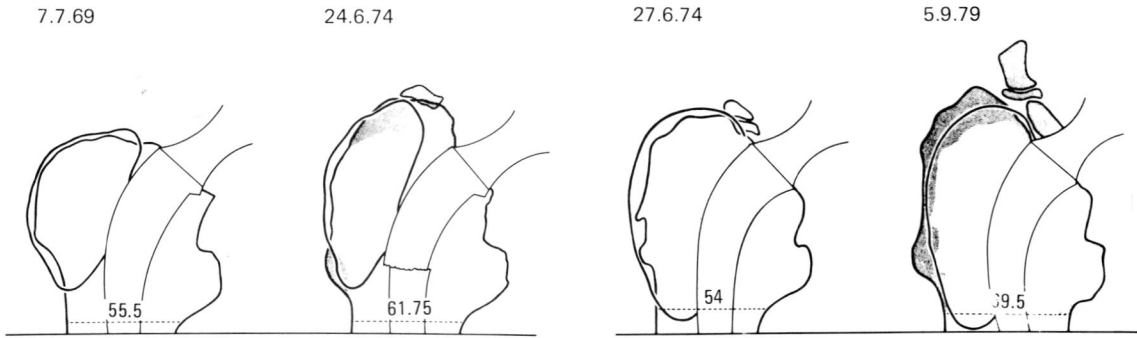

7.7.69   24.6.74   27.6.74   5.9.79

55.5   61.75   54   59.5

Fig. 16.4. Planimetric study of heterotopic ossification and its excision at revision.

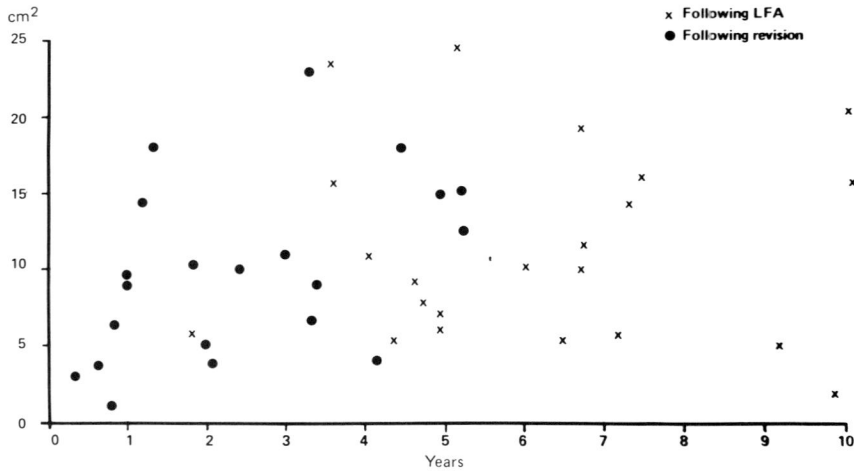

Fig. 16.5. Heterotopic ossification. Its natural course and recurrence after the excision.

intertrochanteric osteotomy, two an arthro-plasty (cup and fluon) and one fixation of a femoral neck fracture. One other patient had had an acetabular fracture treated conserva-tively. The results are summarized in Table 16.3.

Recurrence of ectopic ossification occurred in all except two cases. In the two, negative read-ings suggested that some resorption had taken place. In the other 21 cases, the average area of recurrence (10.1 cm^2) was greater than the aver-age area excised (9.6 cm^2). The study has also suggested that the progress of heterotopic ossifi-cation following excision was more rapid than initial heterotopic ossification (Fig. 16.5).

The findings of this study suggest that in heavy males excision of heterotopic bone leads to its recurrence and is not justified other than

for reasons of exposure. This confirms the find-ings of Lazansky (1973).

Heterotopic ossification around the hip joint following hip replacement is a phenomenon associated with surgery. It is probably correct to assume that the surgery plays a part in its formation, though what part has not been estab-lished with certainty. The study of inclusion of cancellous bone in the operative site, although in a small series, has not produced conclusive results. With periosteal stripping the incidence is higher and the extent is greater.

In order to attempt an explanation of the condition which would take into account all the known facts, not only those associated with total hip surgery but also those associated with the behaviour of the human skeleton in general, we

Table 16.3. Recurrence of heterotopic ossification after excision at revision surgery

Average weight (kg)	Average time to revision (years)	Average bone formation (cm²)	Average area of bone excised (cm²)	Average area of recurrence of ossification	Average follow-up (years) (cm²)
83.5	6.2	11.5	9.3	8–9	2.4

should probably look towards the "quality of bone" in the widest sense, and the response of bone to various conditions and procedures. It is here that the secret probably lies.

Hypertrophic-type arthritis is, by definition, a "bone-forming" condition and any trauma, be it deliberate or accidental, is likely to produce a hypertrophic (as thus heterotopic) response, e.g. early union of fractures, osteotomies or fusions. Any method of prevention or treatment would thus have to be aimed at this basic response, hence the success of radiotherapy and non-steroidal anti-inflammatory drugs. Whether the drug treatment is site-specific or not is uncertain but it is unlikely to be so. A hypotrophic response on the other hand would give not only a low incidence of ectopic ossification but also poorer results in cases of fractures, osteotomies or fusions. The basic response is due to the quality of the bone stock and its metabolism, the surgery being the incidental stimulus.

It is very tempting to speculate even further.

Are we not in fact looking at a much wider problem, that of the quality (whatever that may be defined as) of bone stock and its response to the various and varied conditions, both natural and surgically instituted, the result obtained being largely dependent on the bone rather than the surgeon or his technique (within limits)? If we accept this wider and certainly more fascinating approach, then we should study the "bone response" to the methods of treatment in far greater detail than hitherto. Rather than attempt to force our procedures onto the skeleton we must study its likely response, assess the limitations and results and possibly tailor the treatment accordingly.

This approach would allow a realistic assessment of the chances of success with any method, predictability of the result for an individual patient and the possibility of advancement of methods of treatment, not only in total hip arthroplasty, but in bone and joint surgery in general.

Section II

Practical Approach to Revision Surgery

17 Timing of Revision Surgery

The timing of revision will depend on the surgeon's awareness of the problem rather than the patient's symptoms.

Introduction

Although the clinical success of the operation of total hip arthroplasty can almost be taken for granted the need for revision surgery is not readily realized, appreciated or accepted. On what evidence can we base an assumption that an artificial joint will fare better or last longer than its real counterpart?

The timing of revision surgery must take into account the following: the patients known to be at risk for complications, the radiographic appearances indicating the likelihood of future failure, the asymptomatic nature of some of the complications, the frequent lack of correlation between radiographic appearances, clinical function and operative findings, the progressive nature of the complications, the progressive loss of bone stock and the mechanical effects of socket wear. The dilemma of radiological failure in the presence of clinical success need not exist if the possibility is appreciated both by the surgeon and the patient before the primary intervention.

Problems to be Anticipated at Follow-up

At the follow-up the most important factors for making the diagnosis and planning the management of complications are the continuity of the observer, his anticipation of the problem and good quality serial radiographs showing all of the prosthesis.

Examination of the range of movements of an artificial hip is a gesture more of social benefit than scientific interest. Although of clinical importance it must not override careful study of the radiographs.

Deep Infection

The patients at risk for a higher incidence of deep infection have been identified and include rheumatoid arthritis patients (especially if on steroids), males with post-operative urinary retention requiring catheterization and at times prostatectomy, patients who have had previous hip operations, diabetics and patients with psoriasis. The high risk of deep sepsis following cutaneous infection has been pointed out (Ainscow and Denham 1984). In this context, dental treatment does not seem to be a factor predisposing to deep infection. This may be because so

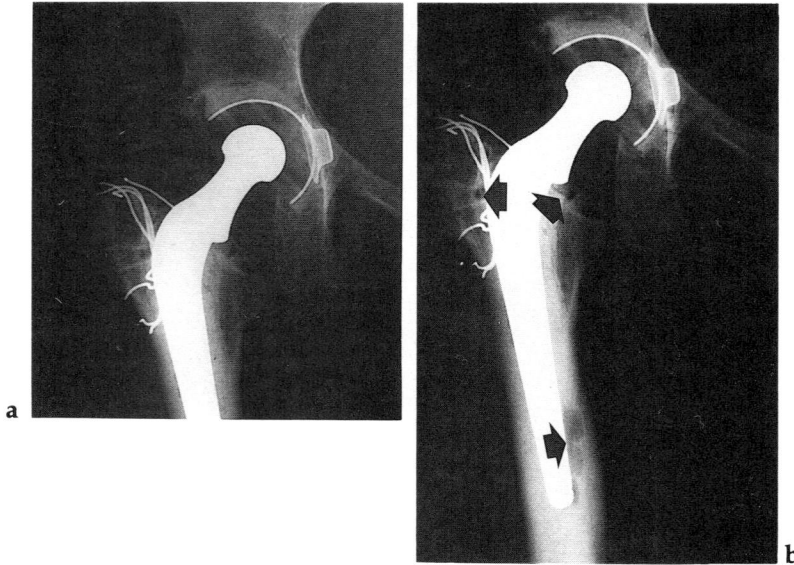

Fig. 17.1. An inadequate radiograph. **a** Trochanteric wires removed because they were thought to be the cause of a painful LFA. **b** Radiograph of the whole of the implant reveals the problem – deep infection. The changes at the medial femoral neck, the trochanteric area and the now-revealed distal stem make the diagnosis obvious.

many of the patients have already lost their teeth by the time they come to total hip arthroplasty.

In the vast majority of cases deep sepsis will usually, if not invariably, be diagnosed within 1 year of surgery, provided carefully kept records and good quality serial radiographs showing the whole of the implant (Fig. 17.1) are available. Any suggestion of an imperfect result warrants a thorough examination and careful scrutiny of the radiographs.

Any of the following findings may indicate deep sepsis: periostitis near the tip of the stem, endosteal porosis, cavitation in any area (but usually near the tip of the stem), early demarcation of the socket, erosion of the inner layer of the stump of the medial femoral neck or unexpected trochanteric detachment (Fig. 17.2).

Dislocation

Shortening, malposition or malorientation of the components may be immediately obvious. Recurrent clicking may indicate subluxation which may lead to dislocation once the rim of the socket has been eroded.

Fracture of the Stem

Healthy, heavy (over 80 kg), active males with a unilateral hip problem or bilateral total hip arthroplasty and with excellent femoral cortex (which is a reflection of their function) often make a rapid post-operative recovery and very soon return to normal activities. In view of the spectacular clinical result, these patients may soon be "lost" to follow-up. This special group of patients must really be followed up indefinitely. The tell-tale signs of fracture of the stem can be seen around 1 year from surgery and include separation of the back of the stem from cement, absent or fragmented cement at the calcar and fracture of the cement at the tip of the stem or at any other level (Fig. 17.3). Endosteal cavitation of the shaft of the femur is rare within 1 year of surgery. Radiographic appearances described above were found in 77.2% of 120 cases of fracture of the stem. These changes, often in combination, were already present within one year of the primary hip replacement. In this group we must include patients who already have had a revision for a fractured stem where the medial femoral neck and the lesser trochanter have not been prepared properly.

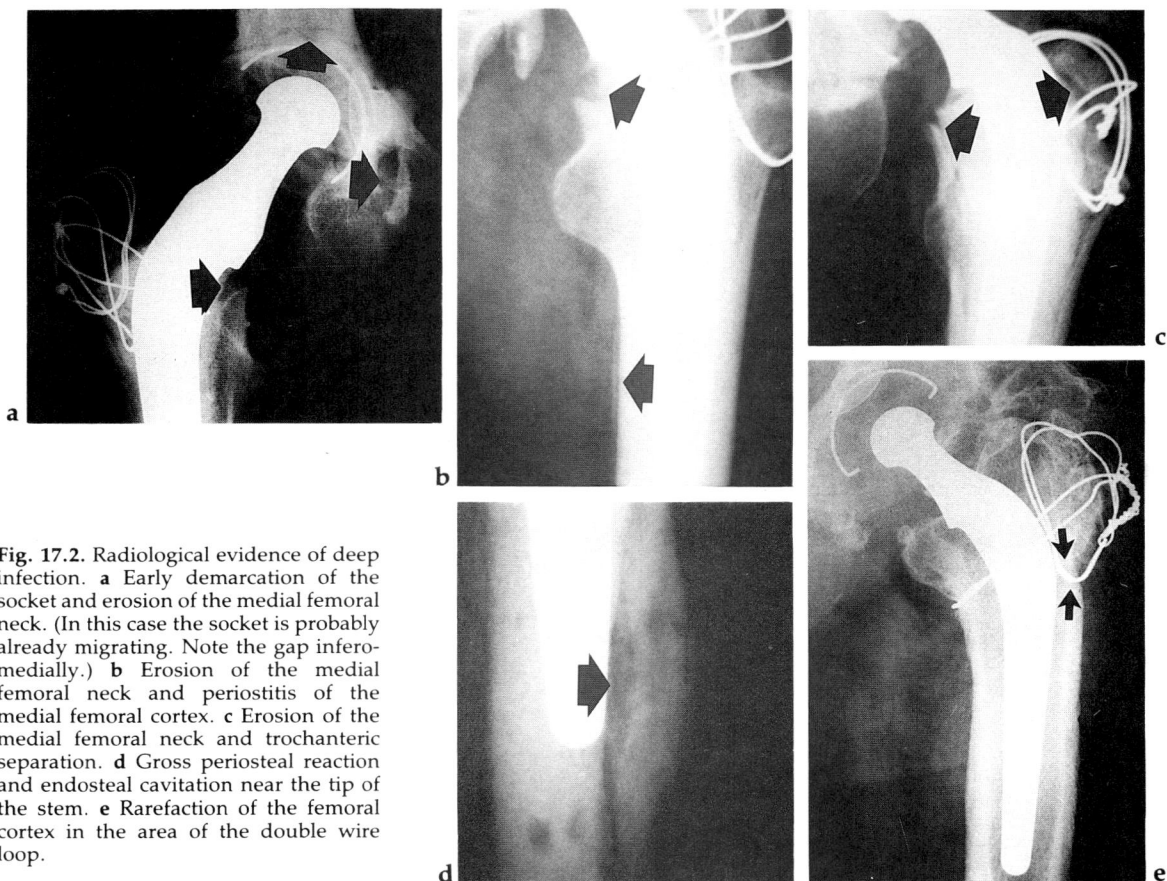

Fig. 17.2. Radiological evidence of deep infection. **a** Early demarcation of the socket and erosion of the medial femoral neck. (In this case the socket is probably already migrating. Note the gap infero-medially.) **b** Erosion of the medial femoral neck and periostitis of the medial femoral cortex. **c** Erosion of the medial femoral neck and trochanteric separation. **d** Gross periosteal reaction and endosteal cavitation near the tip of the stem. **e** Rarefaction of the femoral cortex in the area of the double wire loop.

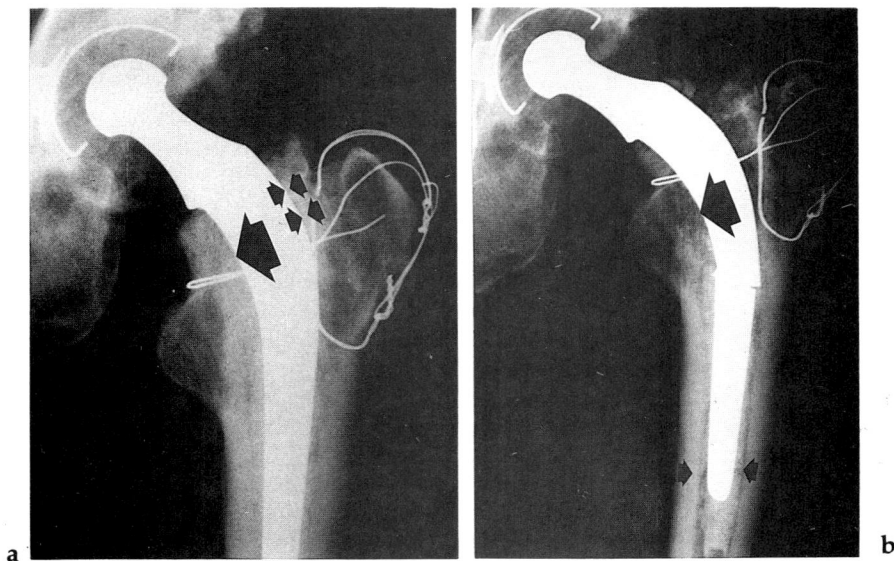

Fig. 17.3. Stem at risk. **a** Separation of the lateral part of the stem from cement. Medial cement proximally rather sparse. **b** Fractured stem. The initial quality of the medial femoral stem support is better appreciated now. The fracture of the cement at the tip of the stem was first noted on the 1-year radiograph.

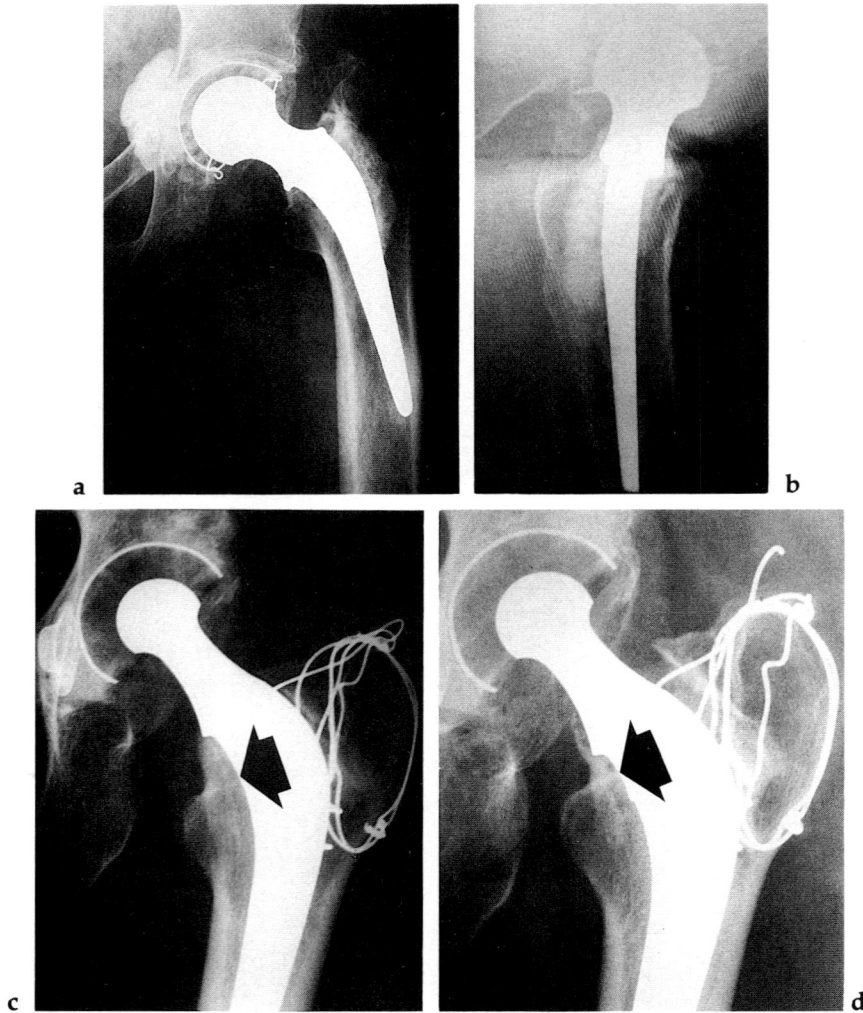

Fig. 17.4. Loosening of the stem. **a,b** Inadequate initial fixation of the stem. Note the amount and the distribution of the cement. **c,d** Early stem subsidence. **e** Early bone–cement demarcation with fracture of the lateral femoral cement. **f** Gross stem subsidence and endosteal cavitation, radiograph at 1 year. **g** Same patient as in **f**, 2½ years later. **h** Delaying the revision of a loose stem.

Loosening of the Stem

Patients with loosening of the stem need not be excessively heavy or active, and in fact they are somewhat lighter (average weight 69 kg) than those with fractured stems. The medullary canal is often wide with a relatively thin cortex and the stem–cement complex may look "lost" within the femur. Some of this is due to inadequate initial stem fixation (Fig. 17.4), some to the poor quality of the cancellous bone. Apart from the signs described under Fracture of the Stem, early

demarcation of the bone–cement complex at its distal part and occasional subsidence or tilting of the stem–cement complex are also risk signs. Viewed retrospectively the signs have been found in 89% of cases that eventually came to revision for loosening of the stem. In this group a large proportion of patients have already had some type of hip surgery, often involving the femur or the medullary canal (Pacheco et al. 1988). The failure here occurs at the bone–cement junction.

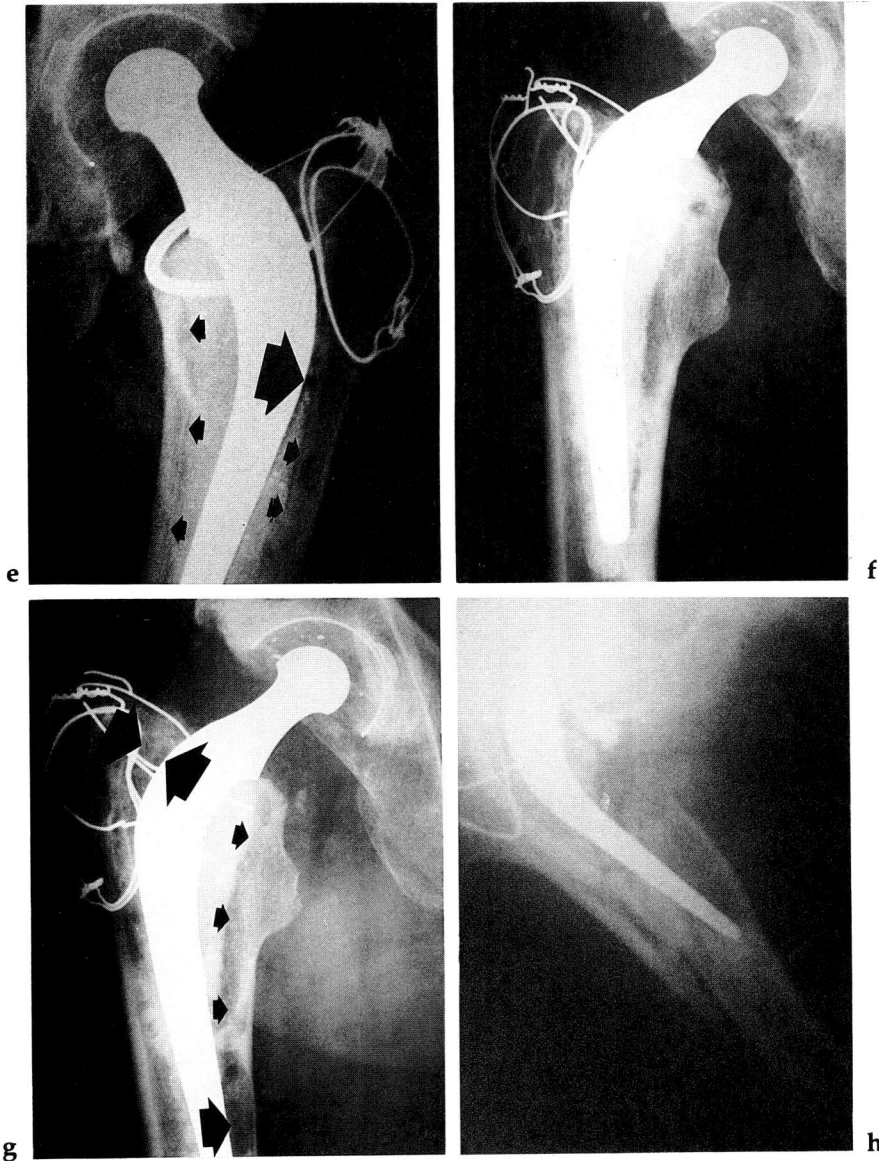

Fig. 17.4. (*continued*)

Under this heading we must include the patients with a narrow medullary canal where excessive or even power reaming had been used to accommodate the stem. Initial results may have been spectacular but in the years to come demarcation of the bone–cement junction and cortical thickening plus discomfort or even pain in the thigh coming on during activity may herald loosening of the stem. A smooth medullary canal is unsuitable for cement injection, and reaming of the medullary canal to the cortex has nothing to commend it. Good planning, a choice of suitable stems and the use of the lesser trochanteric cavity for proximal stem support are recommended, especially in revisions.

Loosening of the Socket

Various grades of socket demarcation and the correlation with the operative findings are discussed in detail on p. 73. With longer follow-up the depth of socket wear will become of increasing importance.

Correlation Between Radiological Appearances and Clinical Function

Both in our training and in clinical practice we are conditioned to treat symptomatic patients. Nowhere is this more apparent than in the management of patients with arthritic joints. How often does the surgeon examine the radiograph before examining the patient? When it comes to follow-up, the clinical result takes priority over the study of radiographs. Although the clinical result of the operation is the essence of our surgical practice, the study of the radiographs is of paramount importance to our knowledge of the long-term results of the method. Clinical success following a well-performed arthroplasty can almost be taken for granted; the radiographic appearances will point to the eventual outcome and the long-term result.

Since the patient and the surgeon are "tied" together for the life of the arthroplasty, there is no reason why the patient should not be made aware of the radiographic appearances of his or her own hip. It will make the planning of any future revision easier.

On the acetabular side, demarcation or loosening of the socket and even prolapse may be compatible with normal or near-normal function. On the femoral side, slow, progressive loosening in a patient slowing down because of advancing years may be assumed to be a normal process. To wait for a patient's symptoms to develop may mean gross loss of bone stock and well-nigh impossible revision.

In cases of deep sepsis the problem may be even more complex. Whether the artificial, and therefore insensitive, joint is lubricated by blood, bursal fluid or pus is of no consequence to the articulating surfaces or the components, provided those are soundly fixed. The only symptoms are due to local or systemic effects of deep sepsis or the eventual failure of the bone–cement junction which leads to loosening of the components. Thus the better the quality of the component fixation the later is the deep sepsis likely to be diagnosed.

For radiological changes to become obvious on serial radiographs, a certain amount of bone stock must be lost. (A simple series of experiments carried out by the author suggested that around 20% of the density of the femoral cortex must be lost before the changes become obvious on the radiographs.) It is true that modern techniques exist to assist in this aspect of assessment. Unfortunately they are only of value more than 1 year after surgery; a keen eye will make the diagnosis from radiographs before then.

The findings at revision as far as the extent of bone stock loss, soft tissue pathology, quality of muscles, extent of bone–cement junction changes or the quality of bone left for component fixation are concerned are invariably more impressive than can be surmised from radiographs. Thus it is an awareness of all these factors that will decide the timing of the revision.

Failure of component fixation and deep sepsis do not improve with time. Although radiographic evidence of deep sepsis or loosening need not be an indication for immediate revision, it invariably becomes so with time. The only indication in this respect for non-intervention can be non-progressive changes in the presence of reasonable function. To wait for the patient's symptoms to become severe is to lose the opportunity for a successful revision.

There are only three possible outcomes of delaying revision until symptoms become severe:

1. The problem will become more difficult technically.
2. The surgeon may improve his knowledge and understanding of the problem and his ability to tackle the problem.
3. The natural causes may provide the solution without the need for surgical intervention.

Only the second outcome is within the surgeon's control. If this is not so then the patient should be referred to others who are well versed in dealing with such problems.

Progressive, although at times slow, loss of bone stock makes late intervention technically more difficult and the chances of longer lasting results less likely, and all this in patients who are older and less fit for major surgery.

On the acetabular side loss of the superior roof or the floor or even disruption of the continuity of the rim will make fixation of the new components difficult or even impossible. On the femoral side loss of the neck down to the lesser trochanter may readily be managed by excavating the cavity of the lesser trochanter. Once this has been lost the straight, and often smooth, tube of the femur will present problems which cannot be tackled by the use of standard hip components. Replacement of the proximal femur carries with it the possible penalty of failure, the result of which is a flail limb or even at times disarticulation.

The dilemma facing both the surgeon and the patient is whether or not to undertake revision surgery for radiographic changes alone, especially in cases where symptoms are minimal or even absent.

It is correct to say, at this stage of the science and art of total hip arthroplasty, that the possible need for revision surgery for radiographic changes alone must be understood and accepted both by the surgeon and the patient even before primary surgery is considered. It is unrealistic to imagine that a patient who has managed to "wear out" his own joints is less likely to do the same to a pair of artificial ones. Once this emotional barrier has been overcome the follow-up and revision surgery, if required, need not be looked upon as anything else but "after-sales service", the need for which the patient has been made aware of before primary surgery and kept informed about at the follow-up. All this requires commitment, the surgeon's specialized knowledge, good facilities and continuing research into this type of surgery. It must be understood and accepted by both the patient and the surgeon that total hip arthroplasty is the beginning of the treatment and not the end. This must also be catered for by the system offering such service.

Excluding emergency cases, the indication for revision will be progressive loosening of components and/or deteriorating function. In its timing revision will be carried out to preserve the maximum bone stock.

18 Assessment of the Patient

Introduction

Assessment of the patient and the accurate recording of the findings should be an integral part of patient management both before primary surgery and at revision surgery. Only in this way can the problem be studied objectively and the findings used with benefit for the future. This aspect becomes even more important at follow-up.

Patient pain is a difficult parameter to assess. Memory of painful experiences is so short as to allow the human race to survive, yet single episodes may be so impressive as to make or break a character.

Patient function is a parameter which would appear to be more easily assessed. This may be so in terms of ordinary day-to-day activities; however, to assess function over time and distance and in terms of the load on the hip joint and velocity and to then translate these results into load and sliding distance at the hip level, is something that has yet to be carried out scientifically, without resort to anecdotes.

Before primary surgery is undertaken accurate records of clinical assessment are essential. In revision cases examination of the range of movements must not take priority over the study of the radiographs.

Assessment of the Arthritic Hip

It is interesting to note how rarely the type and distribution of pain in the arthritic hip is con-

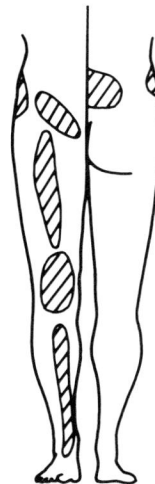

Fig. 18.1. Pain distribution from an arthritic hip joint.

sidered when a patient first presents for surgery. This is probably because by this stage the radiograph has already been examined and the pattern for consultation set. The hip is a deeply seated joint and any pain related to it is distributed, in a referred manner, along the nerves supplying it (Fig. 18.1).

The exact source of pain in the arthritic hip has not been established with any certainty. The theory of increased intramedullary pressure had its protagonists in the era of intertrochanteric osteotomy. The capsule is unlikely to be the source of pain. The capsule is *not* excised as a part of the routine low-friction arthroplasty, yet the pain is completely relieved.

It can be argued that initially the source of pain is the subchondral bone of the femoral head, then the destroyed acetabulum. This is probably true in early cases of osteoarthritis, when cartilage is lost on the femoral head but still remains covering the acetabulum. A cemented femoral endoprosthesis brings dramatic relief of pain until the acetabulum becomes eroded. The pain then presumably arises from the eroded acetabulum. Total hip arthroplasty, again without excision of the capsule, affords complete pain relief.

The recording of the assessment can be adequately made using the d'Aubigne and Postel (1954) method as modified by Charnley (1972). Any method of recording which attempts to combine the clinical examination, radiographic findings as well as subjective assessment of the result of the operation is probably too complex to be of practical value. It also fails to appreciate that with increasing follow-up the radiographic appearances progressively take precedence over the clinical picture. The radiographic assessment, or rather description, of the arthritic hip can usefully and unemotionally be carried out according to the radiographic morphology proposed by Charnley (Wroblewski and Charnley 1982).

Assessment of a Patient with Failed Total Hip Arthroplasty

Clinical History

The clinical aspect of the problem in cases of a suspected failed total hip arthroplasty is no less important than in primary surgery. It is essential to get to know the sequence of the relevant events leading up to and following the primary operation.

Following total hip arthroplasty any problems relating to wound healing must be recorded. Swelling, redness, tenderness, discharge, repeated dressings or prolonged courses of antibiotics, in hospital or after discharge, suggest sepsis. Referral for out-patient physiotherapy in the post-operative period suggests that the arthroplasty never completely fulfilled the patient's expectations. (What is the logic of advocating exercises for a failed arthroplasty?)

Thus a patient who has never been completely relieved of pain is very likely to have a deep infection. A patient who after initial success and a return to normal activities later complains of pain, discomfort, limp, gradual shortening of the operated leg or the need to use support has loosening of the components, usually of the stem. A patient who after several years of spectacular function complains of sudden severe pain is probably telling you that the stem has fractured. Sudden immobility in the early post-operative period indicates dislocation. In the vast majority of cases the likely problem can be predicted provided good quality serial radiographs are carefully examined.

Pain in Failed Total Hip Arthroplasty

A patient with a total hip arthroplasty finds himself in a new situation, with an implant that has no intra-articular sensation. The articular surfaces can no longer be the source of pain. Phantom pain following internal amputation (and total hip arthroplasty is such a procedure) has yet to be described. Whether the artificial joint is lubricated by "synovial" (actually bursal) fluid, blood or pus will make no difference to the articulation itself. Pain will only be present if there are local or systemic effects of the complication involving soft tissues, bone or the bone–cement junction.

That the acetabular side of the articulation does not often lead to the patient's symptoms is not generally recognized. An uncemented acetabular component can function perfectly for many years so there is no reason why a frankly loose socket should be symptomatic. This may be the fact which has encouraged surgeons to perform various types of uncemented total hip arthroplasty without them actually realizing the reason for the apparent short-term success.

The analogy between a normal tooth and a well-cemented femoral stem is probably reasonable. Both can and do support a certain load and can be accepted as being "soundly fixed" for the purpose of the design and function. Both can be extracted with relative ease or made to fail when the load imposed exceeds the level allowed by the fixation or when the fixation has been inadequate. In such situations the symptoms will be produced at lower levels of function. Conversely, with increasing age and decreasing level of activity even inadequate fixation may allow a certain level of function which can be regarded as adequate or even normal.

In a normal femur the load is transferred through the femoral cortex. In a total hip arthroplasty the femur is stressed from inside out by the stem and the cement; this is referred to as "hoop stress". The exact level at which the load is transferred from the stem through the cement to the femoral cortex is not known with certainty in every case. By the very nature of the design and the operative technique load transfer may by-pass the most proximal part of the femoral neck. This may, to a degree, be responsible for the symptoms on the femoral side being referred to the front of the thigh. In some of the cases of sudden severe pain associated with fracture of the femoral stem the author has seen a short longitudinal split in the medial femoral neck. Presumably this is the cause of pain. It is also interesting to note how, over a matter of days, the pain settles almost completely and the patient may even insist that all is well again.

A patient's interpretation of the quality and distribution of pain can often be very vague. The pain is often referred to the front of the thigh, groin or knee. Initially it comes on at the start of activity but improves as the activity progresses. It is usually made worse by walking on uneven ground, or by a sudden unguarded movement such as a stumble or a sudden turn when standing on the affected limb. With time the pain may become more severe, last longer or not be completely relieved by rest. This type of pain is probably related to the changes in hydrostatic pressure within the medullary canal. The stem–cement complex when under load may act as a one-way non-return valve allowing an increase in the intramedullary pressure. On the acetabular side the same situation cannot arise; the changes in pressure can be accommodated because while the superior part of the socket is under compression, the inferior part is under tension. There is a large area of communication between bone–cement and the joint space for pressure equalization to occur. The pelvic bones in general, and the acetabular bones in particular, are not known for their callus formation. There is no reason why their response to an arthroplasty should be different.

Function

If we accept that the quality of the clinical result is directly proportional to the quality of the component fixation, then we must accept that if fixation is marginally inferior, or if the failure of fixation comes on gradually, it may pass unnoticed. Observation of the patient's gait is important. The abductor "lurch" of a patient with a

faulty but mobile joint is typical. The patient "throws" his body over the affected hip joint while load bearing without support. The hip functions in an abducted position in order to reduce the load imposed upon it.

Straight Leg Raising

This is a very useful parameter of assessment and is probably equivalent to putting the weight of the body on the affected joint. It can be carried out by the patient and avoids the sudden movements that can be produced when testing the range of movements passively. It also allows some degree of assessment of the mechanical integrity of the joint, as well as the effective "origin–insertion" distance of the hip-controlling musculature. The relatively limited information that can be gained from examination of the range of movements of an artficial joint has already been pointed out.

Local Examination

Local examination is important when planning any prospective surgery and must not be left until the time when the patient is anaesthetized for the operation. Previous incisions, open or healed sinuses, dehiscence of the deep fascia, areas of tenderness or collections of pus must be noted. Feeling over the femur may indicate an area of cement extrusion or penetration of the femoral cortex by the stem. Opportunity must be taken to search for any areas of sepsis, not only on the affected side but generally, for example in the patients' teeth.

Special Investigations

Of the investigations currently available, good-quality serial radiographs are the most important and form an integral part of investigation of the total hip arthroplasty. Such radiographs must include both hips; the x-ray tube should be centred over the symphysis pubis in order to show the whole of the femoral stem and cement on one radiograph. If a long stem has been used then obviously it must be shown on a separate radiograph. A lateral x-ray is essential to show the position of the stem in relation to the cortex and the distribution of the femoral cement plus any changes indicating loosening or infection.

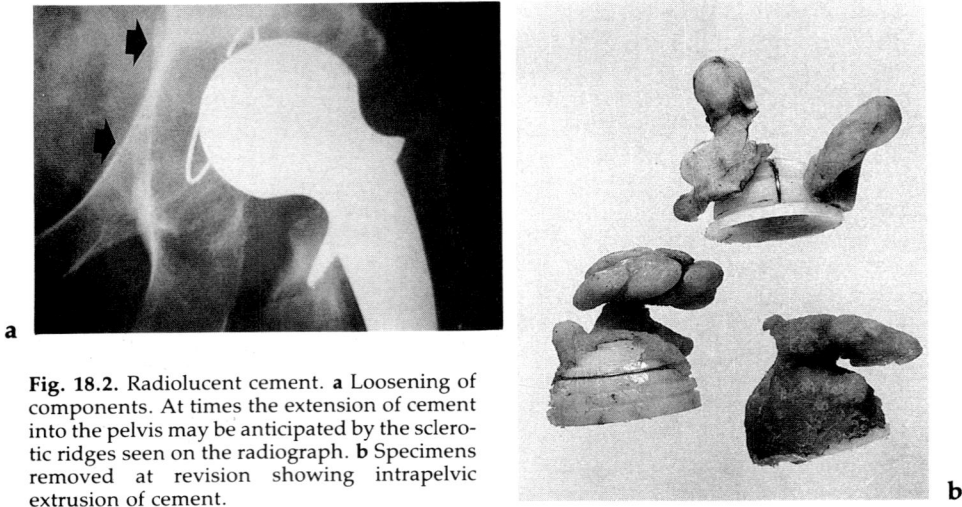

Fig. 18.2. Radiolucent cement. **a** Loosening of components. At times the extension of cement into the pelvis may be anticipated by the sclerotic ridges seen on the radiograph. **b** Specimens removed at revision showing intrapelvic extrusion of cement.

Radiolucent Cement

In this context the use of radiolucent cement must be condemned. It is of no help to the surgeon using it and may be hazardous to the patient when it comes to revision surgery (Fig. 18.2). It is probably correct to suggest that all implants should be easily identifiable and clearly documented in the patients' records. The same applies to any antibiotics included in the acrylic cement.

Scanning Techniques

Scanning techniques have not found favour with the author. By the time they become of diagnostic value, i.e. after 1 year, the radiographic changes indicating the diagnosis, be it loosening, infection or both (Fig. 18.3), are already present. Their use has often delayed the decision-making day leaving little available bone stock for component fixation.

It is unfortunate that at this stage no adequate technique exists for routine investigation of the state of the acetabulum, especially its anterior wall. It is here that surprises are often found at revision surgery, after removal of the socket; the soft tissues are seen prolapsing from the femoral triangle. Any method which would allow estimation of the acetabular bone stock would be a great advance in revision surgery.

Arthrography

This again has not proved necessary although it must be conceded that extensions of tracts of infection have sometimes been apparent on such radiographs. The findings however have in no way affected the plan or the method of treatment.

Sinograms

At one stage these were used routinely and sometimes spectacular radiographs followed (Fig. 18.4). More often than not, however, they are used as a delaying tactic and in the vain hope that the problem is superficial. There are cases where following a sinogram the sinus has dried up and healed, if only temporarily. This presumably is due to the iodine content of the contrast medium.

Aspiration of the Joint

Use of aspiration is only as valuable as the bacteriological back-up facilities that are available. Since there is usually little or no free fluid aspirates do not usually produce a positive result. Biopsy of the granulation tissue is useful and may have to be obtained at open exploration. Thus a competent and dedicated bacteriologist who understands the problems and is

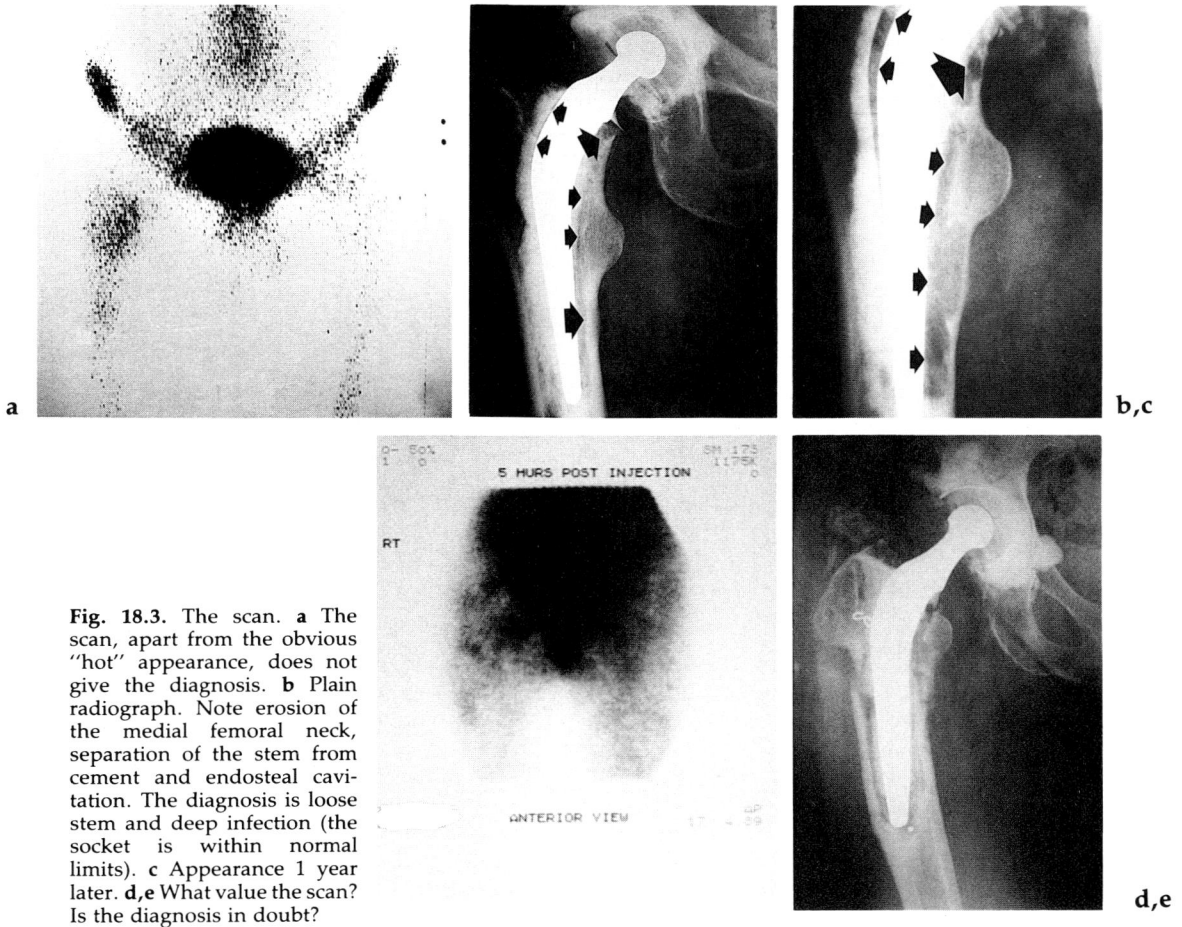

Fig. 18.3. The scan. a The scan, apart from the obvious "hot" appearance, does not give the diagnosis. b Plain radiograph. Note erosion of the medial femoral neck, separation of the stem from cement and endosteal cavitation. The diagnosis is loose stem and deep infection (the socket is within normal limits). c Appearance 1 year later. d,e What value the scan? Is the diagnosis in doubt?

prepared to give all his attention is of the utmost importance. Examination of the specimen cannot be left to a junior technician whose knowledge of artificial joint pathology is limited to a statement "significant" or "insignificant" growth. Whether or not a bacteriological culture is significant is a clinical decision in the vast majority of cases which cannot be left to a non-clinically orientated scientist. What is really needed is collaboration between the two. This becomes more important in cases where the sepsis is obvious but the organisms prove difficult to isolate, or when the surgery has been performed with antibiotic-loaded acrylic cement. In the final analysis it is a combination of all the evidence available and the experience of the surgeon that will allow the final diagnosis of the problem; the treatment can then be planned accordingly. A doubtful diagnosis made on the basis of the results of one test makes no contribution. In cases where doubt exists, if treatment is to be instituted, it should be for the most fearsome diagnosis, i.e. deep infection.

Gram stains and frozen sections are basically of the same value as joint aspirates.

Discussion with the Patient

Publicity in the media associated with total hip arthroplasty is such that there is no reason to withhold information from the patient unless the patient so wishes. Patients' knowledge and understanding of the problem and the treatment proposed will only help to build a working relationship which, after all, must be for life. Unlike other types of surgery the responsibility does not end with primary surgery, it only starts there.

The problems of revision surgery, being often mechanical, do not require the same patient

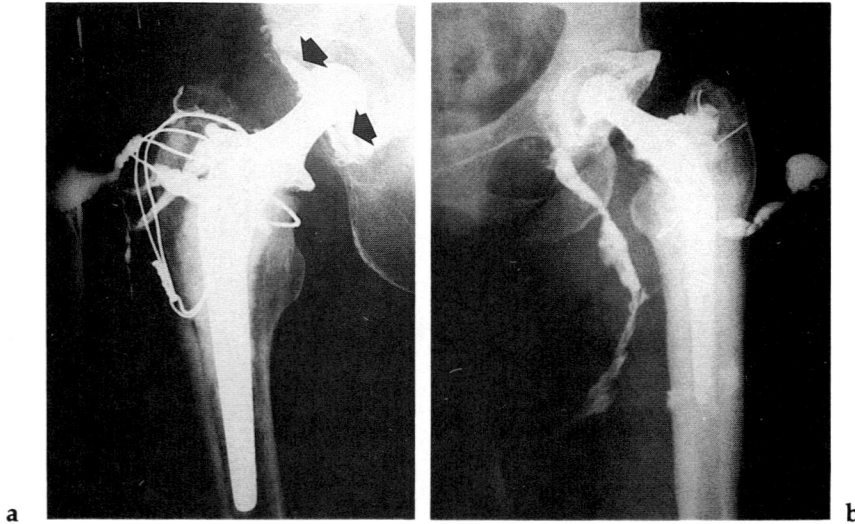

Fig. 18.4. Sinogram. **a** Note the dye extending along the wires to the base of the neck of the stem and to the face of the socket. **b** Another example of a rather extensive sinus.

attitude as does cancer surgery. On the other hand there is a place for broaching the need for revision surgery gently, not necessarily in all cases but when revision may have to be carried out at some future date or for radiographic changes in order to preserve the bone stock.

Some patients would like to know all the details, others have an "I'll leave it all to you" approach. Quoting "percentages" is a simple matter; however, they never apply to an individual once the complication has occurred. The patient must be made aware of the problem and possibly how it has occurred, what is being proposed in the way of treatment and what is the likely outcome. It must also be pointed out that the final decision as to the method of treatment can at times be taken only during the operation and that the surgeon must have the freedom to make that decision. This especially applies to cases where pseudarthrosis is the only acceptable line of treatment.

Every patient when presented with the possibility of pseudarthrosis needs sympathetic and careful explanation of the reasons, the post-operative management, the need for support for ambulation and the rehabilitation which takes so much longer, requires greater effort and produces results that cannot be compared with primary surgery. Printed pamphlets should not absolve the surgeon from the personal contact and responsibility in any case.

Anaesthetic Assessment

It is important that the anaesthetist who is going to be in charge of the patient at the time of surgery should personally assess the patient. The patient's fitness for anaesthesia and any local problems (e.g. intubation) or general problems (e.g. hypertension, steroid medication, diabetes) should alert to the possibility of any likely complications. Unsuitability for hypotensive anaesthesia or any problems likely to result from a longer operative time or higher blood loss must be anticipated. Judicious use of hypotensive anaesthesia greatly helps the surgeon. A gently induced anaesthesia in a well-relaxed patient plus a relatively bloodless field all go to make the surgical procedure easy and enjoyable for the surgeon and safe for the patient.

In primary surgery the clinical assessment of the patient is all important. The radiograph only confirms what has already been established clinically and should be viewed last. At follow-up a normal and an unchanging radiograph in the presence of normal function is the desirable standard. Any departure from a normal appearance must be viewed with suspicion. It will often alert the surgeon to a likely problem. The findings at revision are invariably more extensive than suspected from radiographs.

19 Instrumentation for Revision Surgery

Introduction

Revision surgery is exciting and often leads to most satisfying results as illustrated by the success of individual clinical cases and the patients' gratitude. In the cold light of the operating theatre, however, there can be no room for other than a methodical approach to the problem. It must not be considered out of place or repetitive if the essential points are stressed once more.

The Diagnosis

The problem demanding revision must be clearly established. Apart from the history and the clinical examination, radiographic evidence is essential; there is no substitute for good-quality serial radiographs. There is no place for an exploratory "laparotomy"-type approach, unless full revision is envisaged or indicated.

The Availability of the Instruments and the Components

Surgery is the wrong time to be searching, either inside or outside the operating theatre, for various items needed.

The practical approach must be methodical and unhurried and yet must result in continuous progress of the procedure with all the likely possibilities having been considered and attended to, no matter how exciting or taxing the main part of the operation will turn out to be.

Familiarity with the instruments to be used is important. Most surgeons are familiar with the basic tools of the "do-it-yourself" trade. Somehow their application at surgery, under theatre conditions, brings in a new dimension that is not obvious at bench trials. It has something to do with the exposure and access, as well as the sizes and shapes of various implements. An operating theatre may not be the best place to learn about a new instrument for the first time. The basic premise that "if a new gadget does not work read the instructions" is probably correct in clinical practice as well as in the home.

Familiarity with the instruments goes a long way at surgery to helping maintain the continuity and the momentum of the operation. The instruments are merely the tools in the hands of the surgeon and a reflection of his ability, skill and above all his understanding of the problem being tackled. Power and speed, if used, must be well directed and controlled and must not be equated with progress or a desirable result.

The author's choice of revision instruments (Fig. 19.1) evolved over a number of years and some 500 revisions, and have been used without alterations (although with some additions) for the past 15 years in over 1200 revisions. Although each instrument was designed with a specific aim

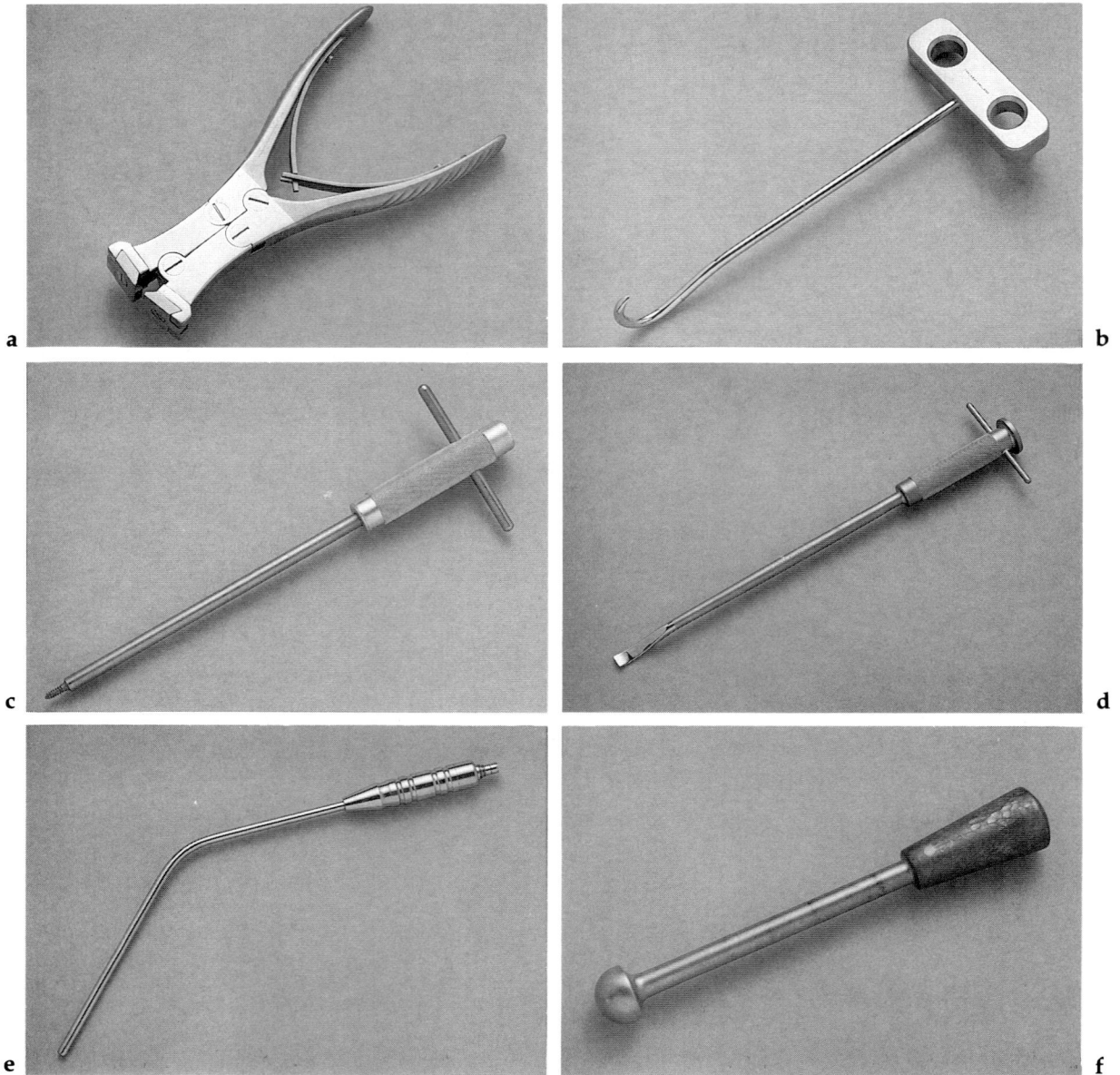

Fig. 19.1. Some of the revision instruments designed and used by the author. (For description see text.) a Wire cutter–puller. b Dislocating hook. c Socket tester. d Socket removal gouge. e Intramedullary illuminator. f Light conical mallet.

in mind it is often in practice the instrument "which makes progress" at any particular stage of the procedure which continues to be used. This most frequently applies to the gauges,

cement breakers and cement drills when working down the shaft of the femur.

The remainder of this chapter will list some necessary instruments.

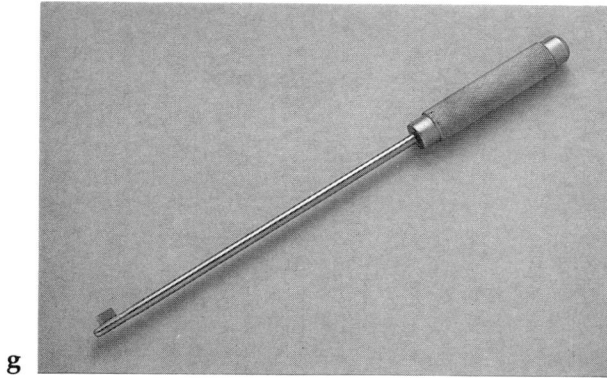

g

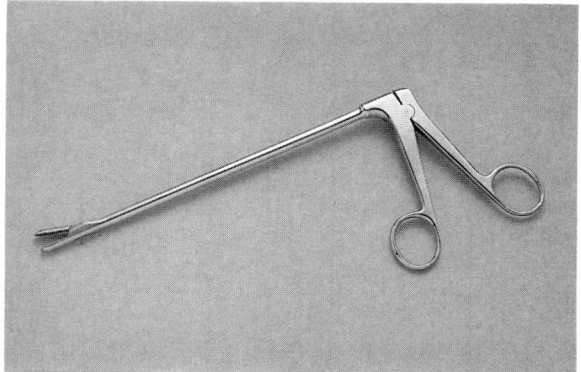

h

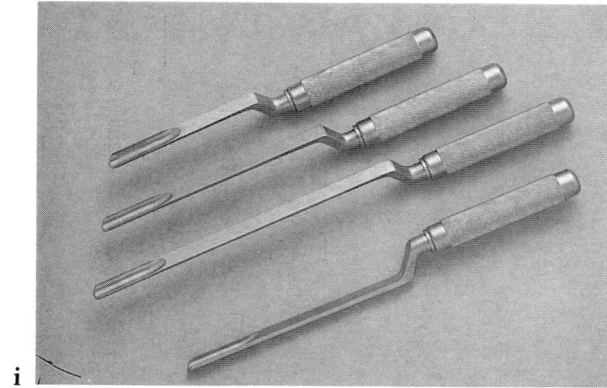

i

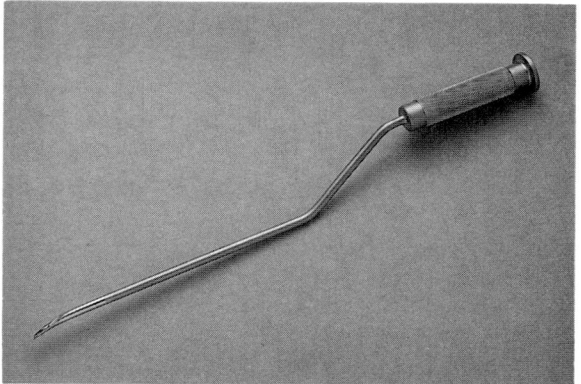

j

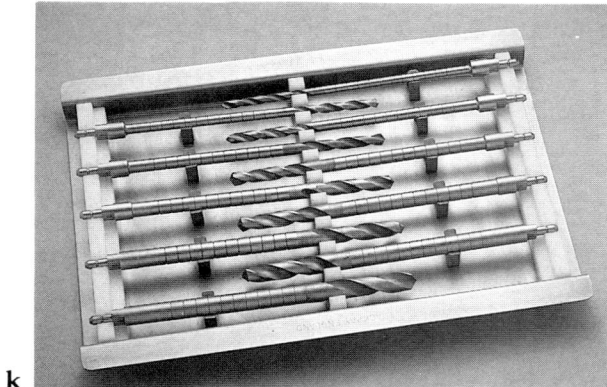

k

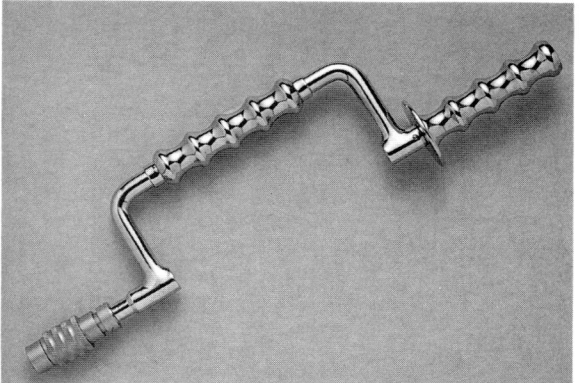

l

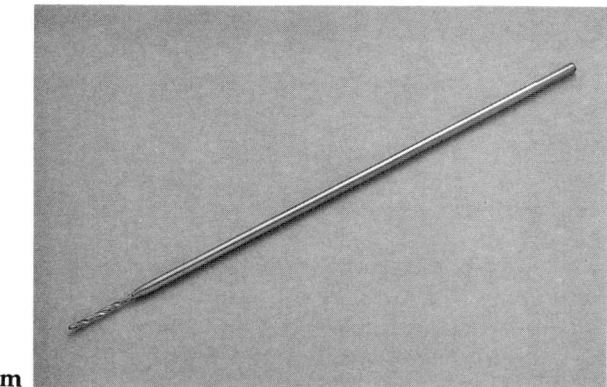

m

Fig. 19.1. (*continued*)
g Cement breaker. **h** Cement grasping forceps. **i** Offset
cement gouges. **j** Long offset cement gouge. **k** Cement drills.
l Short offset throw brace. **m** Distal femoral cement drill.

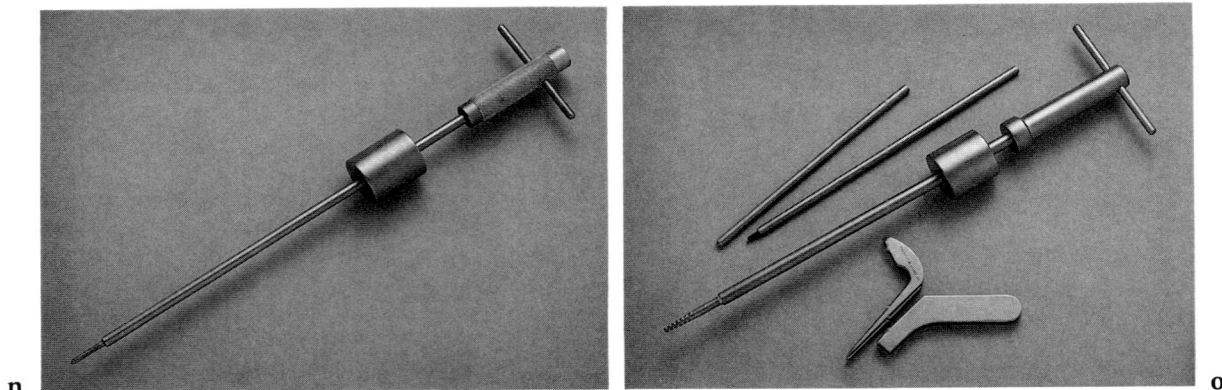

n   o

Fig. 19.1. (*continued*)
n Distal cement extractor. o Fractured stainless steel stem extraction instruments.

Removal of Trochanteric Wires

1. Sharp bone hook.
2. Charnley wire-holding forceps.
3. Wire cutter-puller.

The sharp bone hook is used to elevate wire loops or ends away from the bone and the soft tissue without damaging surgeons' gloves. The exposed wire can then be tackled as appropriate.

Charnley wire-holding forceps are essential for grasping wires, extracting wires by the "sardine can" method or protecting wire ends during the exposure.

The wire cutter-puller is a dual-purpose instrument used for cutting exposed wires or extracting them by the "claw hammer" method.

Trochanteric Osteotomy

1. Trochanteric osteotomy spike.
2. Cholecystectomy forceps.
3. Gigli saw (heavy duty).

The trochanteric osteotomy spike is used to determine the size of the trochanteric fragment and allows a bi-plane osteotomy to be cut after the Gigli saw has been introduced over it with the cholecystectomy forceps. The forceps are used again during mobilization of the proximal femur.

Mobilization of the Proximal Femur and Dislocation

1. Cholecystectomy forceps.
2. Dislocating hook.

The cholecystectomy forceps are used to pick up the soft tissue close to the femur before it is sectioned with cutting diathermy.

Once the proximal femur has been mobilized and the capsule sectioned to expose the neck of the stem, the dislocating hook is put round the neck and the hip dislocated by gentle lateral traction.

Extraction of the Femoral Stem

1. Femoral head protector.
2. Set of Charnley gouges.
3. A small mallet.
4. Stem extractor.

If the femoral stem is to be retained or if it is required for further examination then it is best covered with a femoral head protector to avoid accidental damage. Before the stem can be extracted, the cement over the curved lateral part must be removed to allow unimpeded stem removal. Failure to do this will result in splitting of the proximal femur. The cement is best removed with one of the narrow Charnley gouges. Only when this has been done should the stem extraction proceed.

The jaws of the stem extractor are hooked round the head of the prosthesis, the shaft of the extractor is held in line with the shaft of the femur and the sliding hammer is used to deliver a blow and thus extract the stem. A "slapping" rather than a "pushing" action on the sliding hammer is more effective.

Socket Exposure, Testing and Extraction

1. Pin retractor.
2. East–west retractor.
3. North–south retractor.
4. A set of Charnley gouges.
5. The acetabulum retractor.
6. Socket tester.
7. Socket extraction gouge.

The east–west and the north–south Charnley retractors having been inserted, the face of the socket can then be exposed by excising the soft tissue around it.

The superior lip of the socket is exposed using the largest of the Charnley gouges to remove any soft tissue or protruding osteophytes. If need be, the supero-lateral part of the socket flange may also be removed to expose the bone–cement junction.

The acetabulum retractor is introduced into the obturator foramen to expose the inferior margin of the socket.

The socket tester is inserted into one of the socket holder locating holes and using a gentle rocking and rotating action the quality of the socket fixation is tested.

The socket extraction gouge is used at the socket–cement junction to separate the socket from the cement. The curve of the instrument follows the shape of the socket. The extensions of the cement into the ischium, ilium and pubis demand careful attention. Strong levering should be avoided as it is likely to disrupt the continuity of the acetabular rim. Levering with a Watson–Jones gouge, as previously advocated (Wroblewski 1982a), is liable to lead to fracture of the anterior acetabular rim or the ischium, and is not recommended now.

Removal of the Femoral Cement

1. Intramedullary illuminator.
2. Cement breaker.
3. A set of four offset cement gouges.
4. A long fine cement gouge.
5. Light conical mallet.
6. Cement-grasping forceps.
7. Cement drills and brace.

The principle of femoral cement removal combines good exposure, illumination and methodical breaking up of the cement mantle.

The intramedullary illuminator together with a liquid light guide and source is essential. The handle of the illuminator is held out of the operative field, the light shining along the neck of the femur.

The cement breaker and the mallet are used to break the cement mantle radially, down to the level of the lesser trochanter, the aim always being the thinnest cement layer. This having been done cement gouges are used at the bone–cement junction to separate the cement fragments. The three offset gouges (10, 15, 20 cm) are used to break up and separate the cement from the bone at various depths. The fourth gouge, 15-cm long, allows the removal of cement from the anterior part of the femur.

Cement drills on a light brace are used to break the continuity of the cement mantle only, from the level of the lesser trochanter to the distal end of the stem. Measuring from 8 to 19 mm in diameter they have end and side cutting actions. They must be used with caution on a short throw (6-cm) brace by "feel not force". (Their use is best avoided in the grossly porotic femora.)

The long fine cement gouge is used to tackle small individual cement extensions located distally in the shaft of the femur. The cutting edge is directed outwards, towards the femoral cortex, and can readily penetrate the cortex. It must be used with caution, under direct vision, and never too ambitiously.

Removal of the Distal Cement Plug

1. Distal cement drill.
2. Distal cement extractor.

The distal cement drill should be used only when *all* the cement down to the level of the stem tip has been removed. (It is at times useful to "shape" the distal cement plug into a concavity by using the largest cement drill that will enter without encroaching on the femoral cortex.) Under direct vision the distal cement plug is drilled with the distal cement drill to the full depth of the drill. The distal cement extractor is screwed in fully. The sliding hammer is used to extract the distal cement plug. If the cement plug fractures and only part of it is extracted the procedure is repeated. (When drilling and extracting the distal cement plug, angulation of the drill and the distal cement extractor must be avoided since the drill or the screw may break off the shaft.)

Extraction of the Complete Cement Mantle from the Medullary Canal

1. Cement extractor.

If the femoral cement is evenly distributed and completely loose throughout its whole extent, it can be readily extracted with the cement extractor. The instrument consists of a shaft with a T-handle, a sliding hammer and a screw-in head which comes in three sizes. The size of the head is selected according to the diameter of the cavity within the cement and is mounted onto the shaft and screwed in down the stem tract. The sliding hammer is used to extract all or most of the femoral cement. This instrument must be used with caution. The tapered screw may expand or split the cement or damage the cortex when extensions of the cement, as for example into the lesser trochanter, are being extracted. The instrument, although of value in the early days of revision when the main problem was deep

sepsis of some standing, is rarely used now; a more methodical approach is now favoured.

Extraction of the Distal Fragment of Fractured Stem

1. Fractured prosthesis extractor kit consisting of:
   a. Guide.
   b. Punch.
   c. Drill.
   d. Extractor.

The guide is centred over the distal fragment within the medullary canal. The punch is used to mark the distal fragment and break through the work-hardened metal and serves as a centre point for the drill. The drill is mounted in a power tool, passed through the guide, located in the indentation made by the punch and, using full power, a hole is drilled to about 1-cm depth. Irrigation should be used to cool the drill. The fractured stem extractor is introduced down the hole in the distal fragment and locked into place. It has a left-hand thread. The sliding hammer is used to extract the distal fragment. This method suitable for all stems made in stainless steel. For stems in other metals, e.g. chrome–cobalt or titanium, one of the narrow Charnley gouges can be used at the level of the fracture and not at the tip of the stem. The vastus lateralis muscle is gently distracted at the level of the proximal part of the distal femoral stem fragment. The lateral formal cortex is opened with a narrow gauge exposing the femoral cement and the stem. The gauge is made to bite into the metal using sharp blows with a mallet in the direction of the open neck of the femur. Each blow moves the stem fragment proximally until it protrudes out of the open neck of the femur.

This method was used by Charnley on the first fractured stem revised in 1968.

20 Selection of Components

Introduction

A wide selection of components must be available for revision cases. Each case should be assessed, planned and rehearsed in order to avoid problems, reduce the operating time and offer a better result to the patient.

In the early years of the Charnley low-friction arthroplasty each innovation and development was often viewed with suspicion and resentment. By contrast, the plethora of apparently "newly discovered principles" is so vast that it makes one wonder how it is that 26-year results of the Charnley low-friction arthroplasty still out-perform all others both in the quality of results and the paucity of revisions? The mere fact that new components *can* be inserted must not be equated with the need to use them, let alone with long-term success.

The Acetabulum

The quality of the available bone stock will be the decisive factor when choosing which components or methods are to be used. It must be appreciated that improvement in the quality of the implant has little if anything to do with the quality of the bone stock which is meant to support that implant. The problem is invariably at the bone–implant junction. The acetabular rim is the essential load-bearing part.

The components and instruments necessary for replacement of the acetabulum at revision are as follows: a selection of Ogee-flanged angle-bore sockets; wire mesh and scissors. The Ogee flange, when appropriately trimmed, will provide rim support for the socket as well as adequate pressurization of the acrylic cement and post-operative stability in cases where the incidence of dislocation would otherwise be high.

Ortron wire mesh is very useful in revision cases where defects of the acetabular floor require to be covered in order to avoid the escape of cement into the pelvis. The Ortron wire mesh is cut with the scissors according to the size required, usually into a circular shape. Radial cuts are then made and the gauze "shaped" by bending. Trial will determine if the correct shape and size has been obtained. Once made to fit, the shaped Ortron gauze is partly flattened out. When placed in position and pressed into shape the elastic deformation of the gauze will make it stay securely in its place (Fig. 20.1).

At the time of writing (November 1987) rim-support sockets, although well advanced, are not in general use. They combine the experience of Charnley with the press-fit sockets, the results of revision surgery in the presence of acetabular defects as achieved by the author as well as the present and possibly future developments in bone grafting and supplementation in the widest sense of the term. The sockets ensure rim support of the implant under load while allowing implementation of bone grafting at the same time (Fig. 20.2).

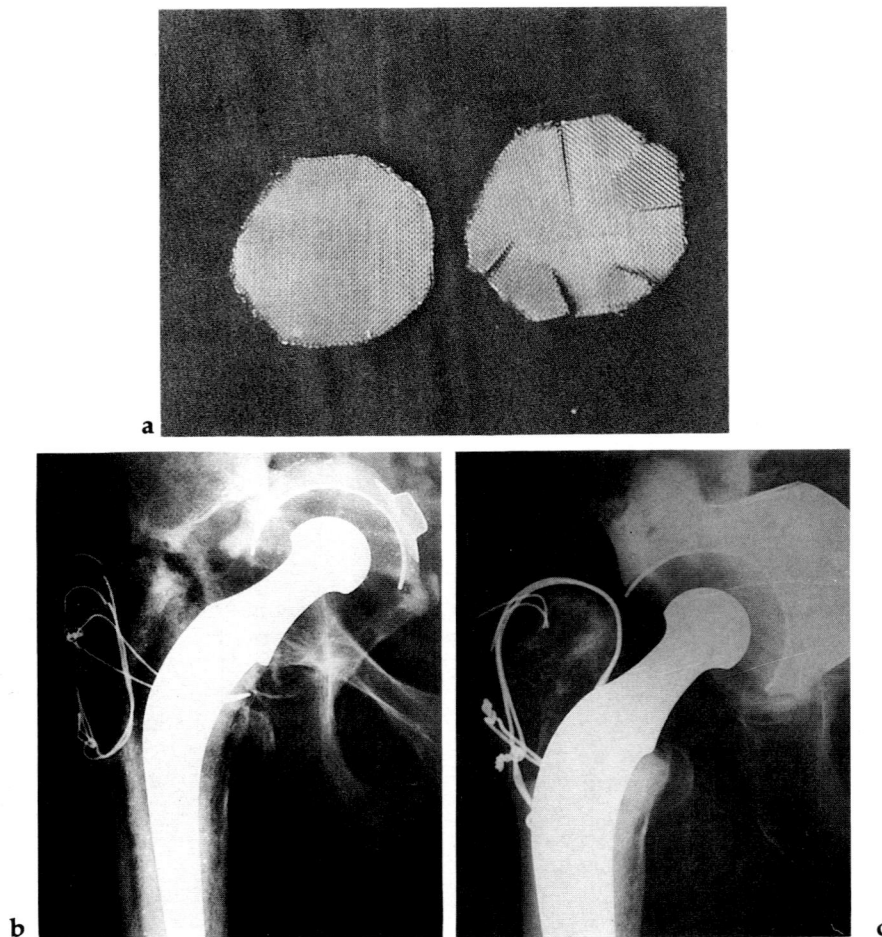

Fig. 20.1. Ortron wire mesh. **a** Wire mesh is cut to size, usually in a circular fashion, then radial cuts are made to allow the mesh to fit snugly into the curved acetabular cavity. **b** Ortron wire mesh in use: central acetabular defect. **c** Ortron wire mesh in use: appearance 8 years after revision.

The Femur

Revision surgery must not be synonymous with the use of ever-longer stems. It has been said that the length of the stem used in revision surgery is proportional to the delay and inversely proportional to the experience of the surgeon. Proximal fixation of the stem is essential but the design will vary with the availability of bone stock.

The following femoral components should be available at revision: standard stems, shorter stems, longer stems, extended neck stems, a modular proximal femoral replacement and a stem–Kuntscher nail combination.

Standard stems, used routinely in primary surgery, probably form the bulk of those used in revisions.

Shorter stems are extremely useful when extraction of all of the distal cement is not essential, or when exposure of the distally closed-off medullary canal is not indicated (Fig. 20.3). The exact length that is acceptable has yet to be determined although information is now being gathered. Experience with shorter stems extends over 5 years and well over 120 cases (both in revision and primary surgery).

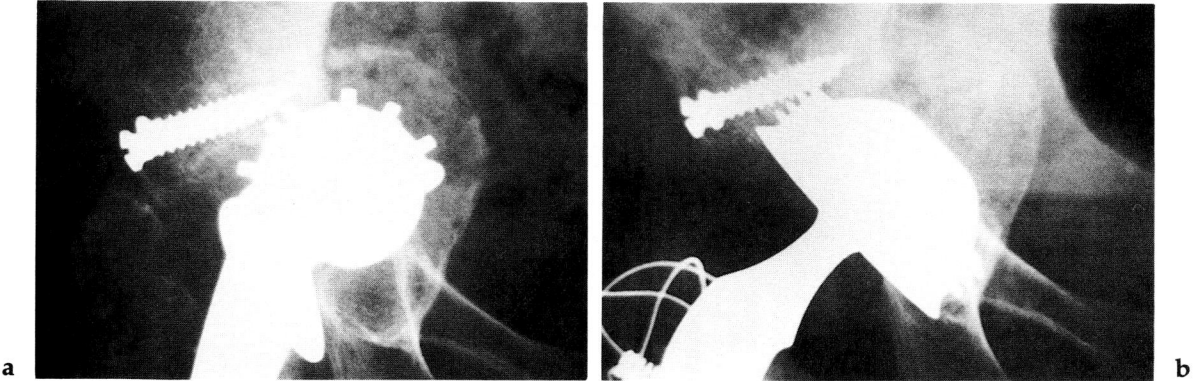

Fig. 20.2. Rim-support socket. **a** Prolapsed socket. **b** Revision with a rim-support uncemented socket. In this particular case bone grafting was used as well.

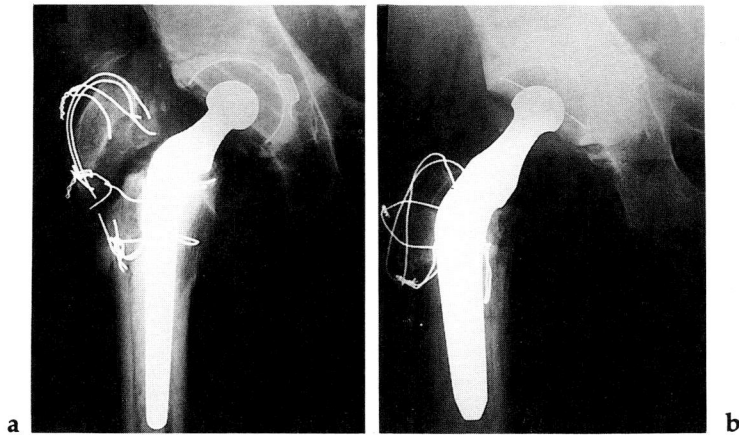

Fig. 20.3. A shorter stem. **a** The problem is recurrent dislocation and trochanteric non-union. **b** Revision using a shorter (long neck, extra heavy) stem, angle-bore socket and compression spring (covered by the stem). Four-year follow-up.

Longer stems are very useful when distal defects or weaknesses of the femoral cortex are to be by-passed. The extra length of some 2 cm appears to be adequate, though in some cases use of a longer stem may be indicated.

Extended neck stems are essential in cases where loss of the femoral neck is the problem. It must be remembered that such stems have a reduced offset and an increased neck–shaft angle. The increase in the length of the extra-medullary portion of the stem may lead to a higher incidence of post-operative dislocation.

Use of the modular stem for proximal femoral replacement is discussed in Chap. 24.

A modified stem–Kuntscher nail combination for the treatment of fractures of the femoral shaft in association with a loose stem is discussed in Chap. 15.

21 Revision Surgery: The Technique

Introduction

Revision surgery can be looked upon as a philosophy, as a state of mind which demands a detailed, methodical approach to a mechanical problem. A cavalier attitude, exploration through a limited exposure or a "laparotomy-type" look, see and deal accordingly approach have nothing to commend them and will only lead to problems. Each case presents problems which can be unique. Knowledge of those problems and their sequential solution are the secret of success. At surgery, lack of progress for whatever reason has a peculiar, very frustrating and dangerous "knock-on effect" and must be avoided at all cost.

By the time the patient is on the operating table the diagnosis would have been established and the details of treatment decided upon. It is the author's practice to discuss briefly with the theatre sister and staff the various steps to be taken during the operation, any likely problems that may be encountered, special instruments or prostheses that may be needed, likely delays (i.e. with the femoral cement) or posssible decisions (i.e. whether revision or pseudarthrosis should be performed). If the suspicion is of deep sepsis then obviously various antibiotics must be prepared and their sequential use noted. In such cases it is nice to clear all clean packs, trolleys etc. from the theatre area.

The theatre sister must be aware where the various items are stored and must instruct the circulating nurse accordingly. Delays here lead to frustration and loss of time and concentration during a procedure which at times is a "one-man show"; few people will have the opportunity to see or be actively involved in extraction of the femoral cement. In short, a brief discussion of the proposed operative procedure while viewing the radiographs (AP and lateral) will make everybody more at ease. The second assistant, the leg holder, must be made aware of any problems likely to be encountered at mobilization, dislocation or preparation of the femur.

Positioning the Patient

The patient's skin will already have been prepared on the ward and again in the anaesthetic room. Before this is done the opportunity should be taken to check the patient's notes and the relevant details which are of interest. These may include the patient's age, the assessment chart, erythrocyte sedimentation rate (ESR), the result of any special investigation or a clear statement of the patient's wishes, i.e. a one-stage revision at all cost, or only one more operative procedure, which may in fact tip the scale towards pseudarthrosis. A further personal contact with the patient, however brief, before the general anaesthesia, will go a long way to creating a relationship.

At this stage, the patient should be positioned, with help, the way you wish to have

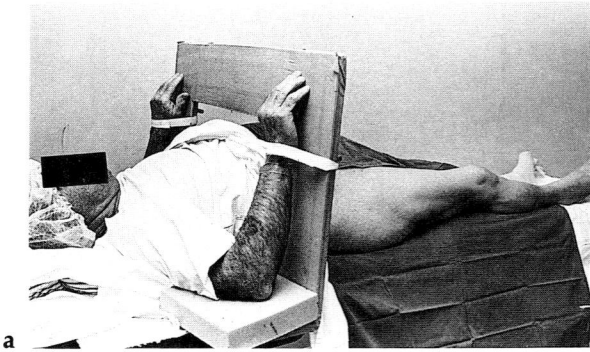

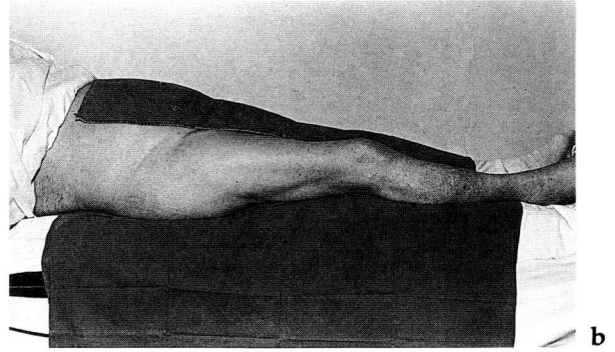

Fig. 21.1 a, b. Positioning of the patient on the Charnley operating table. The patient is positioned parallel to the edge of the table, without overhang of the buttock or adduction of the hip.

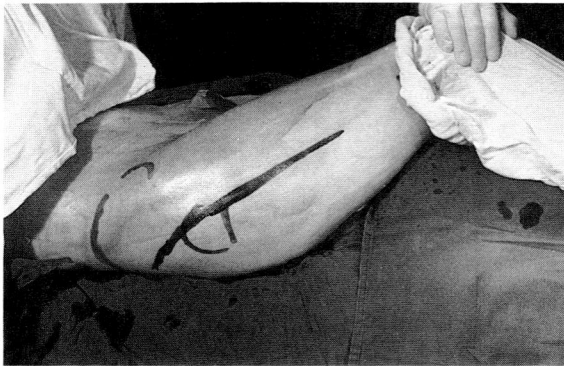

Fig. 21.2. The skin incision. The skin has been prepared with Betadine antiseptic solution. The iliac crest, the anterior superior iliac spine, the greater trochanter and the vastus lateralis ridge have been marked for demonstration purposes only. The incision is from mid-thigh to some 4–5 cm proximal to the line of the anterior superior iliac spine.

them at surgery. Attempting to drag the anaesthetized patient across the table is not much good for the back, the patient's or your own. A supine position and lateral approach are still the best. The patient lies parallel to the edge of the table, level with it and without an overhang of the flesh (Fig. 2l.1). Adduction of the hip must be avoided as it will result in over-lengthening.

A special soft waterproof mattress is essential. Pressure points will be far less likely as a result of what after all is a longer procedure.

The Incision

The patient should be covered by drapes from the rib cage to just above the knee, with the perineum carefully isolated. A transparent plastic drape over the incised stockinette will give a view of scars from previous surgery so that the incision can be planned accordingly. A plastic bag is attached with adhesive below the most dependent part of the hip. This will be used to collect all the washings from the operative site to avoid wetting the drapes and the surgeon's gown. A waterproof plastic drape is fixed to the front of the surgeon's gown to avoid it getting wet and thus contaminated. Suction is not used by the author. The suction tip is readily contaminated and it makes the wound act as a slit sampler by sucking air into it.

With the hip flexed, some 20° adducted and internally rotated by the second assistant (the leg holder) the fleshy thigh and the buttock will fall away posteriorly and allow easier access to the thigh.

The ideal incision gives the benefit of anterior, lateral transtrochanteric and posterior approaches. It is for that reason that the author favours a straight lateral incision, slightly in front of the line of the femur as far as the front of the greater trochanter then curving quite sharply (some 30°) posteriorly and extending some 4–5 cm past the vertical drawn down from the anterior superior iliac spine (Fig. 21.2). The skin incision usually measures about 30 cm.

Scars from previous surgery will have to be noted and the incision modified accordingly. Parts or all of the previous incision may be used, but the new incision should err on the more posterior aspect which will give better access to

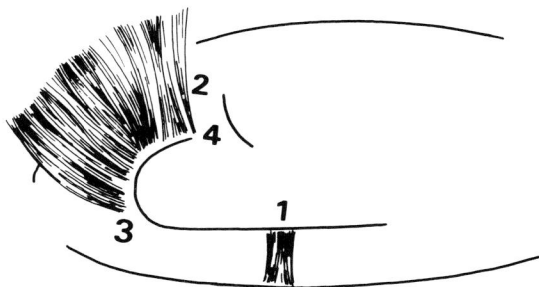

Fig. 21.3. The landmarks at hip exposure. Diagrammatic representation of various points of reference to be looked for routinely at the exposure of the hip joint (right). *1*, insertion of gluteus maximus; *2*, anterior border of the abductor mass; *3*, superior aspect of the greater trochanter and the piriform fossa; *4*, the neck of the stem.

the area above and behind the greater trochanter, and to the socket. To make the incision too anteriorly will create difficulties when delivering the proximal femur out of the wound over the posterior flap of the incision. This may not be a problem in a slim patient but will be a struggle in an obese one.

Incision in the Deep Fascia

The distal extension of the skin incision will depend on the extent to which the femoral shaft needs to be exposed, but will always be distal to the scar of the previous longest incision. This will allow the isolation of the intact fascia lata so that a small incision may be made in it. An index finger may be then be inserted and a sweep can be made proximally and distally deep to the fascia. This will identify the plane and allow extension of the fascial incision proximally; the anterior and posterior flaps which will have to be sutured at the end of the operation can then be carefully isolated. If the fleshy fibres of the tensor fascia lata are encountered anteriorly brisk bleeding will occur; this indicates that the fascial incision is too anterior and a change in direction is therefore needed.

Excision of the old scars does not seem to be essential unless they are in such a position (adherent to the greater trochanter) or so broad and avascular as to make future healing doubtful. Primary skin closure is obviously essential, so skin should not be excised at the outset; any decision to do so should be left until the end of the operation.

A sinus, if present at the incision site, should be excised together with its deep extension; this is always easier in theory than practice. Injection of the sinus may help in identifying some of its ramifications.

The Landmarks

There are four landmarks which are invaluable in cases of revision, more so where the anatomy is grossly distorted. They must be looked for deliberately and identified, no matter how routine the case may be. They are shown in Fig. 21.3 and described here.

1. *The insertion of the gluteus maximus posteriorly.* It indicates that the correct level of the proximal femur has been exposed. The distance from the insertion to the edge of the posterior fascial flap should be some 2–3 cm. If it is more then the incision is too anterior.

2. *Anterior border of the abductor mass.* It may not be particularly fleshy if damaged by previous surgery. The anterior blade of the initial incision retractor will be placed just distal to it after elevation of the trochanteric bursa and the fibrous tissue layer off the anterior part of the abductor mass.

3. *The superior and the posterior part of the greater trochanter.* A gentle sweep of the hand above and behind the greater trochanter at primary surgery will give this part of the exposure so that tissue planes can be easily separated. In cases of revision this may not be easy. Adhesions posteriorly make it difficult, and if trochanteric wires are present then it is easy for the surgeon to puncture his gloves. This part of the exposure may not be fully completed until the Charnley initial incision retractor is put in. Once in place this will put soft and scar tissues under tension and allow their release to get the desired access. Posterior access may be particularly difficult if a posterior approach has been used previously or if tissue is grossly scarred from repeated surgery. Gentle pressure with a sharp osteotome proximally and parallel with the shaft of the femur will allow full exposure and avoid damaging the surgeons gloves. The anatomy of the trochanteric bursa may not be easy to make out in revisions.

4. *The neck of the stem, medially.* If trochanteric osteotomy has been part of the primary surgery then the wires should be removed before pro-

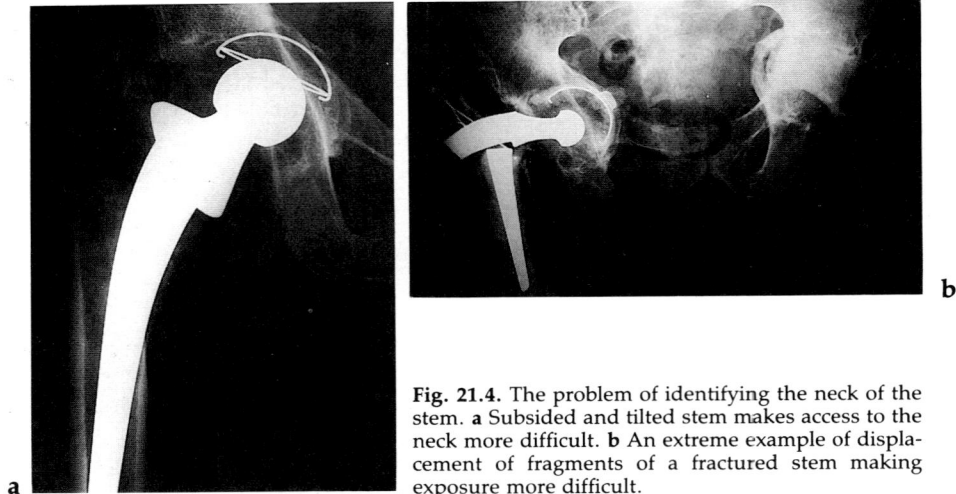

Fig. 21.4. The problem of identifying the neck of the stem. **a** Subsided and tilted stem makes access to the neck more difficult. **b** An extreme example of displacement of fragments of a fractured stem making exposure more difficult.

ceeding with exposure of the neck of the stem. This is best achieved by sharp dissection medially to the anterior border of the abductors. Part of the capsule may have to be deliberately excised. This is usually followed by a small gush of joint fluid (or pus). The metal of the neck of the stem can usually be felt with the tip of the cholecystectomy forceps rather than seen as the capsule is invariably thick. This capsule can be stretched by inserting the cholecystectomy forceps above and below the neck and levering upwards and downwards.

It must be remembered that in cases of gross stem subsidence, the neck of the stem will be very much lower than normal, while with a high fracture of the stem the neck and the proximal fragment may lie transversely to the femoral shaft (Fig. 21.4).

Removal of the Trochanteric Wires

The following instruments are required: a sharp bone hook, Charnley wire holding forceps and the dual-purpose wire cutter–pullers.

At this stage a brief glance at the radiograph will give some indication as to the method of trochanteric reattachment used as well as the number of wires and their likely position, best judged by the number of twisted ends seen on the radiograph. At the time of exposure the wires may be obvious either because they are prominent or because a small fluid-filled bursa surrounds them. If none of the above are of help then palpation over the greater trochanter may give some indication as to their whereabouts. In some cases, usually if the no. 20 SWG wires have been used and some new bone formation is present, they may be completely overgrown by bone and must be deliberately exposed with an osteotome; the easiest wire, i.e. the double wire loop, should be aimed for, distal to the vastus lateralis ridge.

One other very useful method is to use the cutting diathermy needle and divide all the soft tissues as in preparation for the trochanteric osteotomy. Contact of the diathermy needle with the wire will produce a visible spark and an audible crack. The same method may be used cutting the soft tissues over the most prominent part of the trochanter in line with the shaft of the femur until the wires are identified. Care must be taken not to dissect all the abductors off the greater trochanter.

Failing all these methods the wires may have to be disregarded; the Gigli saw or the osteotome will identify them eventually. However, this must be the last resort in cases where wire fragments are present within the bone. The result will be a rather poor osteotomy, a broken Gigli saw and possibly a fragmented trochanter.

Having identified the wires the free ends are held using the wire-holding forceps while the wire strands are elevated away from the bone with the sharp hook. Once the position and number of the wires have been identified the decision is made about which wires are to be removed first and in which direction they are most likely to come out. Thus the wire placed last at reattachment should be the first one to be removed. It seems too obvious to state that kinked, tangled or twisted wires will not run smoothly through the bone and cement, neither will the loop of the double wires. There are two methods of extracting the wires once they have been identified: the "claw hammer" method and the "sardine-can" method.

The Claw Hammer Method

For this dual-purpose wire cutter–puller is ideal. The free end of the wire to be extracted is grasped close to the bone with the blunt side of the cutter–puller and using levering actions is gradually eased out of the bone. Levering is best done against the sturdier shaft of the femur rather than against a porotic trochanter which can be easily fragmented. This is the ideal method for the majority of cases.

The Sardine-Can Method

As the name implies the free end of the protruding wire is grasped with the wire-holding forceps held close to the bone at right angles to the strand. The forceps are locked and then twisted by the handles. By levering against the bone the wire is pulled out and twisted round the jaws of the forceps. This method is best used for short fragments or where access with the cutter–puller is difficult.

Exposure of the Hip Joint

Although there is debate about whether or not trochanteric osteotomy needs to be routinely carried out at primary total hip arthroplasty, the general consensus is that for most, if not all, revision cases, it is essential.

A fair number of technical problems can arise from an inadequate exposure and this aspect is discussed in Chap. 3. Correct exposure is the most important aspect of any revision. It is beyond doubt that, combined with a proper skin and fascial incision, trochanteric osteotomy gives the best possible exposure. Until this is obtained the operation cannot proceed. There have never been any reports to contradict this. Any method which advocates femoral guttering or splitting in order to avoid trochanteric osteotomy is to be viewed with suspicion; it suggests that the point of the revision work in general and of the stem fixation in particular has not been understood.

The argument will no doubt be finally settled when the treatment is replaced by some procedure where skin and fascial incision as well as trochanteric osteotomy become obsolete. Until such time the author offers no excuses for adhering to the method which has given the best possible exposure over the past 20 years and over 5000 low-friction arthroplasties including over 1200 revisions.

Trochanteric Osteotomy

Unlike the situation at primary surgery, the normal neck–greater trochanter junction is absent and so the natural starting point for the Gigli saw is absent. Furthermore, with a subsided or a fractured stem the lateral side of the femur can easily be taken off together with the greater trochanter. This immediately creates three problems:

1. The trochanteric fragment is very big and therefore its viability may be in doubt.
2. Central positioning of the stem within the medullary canal is difficult and the tendency is for the stem to be placed in a varus position with poor medial support.
3. The back of the stem will encroach on the trochanteric bed making reattachment of the trochanter difficult.

In order to retain the advantages of trochanteric osteotomy while increasing the chances of union, the author has introduced a method of cutting a biplane osteotomy with a Gigli saw (Wroblewski and Shelley 1985). The method is based on the work by Debeyre and Duliveux (1954) and more recently by Weber and Stuhmer (1979).

The Method

The trochanteric bursa, if present, must be elevated proximally over the abductor mass. To fail

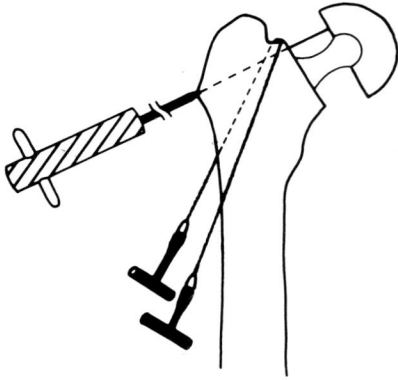

Fig. 21.5. Trochanteric osteotomy. Note the position of the spike and the direction of cut made with the Gigli saw.

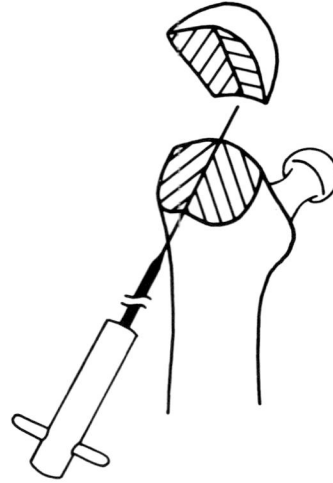

Fig. 21.6. Trochanteric osteotomy completed. Note the position of the spike at the completion of the osteotomy.

to do this is to fail to expose the trochanter and puts the sciatic nerve at risk.

With a hand behind and above the trochanter the size, shape and position of the greater trochanter can be judged. The front of the capsule is opened with the cutting diathermy needle and the neck of the femoral prosthesis identified with the tip of the cholecystectomy forceps. A spike, actually a 4-mm Steinmann pin on a 'T' handle, is hammered in just below the level of the vastus lateralis ridge, mid-way antero-posteriorly, at an angle of some 45° to the shaft of the femur medially and proximally. It emerges somewhere in the capsule at the margin of the pelvis and often rests on the rim of the socket (Fig. 21.5). Cholecystectomy forceps are then inserted over the neck of the stem and the curved tip used to search out the spike. The metal-to-metal contact is easily appreciated. The curved portion of the forceps is then brought over the pin by forcing its handle cranially then posteriorly until it pierces the capsule posteriorly and emerges close to the femoral shaft; care must be taken to avoid picking up soft tissues posteriorly.

In order to check that the cholecystectomy forceps are in the correct position, i.e. proximal to the spike, a simple check can be carried out, using the friction of metal-to-metal contact between the spike and the forceps. While one hand barely touches the handles of the forceps the other hand gently rotates the handle of the spike through some 20°, first clockwise then

anti-clockwise. This manoeuvre will tend to move the cholecystectomy forceps up or down, depending on whether it is the right or the left hip being operated upon. Turning the cholecystectomy forceps laterally, the sharp points will pierce the capsule and emerge close to the shaft of the femur.

The Gigli saw is mounted and brought out anteriorly. The positions of the Gigli saw and the soft tissues between the saw and the back of the greater trochanter are closely inspected to make sure that the sciatic nerve has not been accidentally picked up. A light touch of the saw on the diathermy needle will soon alert the surgeon to possible danger.

With the hip flexed, abducted, internally rotated and held in position by the second assistant, the osteotomy is cut with the Gigli saw. Rhythmic, gentle and unhurried movements alternately cutting at the back and the front will ensure a good trochanteric fragment. The direction of the cuts is along the shaft of the femur, towards the knee. The Gigli saw will strike the spike and cut in front of and behind it, giving a biplane osteotomy, with the spike on the femoral side at the summit of the osteotomy (Fig. 21.6). Since the femoral head and neck are absent, and the trochanter itself may be of poor quality, the spike may not hold very well and may suddenly come out as the osteotomy is completed. To avoid the possibility of the surgeon being struck by the spike, the handle should be held by the assistant.

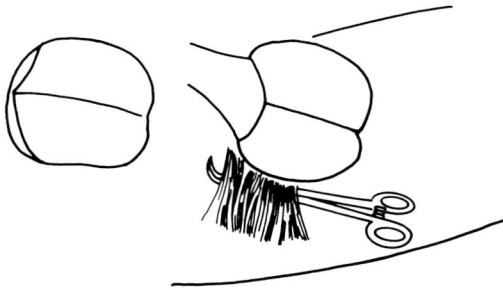

Fig. 21.7. Mobilization of the proximal part of the femur. Diagrammatic representation of the method of mobilizing the proximal femur.

It is advantageous at this stage to mobilize the greater trochanter by dividing the external rotators and part of the capsule. This is easily done with the cutting diathermy needle while tension is maintained by holding the trochanter with the sharp bone hook.

Unlike in primary surgery a truly intracapsular osteotomy cannot always be performed in revision cases; part of the capsule will usually remain attached to the femur preventing a full view of the neck of the stem. The proximal femur must be deliberately mobilized circumferentially.

Mobilization of the Proximal Part of the Femur

This must be done carefully and systematically, always cutting close to the femur. As the first step any remains of the lateral capsule should be excised with cutting diathermy to expose the neck of the stem. This allows the next stage to be carried out with confidence.

With the hip internally rotated, cholecystectomy forceps are used to pick up the tough fibrous tissue and any remaining external rotators at the back of the femur, from distal to proximal. These are then divided close to the femur (Fig. 21.7). Cutting diathermy is used to divide the soft tissue close to the femur. This is done in stages each of which shouldn't be too ambitious. The procedure is repeated laterally, anteriorly and medially until the hand can be placed round the upper end of the femur. Part of the capsule is invariably excised during the exposure. The neck of the stem having been exposed, the remaining part of the capsule is

opened to free the head of the femoral component and allow dislocation.

Dislocation

Dislocation of the hip as in primary surgery, carried out by adduction of the femur by the leg holder, does not usually occur, nor should it be attempted. Levering or rotation is likely to lead to problems. A loose stem acts as an excellent stress riser and may lead to femoral fracture. The medial femoral cortex, which is often shell-like, can easily be avulsed unless that part of the femur has been properly mobilized. With a dislocating hook round the neck of the stem gentle lateral movements are made and traction is applied by the surgeon until the head of the femoral component is brought out of the socket and onto its rim, or at times, just past it. This manoeuvre will place the remaining fibrous tissue, and at times the psoas tendon, under tension and facilitate their division with cutting diathermy. Only when the surgeon can put his hand freely round the head and neck of the stem and the proximal femur should the femur be brought away from the pelvis; this should only be carried out by the surgeon. Before this can be fully achieved the psoas tendon may have to be divided. The stem, even if fractured or grossly loose, should not be removed in a hurry; it serves as a useful lever while mobilizing the proximal femur and bringing it away from the pelvis and out of the wound.

Trochanteric Non-union

Without Trochanteric Migration. The trochanteric fragment is usually of adequate size, the abductors of good quality and the trochanteric wires invariably fragmented. As many of the wires as possible must be removed, some before exploration of the non-union, some after. Tough tissue resembling fibro-cartilage identifies the site of the previous osteotomy. The dissection can then proceed proximally using scalpel and cutting diathermy, or even a sharp osteotome, until the trochanter is fully mobilized. Wire fragments are often found at this stage.

The size and the shape of the greater trochanter have already been determined and everything must be done to preserve its integrity and that of the abductors attached to it.

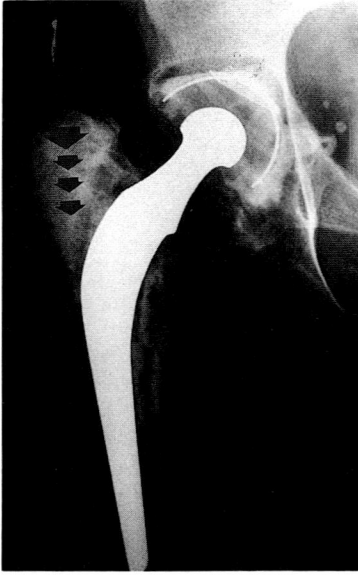

Fig. 21.8. Stem extraction. Although the stem (and the socket) are grossly loose, the cement lateral to the curved proximal part of the stem must first be removed before attempting extraction of the stem. (In this case all the greater trochanter is packed with cement, but note how little of it is present medially).

With Trochanteric Migration. In this case, what is left of the greater trochanter is usually no more than a shell, often identified better radiologically than at the time of surgery, and the abductors are often no more than a mass of fibrous tissue. No attempt should be made to isolate the greater trochanter. It is unlikely that such a trochanter can be brought down into its bed, and it is probably best not to attempt to do so. The fibrous tissues, what is left of the abductor mass, and the trochanteric remnant are isolated by sharp dissection. Nothing is excised, no matter how redundant it may appear, since it will all be useful when it comes to closure.

If the trochanteric fragment is of adequate size then it can be mobilized and dealt with as if there had not been trochanteric migration, but over-ambitious mobilization must not leave the trochanteric fragment isolated.

Complete Absence of the Abductor Mass. Very occasionally on opening the deep fascia the surgeon is presented with a defect where the greater trochanter and the abductors should have been. (This unfortunately is an increasingly common finding because of exposures which pay no respect to the abductors.) The next structure to appear is the neck of the stem and the smoothed-off lateral side of the femur, or even the lateral side of the upper end of the stem. Little can be done to correct the situation although at times some fibrous tissue may be developed by dissection from the abductor area.

Examination of the Components

The Stem

The position of the stem with respect to varus/ valgus orientation will already have been decided from examination of the radiographs.

With the proximal femur fully mobilized and the hip dislocated, the shaft of the femur is positioned horizontally over the opposite thigh while the tibia is vertical. With the head-on view from the surgeon's position, the anteversion–retroversion of the stem can be assessed. The exact orientation of the stem is much more obvious once it has been removed so that the direction of the cement tract can be observed.

Testing of the Stem for Loosening. It must be accepted that any method of testing the stem for loosening at surgery is unlikely to be a reflection of everyday use when the load on the hip can be several times the body weight. It is doubtful if any one of us would be prepared to use such force to test the integrity of the stem fixation at primary surgery, let alone at revision surgery. The very design of the stem and its method of insertion usually allow it to be easily extracted from the cement taper or jammed in by hammering. The soft tissues must be dissected off the sectioned part of the femoral neck to reveal the cement and the stem which can then be tested by a pulling–pushing or rocking movement; any movement at either the stem–cement or the cement–bone junctions should be noted. Being partly extrafemoral the stem may be easily inspected. The decision about whether or not the stem should be changed has usually been made before the operation. However, surprises do occur. If the decision has been made not to change the stem then the plastic protector should be put on early so as not to damage its highly polished head.

Extraction of the Stem. If the decision has been made to change the stem then it should be removed without delay so that the socket can be attended to. It must be remembered that the stem was inserted directly in the line of the femur, before the cement had set. This is therefore the way the stem will have to come out, but the cement on its lateral aspect will prevent this. This portion of the cement is well fixed, as it has never been subjected to load. All of the cement from the lateral aspect must therefore be cleared with gouges (Fig. 21.8). (Failure to do this may burst the proximal femur when the stem is being knocked out.) The jaws of the stem extractor are then engaged round the medial side of the neck. The shaft of the extractor is held in the line of the shaft of the femur and a sliding hammer is used to knock the stem out. The elasticity of any fibrous tissue left at the sectioned femoral neck will tend to hold the stem and make the extraction more difficult; it should therefore be removed at an earlier stage.

The Socket

Exposure. The socket at this stage may be completely hidden from view and its position can be quickly established by feeling the socket bore with a finger. To get full exposure most of the synovium and some of the capsule will have to be excised until at least the area of the superior margin of the acetabulum is exposed.

The Charnley pin retractor is hammered in transversely and above what is estimated to be the roof of the acetabulum. (The position of the pin may have to be changed later if it proves to be too low and intruding into the acetabular cavity.)

The Charnley east–west (E–W) retractor is used next, one jaw resting on the pin retractor, the other on the lesser trochanter. As the E–W retractor is opened the pin retractor will protect the abductor mass and ensure that the area of the exposure is as full as possible by moving the femoral shaft distally. No attempt should be made to get full exposure at this stage; as the operation proceeds the tension on the E–W retractor can be gradually increased if need be.

Most of the synovium and some of the capsule will have to be excised using cutting diathermy. The anterior and the posterior parts are left intact. The former protects the femoral triangle and its contents, more so when the anterior acetabular wall is deficient; the latter protects the sciatic nerve.

A dry swab is folded and placed over the postero-inferior part of the capsule, between the rim of the acetabulum and the lesser trochanter. It will further protect the sciatic nerve from the jaws of the north–south (N–S) retractor which are placed onto it and onto the antero-superior part of the capsule. A swab moistened with Betadine solution is placed over the vastus muscle mass to prevent it from drying, and a further one is placed into the medullary canal and the cement tract in cases of deep sepsis.

With all the retractors in place any soft tissue preventing exposure of the socket is now excised; histology and bacteriology specimens should be collected at this stage as indicated.

The socket is inaccessible at the best of times and will be even more so when it has migrated, especially medially. In order to get a better view of the socket for the purposes of examination or extraction, the superior acetabular rim (often no more than a thin shell of bone) may have to be removed. This is best done with the biggest of the Charnley gouges. The same manoeuvre may have to be used over the ischial part of the acetabulum in order to expose the posterior part of the socket. If a flange is present then obviously this will have to be excised.

Examination of the Socket. The anteversion–retroversion orientation of the socket can be readily assessed, if need be, by aligning the socket holder against its face, the angle open laterally having been estimated from the radiographs. The appearance of the bore of the socket is noted. The area of wear and the ridge demarcating the high wear from the low wear areas can be felt with the finger if the socket has worn to any degree. Inclusion of cement in the socket bore can be easily seen. Any abnormality on the rim of the socket bore is noted, e.g. an erosion indicating recurrent subluxation or dislocation or a smooth, shiny area indicating impingement anteriorly.

The bone–cement junction must be examined carefully over as large an area as possible. This is obviously important where doubt exists as to whether or not the socket will have to be changed. In cases of socket migration the diagnosis is made from study of serial radiographs. Examination at surgery will confirm the diagnosis. The inferior part of the acetabular cavity offers the most useful information and should be examined routinely; this part being most dependent, wear debris, cement particles and granuloma readily collect.

The appearance of a fine, velvety, pale grey–blue granulation (pyogenic) tissue usually indicates that there is more behind the socket. If this

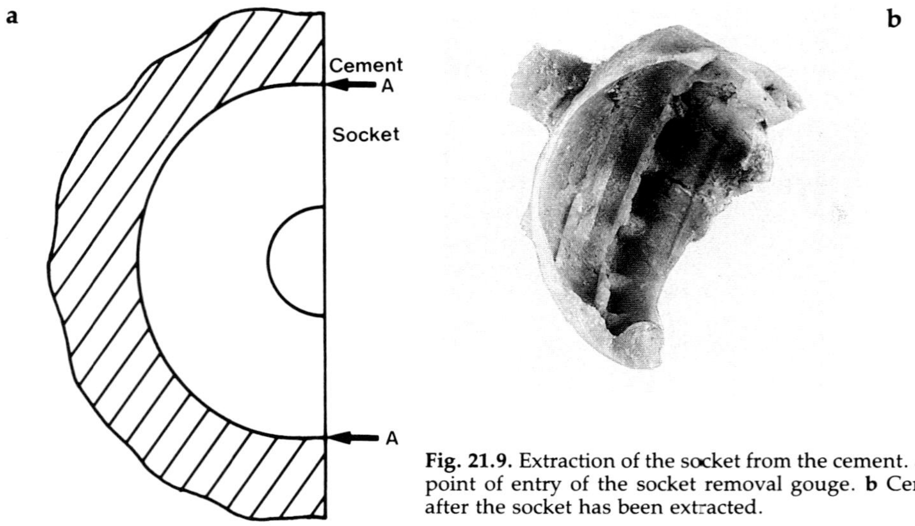

a

Cement
A
Socket
A

b

Fig. 21.9. Extraction of the socket from the cement. **a** A–A, the point of entry of the socket removal gouge. **b** Cement shell after the socket has been extracted.

tissue is dry, fibrous and grey in appearance the problem is probably mechanical loosening. It is usually heavily metal-stained in cases of a fractured stem.

Testing of the Socket for Loosening. The socket is not readily accessible to examination for loosening the way the stem is. Having exposed and examined the socket bore and face and the bone–cement junction a custom-made bone screw on a T-handle is fixed into one of the holes used for the socket introducer. If no such hole is present then it can be drilled without damaging the socket bore. With the screw firmly fixed into the face of the socket gentle pulling–pushing and rocking movements are applied to the handle while the bone–cement junction is observed. Gentle rotatory movements will give more information. Forceful pushing and pulling will produce an elastic recoil of the body, masking any movement of the socket. It must be appreciated that it is possible to deform the plastic shell creating an impression of loosening. If there is a wide demarcation of the superior third of the socket then it can produce the phenomenon of "marginal loosening", the supero-lateral portion of the socket can be seen to deform and move while the rest does not. Such a socket should be changed, especially in a young patient. Once "bubbling" is seen at the bone–cement junction or a squashing noise heard, the socket is grossly loose.

The method described for testing the socket does not claim to represent a physiological test of

a hip under load. Its value rests with its uniformity and reproducibility. With routine use of the method both at primary and revision surgery the surgeon will soon develop a feel for the various "grades" of quality of socket fixation.

Extraction of the Socket. Once the decision has been made to extract the socket there is no going back. If the socket which is about to be removed is to be examined in detail, then it is essential that its orientation within the body is noted. The author's routine is to mark the lateral part of the socket face with a narrow gauge, the anterior part with a scalpel. Unless some such marking method is used, knowledge of the socket site and orientation is soon lost. Sectioning the socket may allow its easy removal but valuable information will be lost.

It must be remembered that while a loose socket is not synonymous with its easy extraction, a prolapsed socket may come out surprisingly easily. Before attempting extraction of the socket, it is important to glance at the radiograph and check for cement distribution, anchoring pegs and extension of cement into the pelvis.

The principles of femoral cement removal apply equally to the socket. The objective is to extract the socket from the cement and then to remove the cement piecemeal. For the purpose of socket extraction the curved socket gauge is invaluable. It is introduced at the junction of the socket and the cement using gentle hammer blows and *always* following the contour of the socket (Fig. 21.9). Once this has been done over the whole body of the socket, gentle rotation can be applied to the fully engaged socket gauge. To use levering at the bone–cement junction with such an instrument as the Watson–Jones gauge is to court disaster, a fracture of the anterior acetabular wall being the likely result. Once the socket has been extracted from the cement, the cement itself can be removed by breaking it into smaller portions and extracting them individually.

Having removed the socket and the cement a careful search should be made for cemented pegs and extrusions.

Extraction of Cement Anchoring Pegs and Extrusions. Unfortunately, radiolucent cement is still being used. The reason for this is not apparent. What is obvious is that revision of cases in which it has been used may be difficult due to extrusion of the cement into the pelvis. The extent of the extrusion cannot be judged except after extraction of the socket and the cement.

Fortunately the majority of cement pegs, their bases having fractured, come out quite easily. For the more stubborn ones gouges may have to be used gently around them before they will come out. Extension of the cement pegs into the pelvis invariably results in mushrooming which makes their removal difficult or even dangerous. In cases of deep sepsis logic dictates that all cement be removed, but at other times the surgeon may have to use his own discretion.

The quickest, easiest and safest method of removing any cement extrusions is by gradually enlarging the defect through which the cement has escaped. This can be done with gouges or a curette. Once the cement can be grasped with the Kocher forceps it can be rocked and rotated gently, for it is the soft tissues that hold the cement. Once the mass of the extruded cement can be spun round several times it will come out without much difficulty. There are situations, however, when any cement extruded into the pelvis is best left alone, except in cases of deep sepsis. The defect thus left will obviously have to be covered with Ortron wire mesh before the new socket is cemented in place.

Exposure and Examination of the Acetabular Cavity

At revision, as in primary surgery, the whole of the acetabulum should be exposed from the tear

drop to the superior acetabular margin and from the ischium to the anterior acetabular wall.

Having removed the socket and the cement and fully exposed the acetabular cavity, the latter should be carefully examined to establish its integrity, the quality of the bone stock, any defects and any fibrous or pyogenic granulation tissue. Visual inspection is essential as is palpation. The feel of the fibrous and pyogenic granulation tissue, the remnants of the cement and the defects of the acetabulum is unmistakeable. Good written documentation of the findings at the operation will give a good record for any future reference.

Preparation of the Acetabulum and Fixation of the Socket

Curettage and vigorous brushing will remove most of the fibrous tissue from the acetabulum. Frequent irrigation with a normal saline–Betadine antiseptic solution (10%) will not only help to wash out free fragments but will also help remove granulation tissue which has an appearance not unlike minute sea anemone. Removal of the fragments individually is a tedious process. If the quality of bone is reasonable in the area then most of them can be removed with the Charnley gouges. There is rarely an opportunity to use Charnley acetabular reamers in revision surgery; they may only be used if the socket has been placed superficially leaving a near-normal amount of acetabular bone. "Cheese grater"-type reamers come into their own in revisions, but care must be taken over the medial acetabular wall.

In preparation of the acetabulum advantage must be taken of every bit of good quality bone, be it cancellous or cortical. The first will allow good cement injection, the second may provide an opportunity to drill some anchoring holes.

The acetabular floor itself, especially if defective, should not be relied upon to serve as anything more than a barrier to prevent the escape of cement into the pelvis. Any defects can be covered either with the Charnley acetabular cement restrictor if they are small, or with Ortron wire mesh cut to size and shape if they are large. The most important part of the acetabulum in revision surgery is its rim. If there is disruption of its continuity then a one-stage revision using a cemented socket is unlikely to succeed. If it is intact, and fortunately it usually is, then it can be used to support the socket. It must be stressed that the technique relies on the socket being fixed on the rim and not merely positioned superficially.

Three areas of the acetabulum demand closer attention, the ischium posteriorly, the superior pubic ramus antero-medially and the ilium postero-superiorly. It is in these areas that better quality cancellous bone may be found for cement injection. Cement is injected into the anchor holes, both the deeper ones and those made in the acetabular margin. The medial portion of the cement probably only acts as a bulk filler; often more than 40 g of cement will have to be used. The cement bulk prevents tilting of the socket. With the socket supported on the acetabular rim, the centre of rotation being medial to it, most if not all the load will be transferred onto the acetabular margin. Although the long-term results of this method aren't yet available, it has proved successful in clinical practice for a number of years now.

The Ogee flange of the socket can be trimmed to fit almost any size or shape. Low-viscosity cement is best avoided but if used in revision surgery its pressurization should be carried out with great caution. It easily escapes through defects even if these are covered with Ortron wire mesh. It is also unreasonable to try to inject cement into non-existent cancellous bone. The cement will usually have to be used at a later stage than in primary surgery, and the pressurizer used less vigorously, reliance being placed initially on the digital packing of the anchor holes and later on the force of the flange of the socket as it is placed into its predetermined position. Any excess of cement appearing round the socket flange must be carefully looked for and removed.

It must be accepted that in a fair proportion of revision cases the acetabular component can never be fixed as securely as it can be in primary surgery. This becomes obvious when the revision has been delayed and bone stock is poor. In such cases the cement is really used as a bulk filler. The radiographic appearances cannot be compared with those that can be achieved in primary surgery. The patient must continue with the use of support for ambulation.

The long-term outcome remains uncertain. In this type of revision serious consideration must be given to any method that augments the bone stock. Findings must be carefully documented and the results objectively assessed for the benefit of future patients.

22 Revision with Trochanteric Non-union: Reattachment of the Un-united Trochanter

Introduction

Although much has been written about reattachment of the greater trochanter at primary surgery, little has been said about management of an un-united trochanter. Volz and Brown (1977) published five cases. In each of these they used a bolt to reattach a painful migrated trochanter. They reported that "pain was relieved and disability reduced" but no mention was made of bony union. Bernard and Brooks (1987) reported 16 cases of trochanteric reattachment for established non-union; none achieved bony union. Since bi-planar trochanteric osteotomy followed by reattachment using a double cross-over wire with a compression spring has achieved an acceptable level of success (98.2%) both in primary and revision surgery (Wroblewski and Shelley 1985), a prospective study was carried out using the same method of reattachment in cases with trochanteric non-union. It must be stressed, however, that trochanteric non-union per se is hardly ever an indication for its reattachment; the latter usually forms a part of revision for other reasons.

The Series

The details of the whole group presented here and the comparison with previous results has

Table 22.1. Details of the series of cases of trochanteric non-union treated by double cross-over wire and compression spring fixation

Indication for revision	No. of cases treated	No. of cases with	
		Bony union	Non-union
Infection	25	20	5
Loose stem and/ or socket	12	11	1
Fractured stem	8	5	3
Recurrent dislocation	7	6	1
Total	52	42	10

been published elsewhere (Hodgkinson et al. 1989b). The method was used on 52 patients with an established trochanteric non-union. The trochanter and its bed were carefully prepared: fibrous tissue at the site of non-union was excised and the new trochanteric bed was prepared according to the quality of bone available. Bone grafting was not used. Post-operatively the patients were mobilized after 3 weeks' bed rest. The details of the series are shown in Table 22.1.

Bony union was achieved in 42 cases (81%) (Fig. 22.1). Neither the duration of the non-union nor the separation gap affected the final

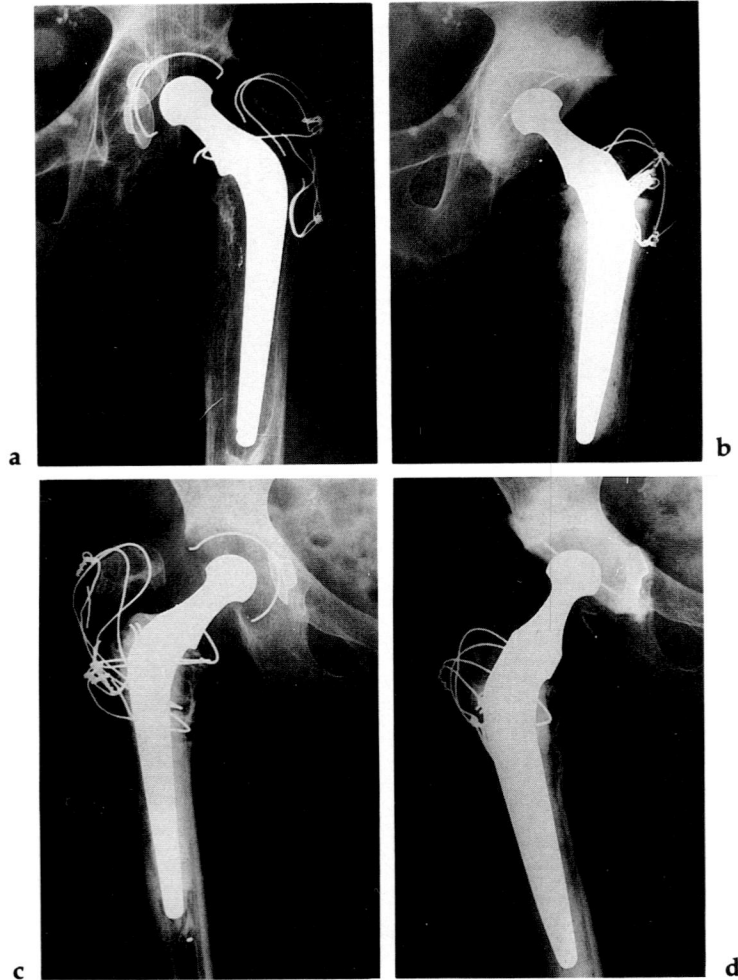

Fig. 22.1. Examples of revision with trochanteric non-union. **a** Trochanteric non-union with loosening of stem and socket. (Loosening of the socket is not obvious because of radiolucent cement. Condensation of the cancellous bone of the medullary canal gives away the secret of the loose stem.) **b** Appearances 2 years after revision. **c** Trochanteric non-union with deep infection and recurrent dislocation. Stem previously revised; socket, with radiolucent cement, was not changed. Cavitation round the wires at the medial femoral cortex indicates sepsis. **d** Two years after revision. The compression spring is partly "covered" by the stem.

result. An observation was also made that intact wires and trochanteric union were always present together, while non-union was always associated with fractured wires. This is in contrast with the experience of Jensen and Harris (1986) who reported 28% wire breakage with union of the greater trochanter. It is likely that the compression spring allows a certain degree of movement yet prevents fracture of the wires and allows bony union.

23 The Femur

Introduction

It must be appreciated that in revision surgery the approach to the femoral side of the procedure, as for other aspects of revision, must follow clearly defined steps. This is necessary to achieve the best possible results for cement removal and stem fixation.

These steps are:

1. Extraction of the femoral component.
2. Removal of the acrylic cement.
3. Removal of fibrous or pyogenic granulation tissue from the bone–cement junction.
4. Removal of a thin layer of condensed cancellous bone.
5. Excavation of the lesser trochanter and stem insertion.
6. Selection of a femoral stem and trial reduction.
7. Distal closure of the medullary canal.

Before attempting a revision it is essential that good-quality radiographs are available showing the whole of the femoral implant and the cement. Antero-posterior and lateral views will give some idea of the position of the stem and the cement distribution and may also at times save embarrassment.

If the cement used was radiolucent, the femur should be palpated carefully, both before the revision and then through the muscle at the time of exposure.

Extraction of the Femoral Component

This aspect of revision has already been dealt with. It is essential however to stress once again that before attempting to extract the stem the soft tissue from around the base of the neck of the stem should be carefully excised and the cement should be removed from above the curved portion of the stem. This having been done the stem extractor with its sliding hammer can be used.

Removal of the Acrylic Cement

At primary surgery it is necessary to achieve good cement injection. At revision extraction of the femoral cement can be the most difficult and frustrating part of the operation unless it is tackled systematically and patiently. Extraction of all of the cement or the stem–cement complex is unusual, except in cases of gross loosening which is usually the result of sepsis of longstanding (Fig. 23.1). In the early stages of the evolution of revision surgery where cases of deep sepsis were tackled late, it was on occasions possible to extract the cement "en masse" with a tapered screw and sliding hammer, but only if the cement was loose and well distributed enough to allow the screw to bite. With time, as revisions were undertaken earlier, this method was abandoned.

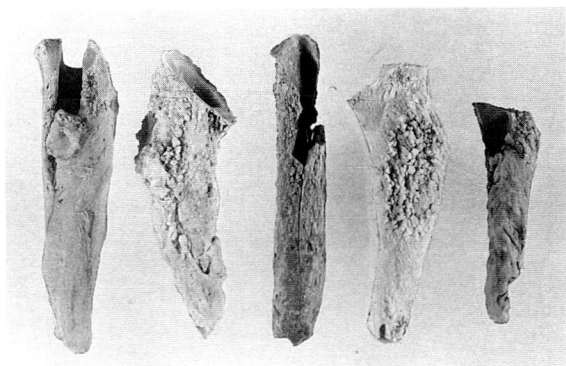

Fig. 23.1. Specimens of femoral acrylic cement removed "en masse" using tapered screw and a sliding hammer.

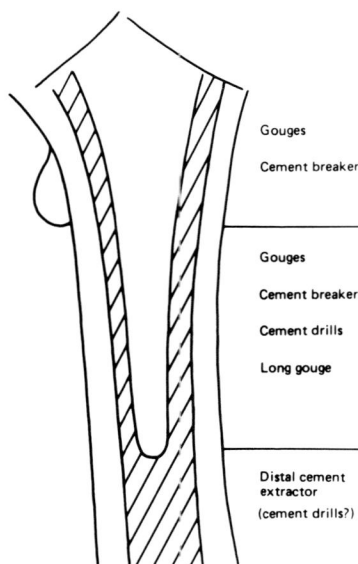

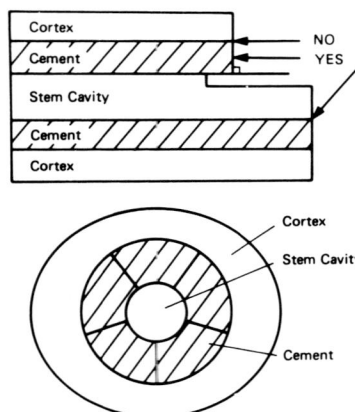

Fig. 23.2. Removal of femoral cement: principles. **a** Consider the problem at three levels: proximal, middle and distal. Each one demands a slightly different approach. **b** Fragment the cement mantle within the medullary canal. Avoid entry into the bone cement space until the cement is fragmented. When fragmenting the cement use gouges at the steepest possible angle. Fragment cement mantle radially then collapse it inwards.

The principle of femoral cement extraction relies on good exposure, illumination and fragmentation of the cement mantle within the medullary canal. Until the latter has been done no attempt should be made to insert instruments between the cement and bone. To do so is to court disaster since the femoral cortex is likely to be penetrated.

For practical purposes the femoral cement can be described as being in three parts, the proximal, the middle and the distal parts. Each one demands a somewhat different approach.

The Proximal Part

This includes the cement within the neck of the femur down to the lesser trochanter. With trochanteric osteotomy the view is excellent. The cement is usually abundant and is often well injected laterally. The cancellous bone may be non-existent, the cortex thin and the trochanteric bed in danger of being disrupted. A no. 1 gauge is used to thin out and fragment the cement starting at its weakest part. Only when this has been done or when the cement layer is relatively thin should the cement breaker be used. The rather obtuse 30° cutting edge of the cement breaker is designed to split the cement without jamming. It is used to cut the cement mantle radially (Fig. 23.2). When this has been done the gauges can be used between the cement fragments and the femoral cortex (Fig. 23.2). The light conical mallet allows rapid, repetitive and untiring action. Only when all the proximal cement has been removed should the middle portion of the cement be tackled.

The Middle Part

This part of the cement extends from the lesser trochanter to the tip of the stem. It is less well seen and usually better injected than the proximal part. The femoral cortex at this level may or may not be of good quality. (It usually is good in cases of fracture of the stem but not so good in

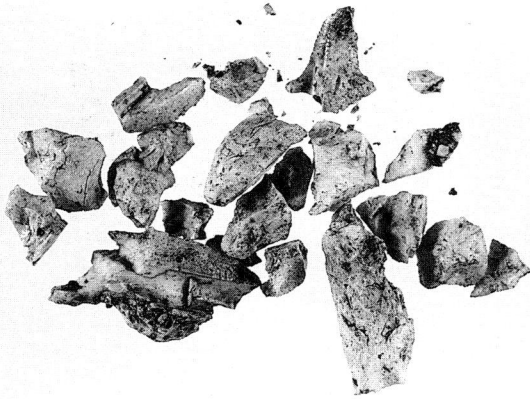

Fig. 23.3. Methodical removal of the femoral cement. Multiple small fragments to show the progress made.

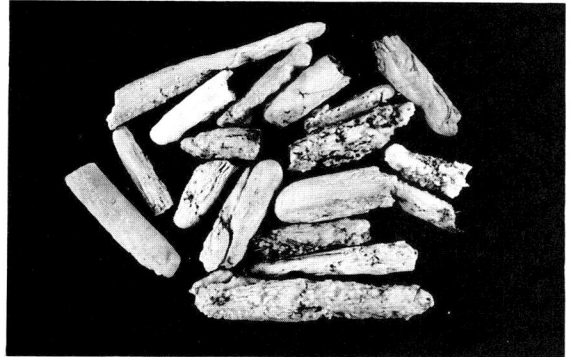

Fig. 23.4. Distal femoral cement extraction. Examples of distal femoral cement plugs extracted with the extractor.

cases of gross loosening of some standing.) The objective once again is to break the circumferential continuity of the cement. Here the cement breaker is used. Radial cuts are made at the weakest part of the cement mantle. If the cement layer is thick then it can be broken up with no. 2, 3 or 4 gauges used at as steep an angle to the femoral shaft as possible (Fig. 23.2).

Frequent irrigation is essential to remove free cement particles and to show clearly the cement crescent to be cut into. As the continuity of the cement is gradually broken up gouges can be used cautiously between the cement fragments and the cortex. Progress need not be slow if the whole procedure is carried out methodically. If the femoral cortex is of good quality then cement drills can be used with confidence. They are meant to be used to break the circumferential continuity of the cement and *not* to drill out all the cement. Being end and side cutters, they will tend to progress distally rapidly, especially if pressure is applied. They are not directed by a guide or a jig, and as they are self-seeking within the stem tract they will cut through the cement offering least resistance. It is for these reasons that they must be used in 1-mm diameter increments on a short offset brace. They must be used gently and not with force, starting with the smallest drill and cutting from distal to proximal, the parallel cutting edge cutting within the taper of the cement mantle. During this stage of the procedure copious irrigation and frequent visual checks of the progress are essential.

Once the continuity of the cement mantle has been broken, usually somewhere around the 13-mm diameter drill, the cement breaker and the gauges can be used. Free cement fragments can be lifted out with the cement-grasping forceps. Removal of small individual fragments still adherent to bone can be done with the long gouge. Note that the direction of the cutting edge is towards the femoral cortex, so it should be used very cautiously.

It is a well-directed, positive, repetitive action that leads to progress rather than ambitious attempts to remove large parts of the cement all at once (Fig. 23.3).

The Distal Part

Only when all the proximal and middle parts of the cement have been removed should an attempt be made to extract the cement which is distal to the stem. Any attempt to do so before all the middle part of the cement has been removed will end in disappointment. The distal cement plug is drilled, either under direct vision or down drill guides, in order to enter its strongest part. The screw of the distal cement extractor is screwed in to its full depth until it stops at the shaft of the extractor. The sliding hammer is used gently to dislodge and extract the cement plug (Fig. 23.4). If the cement breaks and only part of the plug is extracted then the procedure is repeated. If the cement thread strips or the cement breaks up too much then the plug can be drilled out using cement drills.

Femoral Cement Restrictors

If an intramedullary bone block has been used at primary surgery then it is usually incorporated

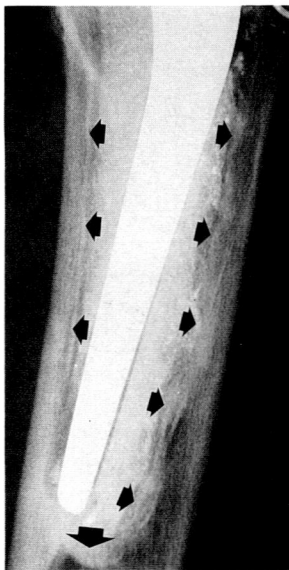

Fig. 23.5. Condensation of the cancellous bone. Stem–cement complex has subsided within the medullary canal. The condensation of the cancellous bone is almost continuous in the areas and very prominent at the tip of the stem.

in and closes off the medullary canal. Exploration past it is not required. If any other type of cement restrictor has been used, be it cement or plastic, it should probably be removed. Cement restrictors should always be removed in cases of deep sepsis. Cement and solid HDP plugs present no problems. The HDP shuttlecock-type restrictors are difficult to grasp or drill out and because of their design they tend to migrate further down the medullary canal as attempts are made to extract them.

Removal of Fibrous or Pyogenic Granulation Tissue from the Bone–Cement Junction

This very definite structure is most obvious in cases where loosening, whether with or without deep sepsis, is of some standing. In such cases the whole lining can be literally dissected out by using the gauges to strip the fibrous tissue off the bone. In cases of deep sepsis these areas of fibrous tissue may be relatively small and scattered and should be searched for deliberately.

Any area of endosteal cavitation must similarly be explored, from the inside of the medullary canal, in order to remove the fibrous membrane and prepare the bone for cement injection.

Removal of a Thin Layer of Condensed Cancellous Bone

This layer (Fig. 23.5) is most obvious in cases of large medullary canals, where the stem–cement complex forms a relatively small part. It is formed by condensation of the cancellous bone which is subjected to stress low enough so as not to lead to its destruction. It is a continuous process but only becomes radiologically obvious when the bone reaches a certain density as compared with that of the femoral cortex, and thus is able to "appear" through it. Because of this it may not be present on the radiographs but becomes obvious at surgery. Cement cannot be injected into this smooth layer of bone. Wherever possible this thin layer of condensed cancellous bone should be removed to expose areas of good cancellous bone which after careful preparation will allow good cement injection. Failure to remove this layer will lead immediately to a loose stem.

Excavation of the Lesser Trochanter

In the development of the proximal femur the lesser trochanter is formed by the traction of the ilio-psoas which separates the femoral cortex into two layers, the outer cortex and the inner, thinner layer, the femoral calcar. The femoral calcar extends from the femoral cortex below the lesser trochanter, covers the cavity of the lesser trochanter, then merges with the medial femoral cortex postero-medially to form the medial femoral neck, erroneously called the "calcar" ("surgical" calcar it may be, "anatomical" calcar it is not). Its presence may be demonstrated on the pre-operative radiographs using oblique views (Fig. 23.6). With increasing age the calcar is thinned out and lost and this probably contributes to the increasing incidence of femoral neck fractures with the postero-medial comminution.

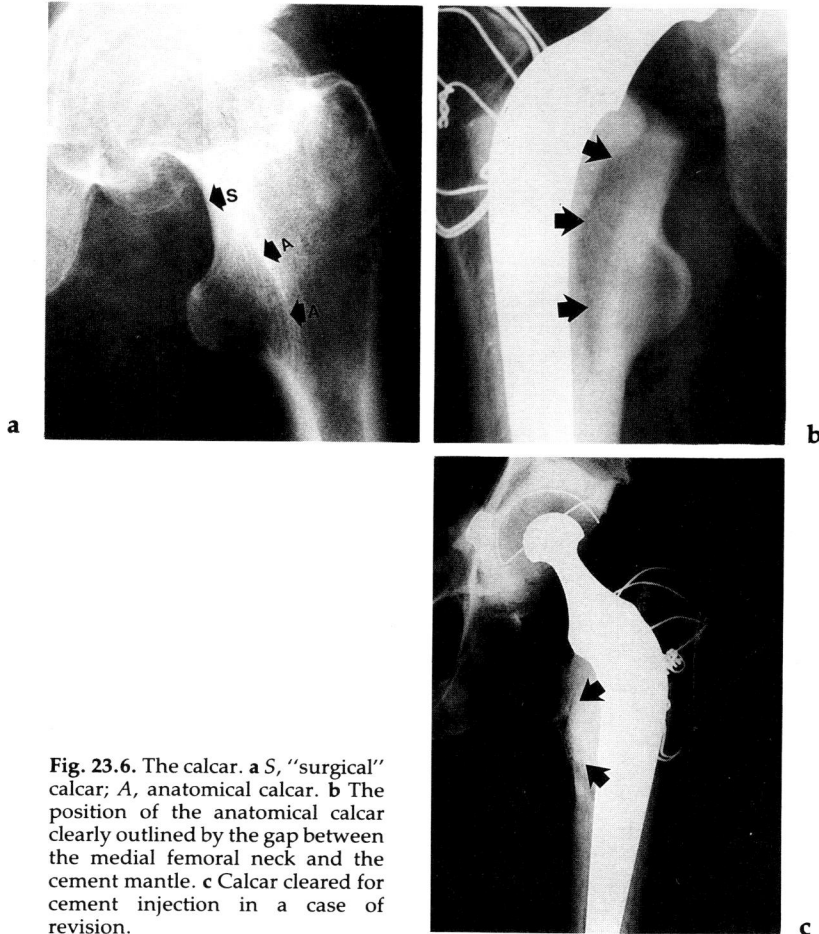

Fig. 23.6. The calcar. **a** *S*, "surgical" calcar; *A*, anatomical calcar. **b** The position of the anatomical calcar clearly outlined by the gap between the medial femoral neck and the cement mantle. **c** Calcar cleared for cement injection in a case of revision.

At revision surgery the anatomical calcar should be removed by excavating the lesser trochanter and thus allowing cement injection into strong cancellous bone. This technique offers support to the head and neck of the stem postero-medially (Fig. 23.6). It is there that support is needed most since the load on the hip is from the antero-superior direction (i.e. the hip is loaded in flexion). It becomes obvious that in deciding on the timing of the revision this aspect must be kept in mind. Revision should not be put off for too long; loss of the proximal femur beyond the lesser trochanter creates problems that demand use of a different technique. Failure to prepare that area carefully will result in

immediate lack of proximal support of the stem and the likelihood of a future problem.

Selection of a Femoral Stem and Trial Reduction

Selection of the length of the stem in primary surgery has followed Moore and Thompson by tradition rather than on evidence. That a 10-cm length intramedullary portion is sufficient provided it is well fixed has already been mentioned.

The use of ever-longer stems has, however, found its advocates. The argument is that better bone distally will offer better fixation of the stem. This may be true only as far as the isthmus of the femur. Distal to the isthmus the negative taper of the medullary canal is unlikely to contribute much to stem fixation. It cannot be denied that long stems have to be used but only to make up bone loss or to bridge bony defects. What *is* needed is proximal support for the head and the neck of the stem. Using a long stem will not achieve this; it is likely to lead to problems and will certainly make any future revision more difficult. There is no single stem which will fulfil the criteria of adequate length of neck and/or stem and of a suitable offset to cover the many possibilities. The ideal is for a collection of stems to be available. In cases where the femoral neck is deficient but the medullary canal is closed off or some of the cement can be safely left, then a shorter stem is very useful. In fact the author now has a full selection of standard stems shortened by 2 cm. These come in very useful indeed. In practice, the most bulky stem that can be inserted comfortably is invariably used.

Once the femoral neck or the proximal femur is lost, the critical level being the loss of the lesser trochanter, then the stem design needs to be radically different. The offset is now fully extramedullary and the fixation of the stem is now in a relatively symmetrical tube of the femur. The taper of the stem becomes of vital importance. The end-weight bearing on the cut surface of the femur is essential and a collared stem should be considered. This creates a problem, i.e. the need for a variable length extramedullary portion. So far this has meant producing custom-made stems from the radiographs. The delay, the cost and the need to be accurate with the design and the level of the femoral section are major drawbacks. In order to overcome all these problems a modular stem has been designed. Its use is discussed in detail in Chap. 24.

Trial Reduction

At trial reduction it must be ensured that the positions of the stem within the medullary canal and of the head and neck outside it are those which will pertain at stem fixation. Only then can the stability, the leg length and the position of the greater trochanter be checked with confidence. (Stability takes priority over leg length.) Although there are several ways of doing this, the Charnley ATP really comes into its own here,

ensuring stability of the stem at trial reduction and reproducibility of the position at the time of stem fixation.

Distal Closure of the Medullary Canal and Stem Insertion

In a large proportion of cases either of deep sepsis or mechanical loosening, the medullary canal is closed off by a condensation of cancellous bone (Fig. 23.5). Unless there is a compelling reason why a longer-than-standard stem need be used, the medullary canal need not be opened distally, provided good support for the stem can be obtained proximally and any defects by-passed. Advantage should be taken of this fact. If this precludes using a standard-length stem then a shorter one can be used. If the medullary canal needs to be closed off then a cement restrictor can be used. The author has so far avoided using HDP restrictors for fear of producing HDP granuloma in cases where the rate of loosening of the components is expected to be higher than in primary surgery.

Before inserting the cement the medullary canal is vented proximally. Often more than 40 g of cement will have to be used. If low-viscosity cement is used with a pressurizer, care must be taken to ensure that no cement escapes into the soft tissues. In fact it is a sound practice, and one not to be ashamed of, to feel the femur through the muscle routinely once the cement has set. If any cement has been extruded then it can at least be removed at this stage.

Reattachment of the Greater Trochanter

The method and the results for reattachment of the greater trochanter have been previously published. A double cross-over wire with compression spring is used routinely. The wires are meant to hold and compress the trochanter onto its bed and must not be used to pull it down.

In cases of trochanteric non-union both the trochanter and its bed must be carefully prepared to expose as much of the cancellous bone as possible. Both can at times be shaped to achieve a reasonable resemblance to a biplane shape. Gauges and a sharp narrow osteotome are very useful for this purpose. If the trochanteric fragment is excessively large then it can be reduced to size and shaped with a Gigli saw in the following manner: while holding the troc-

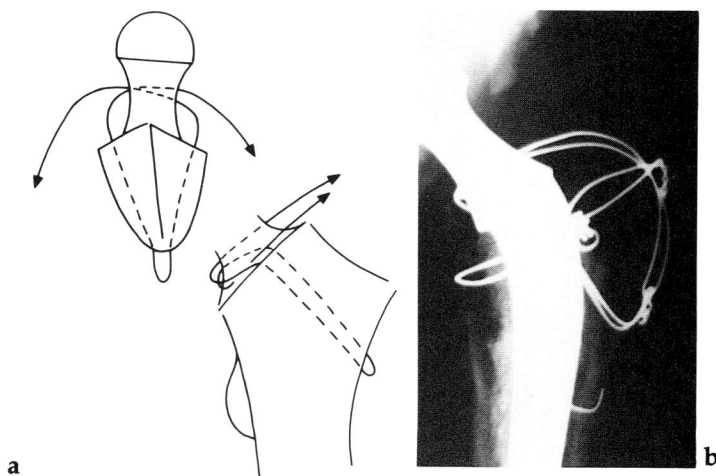

Fig. 23.7. A method of trochanteric reattachment when the stem is not being changed. Long free loops are prone to fatigue failure. **a** Diagram to show the position of the double wire. **b** Double wire and compression spring in place.

hanter in the Charnley trochanteric holder the spike is introduced through the middle of the trochanter (distal to proximal) until it emerges at the top of the trochanter. A Gigli saw is put round the spike which can then be tapped into the pelvis above the socket. While the first assistant holds the trochanter in the holder and restrains the handle of the spike, cutting begins. The result is a reduced size biplane-shaped trochanter. The trochanteric bed can then be shaped to match it.

If trochanteric reattachment is not possible then the soft tissues over the greater trochanter are sutured to the periosteum and fascia of the vastus lasteralis. An unabsorbable suture material such as polypropylene should be used.

Reattachment of the Greater Trochanter when the Stem has not Been Changed

It is not uncommon for the socket alone to have to be changed. Judging by the information concerning revision surgery there is little doubt that this procedure will have to be performed even more frequently in the future. Therefore, it may not be out of place to describe a simple method for trochanteric reattachment when trochanteric osteotomy has been performed but the stem did not have to be changed.

The Method

A double-looped wire and a compression spring are used. A drill hole is made about 1 cm distal to

the middle of the trochanteric bed. From the same point of entry two separate holes are drilled, one in front, the other at the back of the base of the neck of the stem. The anteriorly emerging wire is passed round the base of the neck of the stem to emerge posteriorly, while the posteriorly emerging wire is passed round the base of the neck of the stem to emerge anteriorly. They are then crossed over so that the posteriorly emerging wire will pass over the anterior part of the trochanter, while the anteriorly emerging wire will pass over the posterior part of the trochanter.

The compression spring wire is passed through a drill hole medial to the stem, usually through the base of the lesser trochanter (Fig. 23.7). The wires are then tightened as in primary surgery.

There has not been a sufficient number of cases using this method of trochanteric reattachment to evaluate its efficiency. Because the wires are not adequately anchored in the cement within the medullary canal and the free loops of wire are relatively long, it can be expected that the results will not be as good as they would have been otherwise.

The alternative method is to remove the stem, insert the trochanteric wires and then use extra cement and a narrower stem. Theoretically this is a very attractive method; the problem may be the discrepancy in the cement tract created by the introduction of the trochanteric wires.

24 Loss of Bone Stock

Introduction

The problems of diminishing return apply to revision surgery very aptly. On the one hand is the inability to eradicate infection with various antibiotic combinations, while on the other is the ever diminishing bone stock for component fixation. Although pseudarthrosis still is, and must be accepted as, the inevitable outcome in some cases, every effort must be made to preserve or even increase the bone stock. In order to preserve bone stock, revisions need to be timely, while efforts to improve the bone stock may be made at the time of surgery. It is correct to say that at this stage the author's experience with bone grafting in revision surgery is rather limited, for several reasons. Revisions are undertaken early whenever possible. On the acetabular side the concept of "rim support" for the socket has been actively pursued for a number of years, with some success. On the femoral side excavation of the lesser trochanter for stem support postero-medially has been carried out routinely in revisions. It is the loss of bone stock beyond the level of the lesser trochanter that demands alternative stem designs and methods of support.

Bone grafting in revision surgery, be it on the acetabular or the femoral side, has not been pursued with much enthusiasm. A possible mixture of dead bone, cement and at times bacteria would not be a sound basis for revision. It must not be thought that an increase in the bone stock is not to be aimed for or that use of cement in revisions is mandatory. The whole concept of bone grafting in revision surgery demands clearly thought out principles and methods. When bone grafting is put into practice the results must be carefully assessed and communicated in a scientific manner. The problems associated with autogenous bone grafting are few, and are mainly concerned with the availability of suitably sized bone grafts. It may be possible for the patient to keep his own femoral head grafted somewhere in his anatomy for future use.

Allografts, although in almost unlimited supply and not too difficult to handle, pose an increasingly important problem, i.e. selection and testing of donors. What about the possibility of alternative and simpler methods, e.g. the use of bone substitutes and bone-stimulating collagens? If bone grafting is used then it is essential that the component is supported by the skeleton rather than the graft, yet some loading of the graft is essential to stimulate its incorporation.

Acetabular Defects

The principle of sound component fixation, so often mentioned, applies equally in cases of revision in the presence of acetabular deficiencies. There is, however, one aspect of the method that may at first appear illogical, i.e. sound fixation of the socket is not essential to achieve clinical success but movement at the

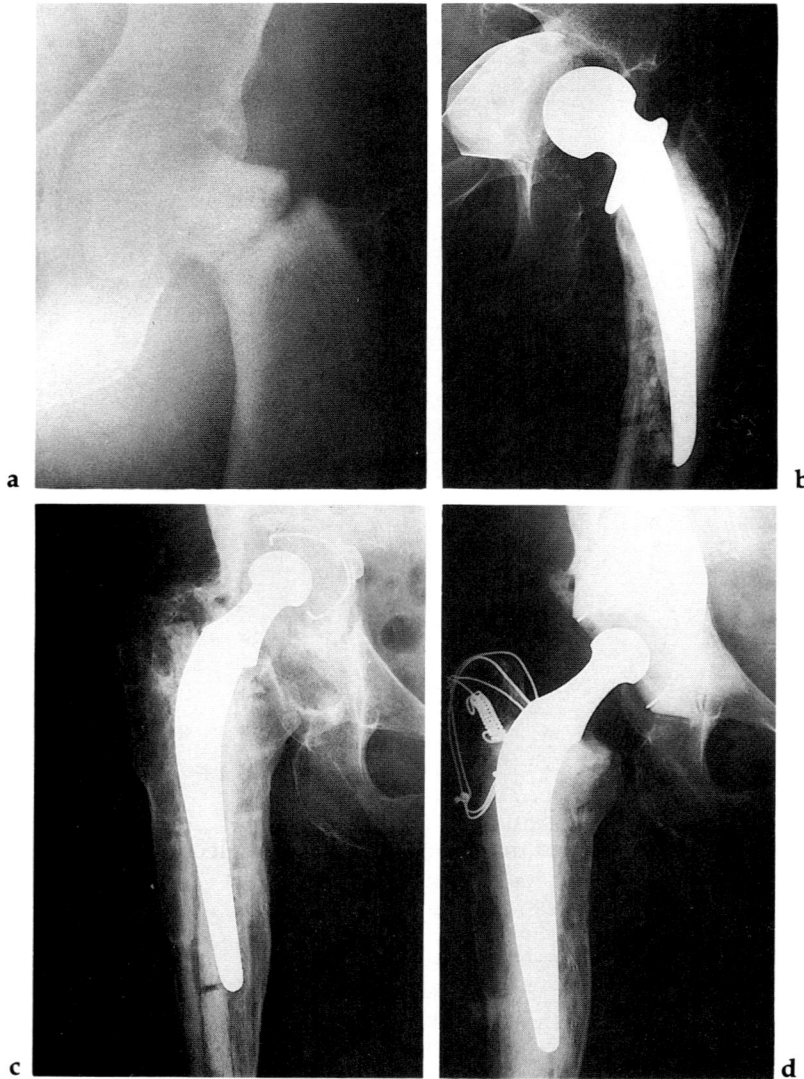

Fig. 24.1. Central acetabular defect. **a** Fracture of the femoral neck. **b** The result here is probably due to a limited exposure and failure to appreciate the principles of total hip arthroplasty. **c** One-stage revision for deep infection. **d** Appearance 7 years later. Ortron wire mesh covering acetabular defect.

implant–bone interface is likely to result in a clinical failure. Thus what is essential is maintenance of the position and avoidance of movement rather than fixation of the implant.

Three main types of acetabular deficiencies present for practical solution: central deficiencies, superior deficiencies and disruption of the acetabular ring.

Central Acetabular Deficiencies

These may result from over-enthusiastic preparation where the acetabular floor is normal, as in cases of fracture of the neck of the femure, or in protrusio-type osteoarthritis (curettage is usually sufficient) (Fig. 24.1). Similar problems may arise in cases of deep sepsis (Fig. 24.1c,d).

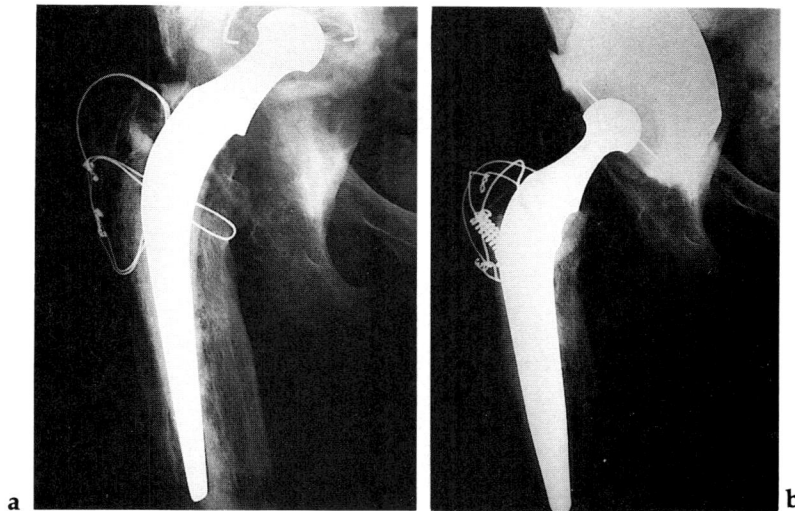

Fig. 24.2. Central acetabular defect. Rim support for the socket. **a** Central defect with socket prolapse. The stem was loose as well. **b** Following revision. Clinically successful at 4 years.

Probably all of them have a common pathology, that of load transmission through the acetabular floor rather than the rim. Progressive, and often asymptomatic, socket migration must not divert the surgeon's attention away from the real problem, which is an increasingly difficult revision. Sooner rather than later the problem will have to be tackled. After extraction of the socket the acetabular rim and the floor must be carefully inspected to assess the quality of bone remaining and the extent of the defect.

It is probably correct to say that the central defect, irrespective of its size, can be covered with a wire mesh to prevent the escape of cement; the mesh is not meant to serve any other purpose.

The acetabular rim is carefully prepared with curettes and small anchor holes are drilled for cement injection. The flange of the Ogee-flanged angle-bore socket is trimmed accurately to ensure that it rests on or just within the rim of the acetabulum. The cement pressurizer, if employed, must be used with great caution. It is an advantage to use the cement slightly later than in primary surgery in order to prevent its escape into unwanted areas.

No claim is made that this method gives socket fixation, however, it certainly does give socket support as judged by some of the results (Fig. 24.2).

Superior Acetabular Defects

These are fortunately rare and are usually the result of post-traumatic disruption of the acetabulum or neglected superior socket migration. In some cases there may just be sufficient bone stock for socket fixation; in others the defects are so gross that the only possible method available is the bold use of masses of cement (Fig. 24.3). It is in such cases that massive bone grafting may hold a promise.

Disruption of the Acetabular Rim

The bones of the pelvis, being relatively elastic, must deform under load to quite a degree. It has always been maintained that with a disrupted acetabular rim a cemented socket, however supported, is unlikely to hold for any length of time. Although a handful of them have remained in situ, most have not. Furthermore, the quality of bone remaining, often together with sepsis, has mitigated against revision; pseudarthrosis is usually carried out instead. This is still probably the correct line of treatment in cases where repeated revisions, recurrent sepsis and loss of acetabular bone stock are such that it is in the patient's interests to cut the losses rather than endanger the limb, if not life.

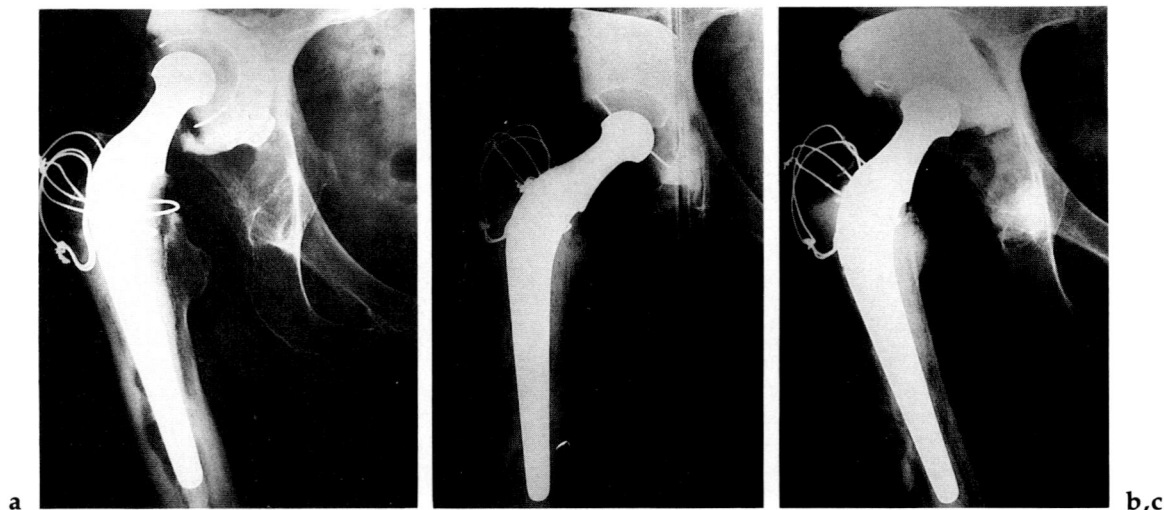

a   b,c

Fig. 24.3. Superior acetabular defect. **a** Postero-superior fracture dislocation of the hip with failed open reduction treated by LFA; complicated by deep infection. Patient referred for treatment at this stage. **b** Superior defect covered with wire mesh in order to contain the cement. **c** Five years after revision. Socket obviously migrated but the infection has been controlled. Limp and shortening present; use of a stick for support needed. Patient felt greatly improved.

Support and Reinforcement Rings

Support and reinforcement rings probably have a role in revision surgery, though what the indications are is not exactly clear. Failure occurs at the bone–implant interface. Thus there are two aspects of revision that must be considered carefully: the quality of the bone stock and the type of implant used. There is almost no limit to the improvements that can be made in the quality and strength of the implant (the socket and the cement etc.). This however does nothing to improve the quality of the bone stock which is meant to support the implant. It is not correct to assume that the quality of fixation depends on the implant, on the contrary it almost entirely depends on the quality of the bone stock and of course the surgical technique. If support and reinforcement rings are to be used then their function must be clearly understood; they must not be an apology for an inadequate technique, absent bone stock or delayed revisions (Fig. 24.4).

Future Developments

There is little doubt that revisions for socket loosening and acetabular bone deficiency are on the increase and are likely to increase still further. Some of the increase is due to the longer follow-up now available, some to the ever-

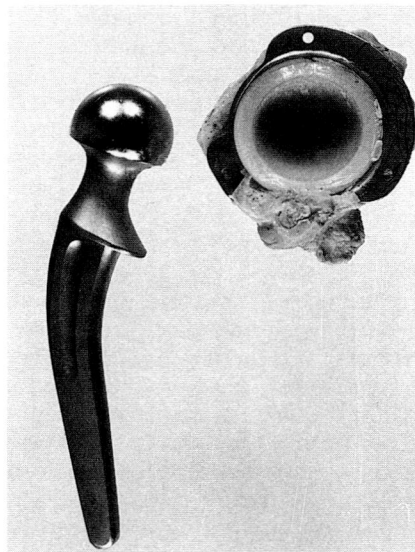

Fig. 24.4. Acetabular reinforcement ring. Note that the ring and cement came out "en masse" indicating that the failure was at the bone–cement interface. The ring has "reinforced" the cement but offered no "support" to the socket.

increasing numbers of younger patients being accepted for surgery, but most of it is probably, and sadly, due to the failure to appreciate that a loose and migrating socket may be asymptomatic and can be compatible with normal or near-normal function. This leads to delay in revision surgery and progressive loss of bone stock.

Timely intervention using the methods applied to primary surgery may salvage a number of cases. There is increasing evidence now that every effort must be made to improve the quality of the bone stock, especially in cases where life expectancy of the patient is likely to be greater than that of the arthroplasty. How this is done is probably immaterial as long as the method used to supplement bone stock allows a certain level of function so that the bone is stressed and thus has an opportunity to respond to function (bone responds to function). However, it must be fixed sufficiently well to avoid it being over-stressed or disrupted. This field offers a challenge for design, surgical technique and the development of implant materials. The results are likely to be rewarding.

Femoral Defects

Femoral defects do not, by and large, produce problems of the same magnitude as do acetabular ones. This may be so for several reasons. Femoral component loosening is better understood and is more widely reported. It is more easily diagnosed radiologically, the changes being primarily distal migration and movement into the varus position, although there are exceptions. Radiological points of reference are more obvious and are readily used with relative accuracy. A loose stem is almost always symptomatic and this, probably more than any of the other factors, brings the problem to the surgeon's attention early.

The problem of loss of bone stock really starts if there is a delay in undertaking the revision or if the revision is carried out without understanding the problem or the aims of the operation. Repeated inadequate revision will result in progressive loss of bone stock and the abductor musculature, making any subsequent revision even more difficult technically and less likely to succeed mechanically. It should not be out of place to point out once more that revision for a loose stem demands removal of the stem and the acrylic cement as well as the fibrous layer so often present between the bone and the cement. A thin layer of condensed cancellous bone, formed as a response to loosening and not always identifiable on radiographs, must also be removed exposing strong cancellous bone whenever possible. To ream the medullary canal to the cortex is to reduce the area of contact and keying for the acrylic cement and to invite loosening at some, often early, stage.

The cavity of the lesser trochanter must be excavated so that when it is filled with cement it will offer support for the stem in its postero-medial part proximally. Any defects or areas of weakness must be by-passed using a longer stem though this must not be carried to extremes. Routine use of long stems in revisions has little to commend it. In all this the possibility of deep sepsis must not be overlooked.

Minor Femoral Deficiencies

Loss of the femoral neck down to the lesser trochanter can readily be compensated for by the use of extended neck stems. This, combined with the availability of somewhat longer shafts of the stems, means that the vast majority of problems can be solved without much trouble. In this context slightly more bulky stems may also be advantageous. Use of cement to support the extra-femoral portion of the stem has nothing to commend it.

Major Deficiencies of the Proximal Femur

Technical problems really begin when the proximal femoral deficiency extends past the lesser trochanter. The reasons for this are threefold. Firstly, the anatomy of the remaining part of the femur is so different that the standard stem design can no longer be of practical use. The almost symmetrical tubular portion of the femur demands a different type of stem support. Secondly, the variability of the deficient segment is something that, although surmised from the pre-operative radiographs, can only be accurately assessed at the time of surgery. This makes stem selection difficult. Finally, on extended proximal femoral deficiency carries with it the likelihood of the loss of the abductor muscles and with this their stabilizing action for

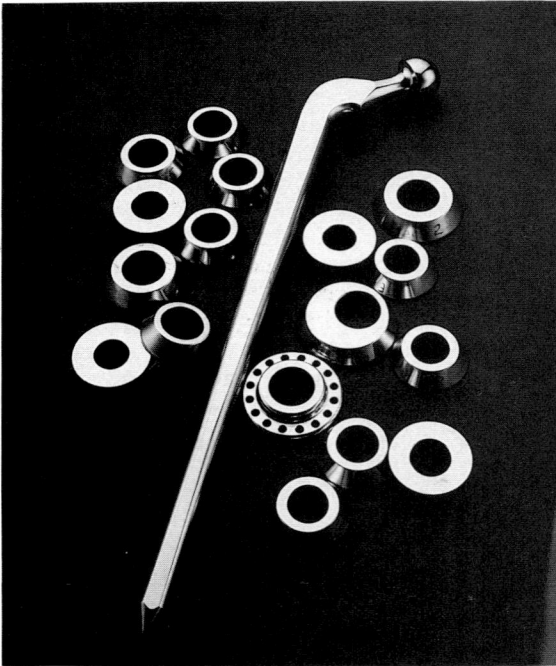

Fig. 24.5. The modular proximal femoral replacement stem system. The stem, support rings and perforated ring for the maintenance of continuity between the abductors and the vastus lateralis fasciae.

the arthroplasty. The result is a positive Trendelenburg gait, an increased load on the joint as well as a greater possibility of post-operative dislocation.

Practical Approach: The Modular Stem System (Fig. 24.5)

The chances of successful revision have been improved by the use of the modular stem design to overcome the problems of variable deficiency, altered load transmission and stability of the arthroplasty. The variability of the deficiency is overcome by the use of rings which fit very precisely at various levels of the stem shaft from 2 to 10 cm in 0.5-cm increments, thus allowing the correct adjustment for tension, leg length and stability at the time of trial reduction. The load transmission being now exclusively on the taper of the stem must be transferred to the proximal part of the femur. This is done by the careful preparation of the proximal femur with special cutters to allow accurate seating of the appropriate collar.

The stability is enhanced by provision of a

perforated ring which is placed proximally on the shaft of the stem and to which the abductors can be sutured through the fibrous aponeurosis, thus maintaining the continuity between the abductors and the vastus lateralis. The prevention of excessive rotation improves the stability and reduces the likelihood of post-operative dislocation. Despite this, a tibial anti-rotation pin may still be necessary and preferably should be used routinely for 3 weeks post-operatively.

The modular stem design has been used now for over 4 years and the number of problems treated is relatively small; the results have been most encouraging (Fig. 24.6). (The design has been subjected to intensive mechanical testing far in excess of the British Standards Institution. At 10 cm unsupported (except by the collar) the stem has withstood 70 million cycles at 700 kg without failure.)

When considering this or any other method of proximal femoral replacement it must be remembered that the penalty for failure may be a flail limb. Ambulation under these circumstances may be difficult and amputations have been reported. This possibility must be taken into account and may well decide the line of treatment. Finally, pseudarthrosis may still be a reasonable choice of method when the alternatives are carefully considered.

Future Developments

It is probably correct to say that a better understanding of stem fixation at primary surgery and early and well carried out revisions will, in the long run, pay better dividends than an ever-increasing dependence on the replacement of bone with whatever happens to be available. In this context any method which attempts to increase the bone stock must be given the consideration it truly deserves. Any such method should be encouraged, but this also demands objective reporting of the results other than by anecdotes.

One other aspect of the ultimate results of stem fixation merits very careful study and that is the alteration of normal stresses in the femur (stress protection and stress concentration). This may not be an important issue in cases where the arthroplasty outlasts the life of the patient, but will become increasingly important as ever-younger patients are accepted for surgery. Their life span, life style and bone turnover are such as to make the study of this aspect of total hip arthroplasty essential.

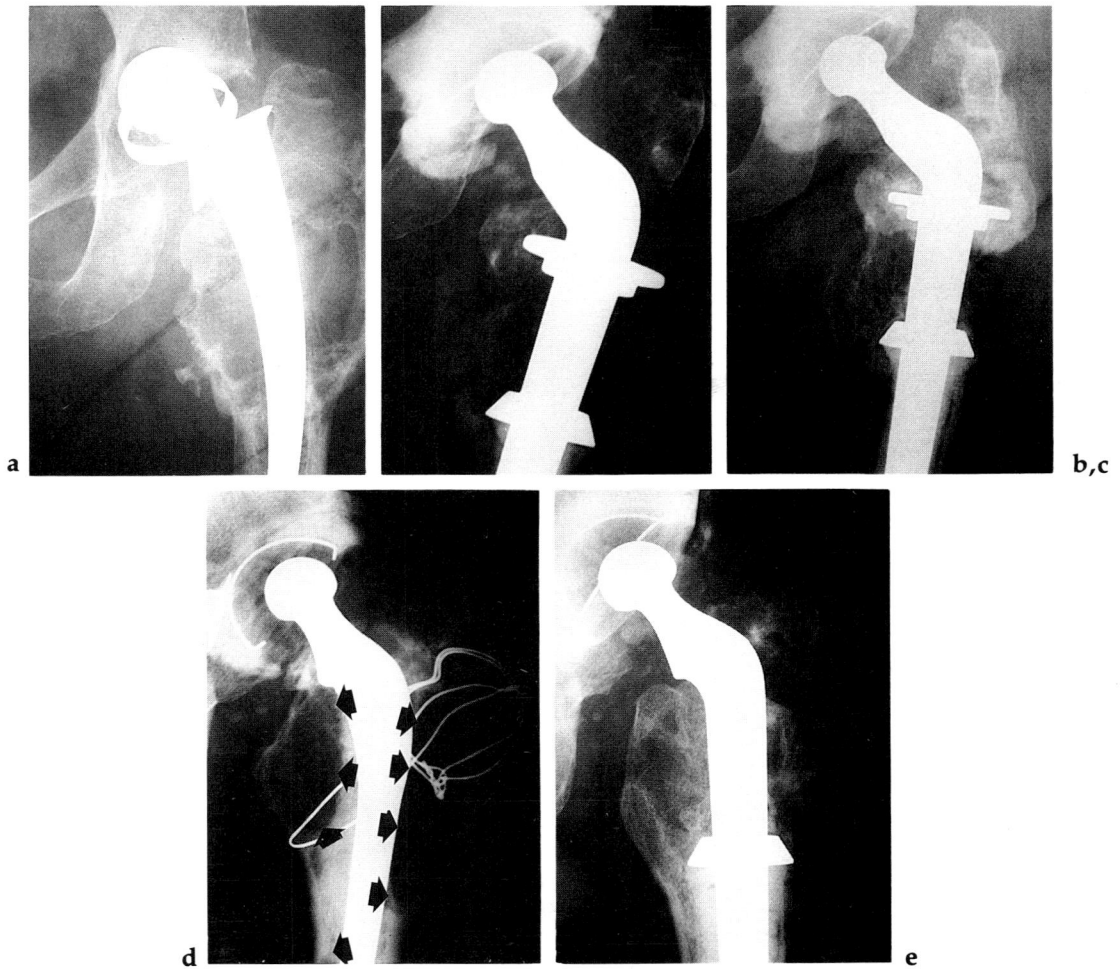

Fig. 24.6. a–c Proximal femoral replacement modular stem in practice. **a** HDP femoral head replacement arthroplasty. Note the tumour-like destruction of the proximal femur due to HDP wear particles and movement of the loose stem and the erosion of the acetabulum. **b** Immediate post-operative appearance. **c** Improvement of the quality of the bone 2 years after revision. (Bone graft not used.) **d** Charnley LFA in a young active male. Loose socket and stem. Massive cavitation of the lesser trochanter and the greater trochanter to the mid-shaft of the stem. Cavitation at the tip of the stem. **e** Appearance at 1 year following revision; abductor ring not used. (Bone graft not used.)

25 Wound Closure

Introduction

It is of practical value if the whole of the operative procedure of total hip arthroplasty is considered in layers. Attention to detail at each layer will ensure a methodical approach to the procedure as a whole, both at the time of exposure as well as at closure. Any tendency to disregard this layer-by-layer methodical surgical approach may lead to problems. This aspect is even more important in cases of revision where dissection of various layers may be difficult. These layers are:

1. The acetabulum, femur and total hip components.
2. The capsule, the abductors, the greater trochanter and the vastus group of muscles.
3. The deep fascia.
4. Subcutaneous fat.
5. The skin.

The Acetabulum, Femur and Total Hip Components

The need for attention to detail at preparation, cement injection and component fixation has already been pointed out. The object here is to achieve fixation and thus enable the components to function as an integral part of the skeleton.

The Capsule, the Abductors, the Greater Trochanter and the Vastus Group of Muscles

This layer must effectively cover the implant while the integrity of the muscles is retained. Thus correct handling of the abductors is necessary at all times. Fixation of the trochanter must be deliberate and secure.

The Deep Fascia

This is the most important layer as far as sepsis is concerned. Its careful closure will effectively allow a watertight separation between the implant and the superficial layers, between the vital and the problem layers of the total hip arthroplasty. It is to achieve this clear and effective separation that non-absorbable polypropylene sutures on a curved 1-0 needle are used. Closure should start distally and proceed proximally. The initial knot is made deep to the deep fascia in order to avoid its prominence in a thin patient. The stitch is a continuous one, with about 1 cm between each loop. Every second or third loop is locked, the locked stitch always running to the front (the direction of the next loop), thus avoiding the likelihood of fracture of the polypropylene. From the greater trochanter proximally care must be taken to pick up the fascia only, and not the fleshy fibres of the tensor fascia lata. (Care must be taken to avoid picking up the deep drains with the stitch.)

Subcutaneous Fat

This is the problem layer. Fat necrosis, buried foreign material and haematoma close to the skin may all predispose to infection. The layer itself is relatively avascular and has not the substance to hold stitches effectively. One of the solutions offered was use of the compression foam pads and pull-out sutures advocated by Charnley which effectively close the dead space and avoid buried foreign material.

The time required for a fat layer to heal has not been established accurately. Suggestions have been made that provided the layer is well drained there is in fact no need to suture it. Following this the author has not sutured the fat layer, either at primary or revision surgery, for 20 months. During this time six haematomas in some 340 LFAs occurred. The three in primary surgery were infected and required evacuations. So far none have led to deep sepsis. This compares with three infected haematomas over an 11-year period and some 2500 cases. The pull-out fat sutures are being used once again. (On the plus side has been the reduction of the operation time by about 10 min per case.) Since the pull-out suture is continuous between deep fascia and skin there must be a possibility, at least theoretical, of an increased incidence of deep infection. This certainly does not appear to be so. Without this suture the incidence of superficial haematoma has certainly been unacceptable.

The Skin

It is probably correct to say that a uniformly satisfactory method of skin closure of the hip has yet to be suggested. Each surgeon will find his favourite method which he will perfect for his own use. The ideal stitch should approximate the skin edges without tension, allowing their gentle eversion, while at the same time avoiding repeated piercing of the skin. The subcuticular stitch has much to commend it provided a strong subcuticular layer is present. It is obviously less

suitable for patients whose skin has been affected by disease or steroid medication. Skin edge necrosis can readily be produced if the tension is too excessive.

The recent advent of skin staples is appealing because of speed, rather than because of results or cost. Since by their design the depth to which the clips close is predetermined, care must be taken when picking up the skin edges. The "volume" of the tissue picked up must remain constant with respect to the clips but variable with respect to the tissue quality.

The author's preference is for a continuous blanket stitch, the tension being adjusted by the surgeon himself. The aim of this method is to avoid strangulation of the skin edges by allowing some "self-adjustment" of the tension of the stitch which acts almost like a self-adjusting spring. Because in revisions there have been previous skin incisions it is probably advisable to leave the skin sutures in for about 12–14 days.

The Use of Drains

Drains are used to prevent the collection of blood in the cavity of the joint and also in the fat layer of the thigh which may otherwise lead to haematoma and deep infection. Four drains are used routinely, two deep ones around the neck of the stem and two in the subcutaneous fat layer. They are introduced using drain introducers, from inside out, and are not handled once out of the skin. Their ends must be carefully placed in the position required so that they run smoothly at the time of extraction. It must not be assumed that drains will function no matter how or where they are placed. For a drain to function effectively it must be placed in the most dependent part of the cavity where the blood is likely to collect. It must be free from kinks, twists, knots or bends. These can easily occur if the drain is bent over a drainage hole. The drainage holes must be patent and must not be occluded by debris such as bone marrow or fat, or be compressed between the tissues of the buttock and the bed.

None of the drainage holes must be outside the skin and the drain must not be kinked after exit from the skin. All the connections must be air tight. The suction pressure used must be continuous and at such a level as to allow suction of blood while avoiding suction of fatty tissue. There must be a watertight separation between cavities to be drained and the skin. When all this has been achieved there is usually only one hole of a drain which will drain effectively one closed cavity.

Any break in the system may lead to a haematoma. Thus it is most essential that attention is paid to every detail of drain insertion. Even with positive suction, advantage should be taken of the hydrostatic effect of the column of blood within the drain by placing the drainage bottles in the lowest possible position. It is also advisable that the drains are gently pulled out by some 2 cm when the drainage has ceased but while suction is being maintained. This may have to be repeated several times, especially if after each "pull" drainage continues. Eventually, as oozing from the raw surface ceases and the blood clots within the drains, suction stops being effective and drains can be removed. Experience has shown that in revision surgery this is usually some 60 hours after the operation, although very occasionally it may be longer. Before the drains are removed the suction pressure must be increased or the drains clamped to avoid the clot within the drain being sucked back by the negative pressure effect. The drain exit holes should be covered with a clean dressing as some oozing often occurs.

26 Post-operative Management

Post-operative management must be tailored to the needs of the individual patient as dictated by the problem leading to the revision, the state of the bone stock and the quality of the component fixation possible. All of these must be carefully documented in the patient's records.

In the cases of revision for recurrent dislocation the routine is 3 weeks' bed rest with an abduction pillow. In revision for deep sepsis also 3 weeks' bed rest seems to pay dividends. The wound heals well, oedema of the leg is often avoided and the patient mobilizes readily in bed. In fact patients are usually ready for discharge within 1 week of getting up. The fear of pulmonary embolism in such cases is probably more theoretical than real (see Chap. 28). When the problem has been loosening of the components then 2 weeks' bed rest is usually sufficient, but some patients may be mobilized earlier.

In each case the patient is under the supervision of a physiotherapist, both when in bed and while mobilizing, and remains weight bearing with the support of elbow crutches for not less than 6 weeks after discharge. In cases where the bone stock is poor or the patient is young, 12 weeks' partial weight bearing is indicated. In all cases of revision the use of support is encouraged though not always accepted.

The Ultimate Challenge of Surgery

27 Girdlestone Pseudarthrosis for a Failed Total Hip Arthroplasty

Introduction

A well-timed pseudarthrosis may still be the only acceptable outcome for a failed total hip arthroplasty. That comparatively little has been written on the subject is probably a reflection of the fact that few surgeons have treated sufficient numbers or have the enthusiasm to be an authority on a subject which, after all, is regarded as the ultimate failure of total hip arthroplasty.

It was with an awareness of this possible outcome, and no doubt conscious of the "Teflon experience", that Charnley used the "pseudarthrosis test" before accepting patients for surgery. Even in later years the test was still used (Charnley 1979b p. 348). In fact a review of the patients with the longest follow-up and the records of the histological examination of post-mortem specimens shows this aspect quite clearly – it is unusual to see a patient whose pain was recorded as grade 4 or above; it was invariably grade 3 or even 2. The test was carried out to ensure that even if the total hip arthroplasty did fail the patient was not made worse by a pseudarthrosis, and possibly even improved. After all, the Girdlestone pseudarthrosis was found to be a reliable procedure and was recommended for cases of unilateral osteoarthritis (Taylor 1966).

With the increasing numbers of people having total hip arthroplasties and particularly of young patients being accepted for surgery, it has no doubt been realized that at least a proportion of them will have to have the implant removed from one reason or another. It cannot be hoped for that a revision in one form or another will always "save the day". In fact it should be accepted that a well-timed pseudarthrosis is preferable to repeated surgery, diminishing bone stock and loss of limb length in the presence of sinuses and in the face of the ultimate alternative, amputation.

Indications for Pseudarthrosis

It is not possible to state categorically the indications for a pseudarthrosis. The final decision must be left to the surgeon and the patient concerned and can only be made in the light of the information available on the particular case, the current state of the art and science of revision surgery and the findings at surgery. It is for that last reason that the decision will have to be left in the hands of the surgeon. Critical assessment of the various possibilities is often best made at the time of the operation. This aspect should be made clear to the patient, for at that stage there is no chance for a further discussion.

The author's indications for the procedure have not altered from those put down in 1984 (Wroblewski 1984a). These were, and still are:

1. Inadequate bone stock for component fixation using current methods of revision technique.

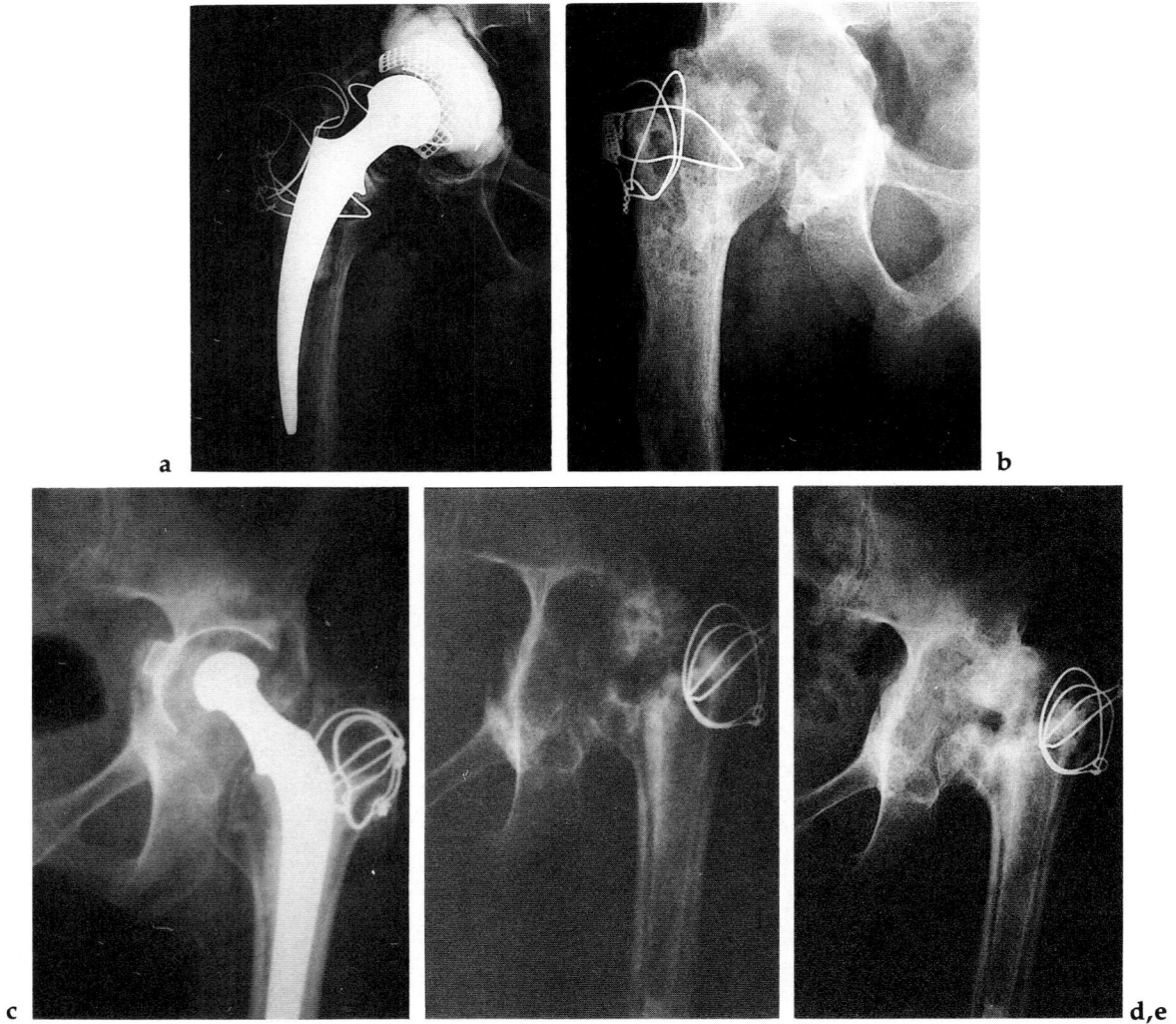

Fig. 27.1a–e. Examples of stable pseudarthrosis. The shaft of the femur is close to the acetabulum offering stability and freedom from telescoping. (Note the improvement in the quality of the femoral bone stock with function.)

2. Repeated surgery in the presence of gross sepsis, scarring and abductor muscle loss.
3. Extensive soft-tissue infection with mixed or antibiotic-resistant organisms.
4. Patient's general health or desire to avoid the possibility of, or the need for, repeated surgery.

Usually a combination of these factors has to be taken into account.

Pre-operative assessment should be no different from that already described but the aims, the post-operative management and the long-term progress and prognosis must be clearly outlined.

The slow progress, the need for support, permanent in most cases, and the "mechanics" of the pseudarthrosis must be sympathetically explained. The patient's fear of the leg almost hanging free in space or of it being stiff (how marvellous if it always was so!) must be dispelled. (A recent remark from a patient brings some humour to this aspect of revision surgery: "My surgeon said 'I will take the hip out and *put a Girdlestone in!*' ")

Post-operative mobilization may be made easier if other aspects interfering with mobility are tackled first. In this context the arthritic contralateral hip often comes in for discussion. If there is an indication for a total hip arthroplasty then it probably should be carried out first; the fear of the possibility of metastatic infection appears to be unfounded (del Sel and Charnley 1979) though antibiotic cover is mandatory. The femoral head serves as a useful graft and has been "carried" by the author from one hip to the other, in the same patient, thus making fixation of the components more sound on the side of revision.

The Operative Procedure

This is basically the same as a one-stage revision for deep infection up to the point of insertion of new components, with one exception: the soft-tissue dissection and excision should not be as extensive in order to avoid producing excessive laxity and telescoping.

The psoas tendon should probably be left intact if possible; this may be the only structure that keeps the femur closely apposed to the acetabulum. The cases where this has been done give a very much better result as far as stability and lack of telescoping is concerned.

Guttering of the femur as suggested by Clegg (1977) has never found favour. Although carried out in some cases initially, it was obviously weakening the femur and making any future revision impossible. Every effort must be made to leave the anatomy of the hip, including that of the abductors, as near normal as possible since the possibility of future interventions must always be considered (Fig. 27.1).

Post-operative Management

Much has changed in the past few years. Traction is no longer being used post-operatively by the author. It did not contribute much to the eventual leg length or stability. Given a choice patients invariably preferred to be treated without traction. The routine now is to keep the patient in bed, with an abduction pillow, and mobilize with support when the patient feels ready which is usually within 1 week of surgery.

If there is a tendency for gross external rotation to occur then a tibial pin and overhead suspension while the patient is in bed will help to correct it. This is continued for about 3 weeks while the patient mobilizes, walking with the tibial pin in situ. The type of support used will depend on the patient and will vary from pulpit to elbow crutches. Some eventually will be able to manage with two sticks or even one; a few will manage a short distance without any support.

Clinical Results

Provided the patients are carefully selected for primary surgery with pain being grade 3 or 2, then they are unlikely to be made worse by the procedure. Their mobility is unlikely to be improved, however. This aspect puts more stress on the careful selection of patients at primary surgery.

Conclusion

These have already been presented (Wroblewski 1984a) and have not changed since:

Pseudarthrosis following a failed total hip arthroplasty may be an inevitable outcome in cases of deep sepsis, gross loss of bone stock or patient's unwillingness to accept repeated surgery.

If the patients selected for the original operation have severe pain and are grossly disabled, they are unlikely to be made worse if the operation fails.

The improvement in the pain relief will be more obvious than the patient's mobility. This will be achieved at the expense of higher mortality and morbidity, repeated surgery and longer hospitalization.

If pseudarthrosis is inevitable, then a method to achieve the best result quickly is yet to be established. What is required is the stability of the pseudarthrosis without recurrence of infection.

28 Pulmonary Embolism

Introduction

The literature on the various aspects of pulmonary embolism is so vast and complex that it is outside the scope of this work to attempt to summarize even some of it. The study of methods of prevention, diagnosis and management of deep vein thrombosis is best left in the hands of the specialized, the equipped and the interested. For a practising orthopaedic surgeon the question remains "Can the possibility of fatal pulmonary embolism be predicted or prevented?"

There is sufficient evidence to suggest that a swollen leg does not necessarily indicate a deep vein thrombosis. Even if it did it can be argued that the obstruction to the venous return is likely to prevent the migration of a solid clot. It is the normal-looking leg which should be viewed with suspicion; it may be harbouring a thrombus "swaying" in the good flow of the venous stream which could become detached at any moment. The rationale behind the elevation of the foot of the bed is to prevent venous stasis but it may also keep the vein walls collapsed, reducing the likelihood of clot migration.

It would be of great interest to identify the circumstances leading to thrombus migration. The causes are probably purely mechanical and related to the changes in volume, pressure and flow rate.

In the practical approaches to pulmonary embolism three aspects are usually discussed: prediction, prevention and treatment.

Prediction

Here the history of previous episodes is probably the most important factor, although obesity and the likelihood of post-operative abdominal complications are also said by some to be highly predictive.

Prevention

This can be either mechanical or medical. Elevation of the foot of the bed, leg bandaging and elastic stockings seem logical. Calf stimulation or any method which improves venous return or improves circulation may be of help *before* thrombus formation, but probably not after it has formed.

Medical methods of prevention have always centred on reducing blood coagulability and various associated aspects. Anti-coagulants, aspirin and many other drugs have been advocated at various times. The effectiveness of any of the methods is well nigh impossible to establish. It is no more possible to assess something that has not occurred than it is to convince a clinician to use mortality statistics when his interest lies in establishing the diagnosis by methods other than post-mortem examination.

What is needed is a vast, well-conceived, prospective, multi-centre study. The desirable

Table 28.1. Prophylaxis of pulmonary embolism in the Centre for Hip Surgery, Wrightington Hospital (after Johnson and Loudon 1986)

Method of prophylaxis	No. of cases	Pulmonary embolism		Treatment-related mortality (%)
		Fatal (%)	Non-fatal (%)	
Nil	1967	1.8	12.5	—
Dindevan	450	0.9	6.5	0.7
Heparin				
Intravenous	137	0.7	9.5	—
Subcutaneous	47	6.4	6.4	2
High-molecular dextrans	4096	1.1	8.2	—
Hydroxychloroquine				
600–800 mg	2486	0.5	2.6	—
1200 mg	1830	0.1	2.3	—
1600 mg	52	0.0	1.9	—
Hydroxychloroquine 600–800 mg plus Dextran 70	1300	0.4	4.6	—

methods of investigation are very likely to outweigh the benefits of the study. Thus prevention is being used empirically on the assumptions that "to do something is to do good" or "to do nothing suggests negligence".

Treatment

This usually includes various forms of anticoagulant therapy. Whether this is either logical or effective can be questioned. Pulmonary embolism, if fatal, is invariably so within minutes rather than hours or days. This is far too fast for any anti-coagulant to be of effect, the cause of death being mainly mechanical i.e. sudden obstruction of pulmonary arterial flow. The majority that do survive are unlikely to die subsequently. Thus the effectiveness of anticoagulant treatment cannot be assessed with any confidence. If it works by stimulating resorption of minor pulmonary emboli why can it not do the same to leg vein thrombi, thus increasing the likelihood of their migration?

The experience from the Hip Centre with various methods of prophylaxis has been succinctly summarized by Johnson and Loudon (1986). A quick glance at the various studies highlights the problems of trials and interpretation of the results (see Table 28.1).

The author's practice is to routinely use hydroxychloroquine, 200 mg three times a day, from the day of admission and usually continuing for 2 weeks after discharge. The contraindications would be a known sensitivity presenting either as a skin rash or blurred vision, gastrointestinal upsets such as indigestion or very occasional bleeding, either gastric or from the operative site.

Reviews of Pulmonary Emboli Trends

The difficulties in diagnosis, the differences in methods of treatment and the disagreements in interpretation of cases of deep vein thrombosis and pulmonary emboli are too obvious to repeat. Thus any study reporting results of clinical and post-mortem diagnoses is bound to be viewed with suspicion. However, the sheer volume of the material available from the Hip Centre is such that it demands presentation and interpretation. It is accepted, and indeed hoped, that constructive criticism will follow.

Four findings need further detailed studies:

1. Yearly variations in the incidence of pulmonary emboli.
2. Seasonal variations in the incidence of the complication.
3. Variations in the incidence between different patient groups.
4. The incidence of fatal pulmonary emboli during the post-operative period.

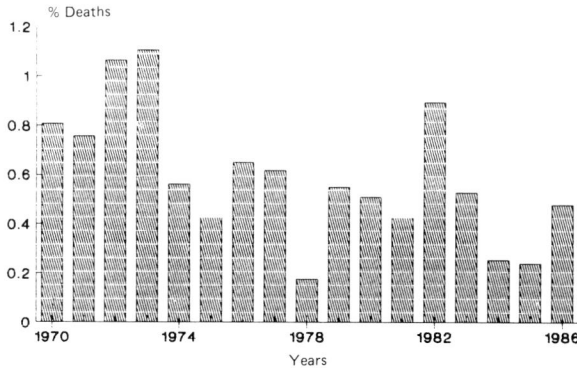

Fig. 28.1. Yearly variations in the death rate from pulmonary embolism. Note the gradual reduction in 1974.

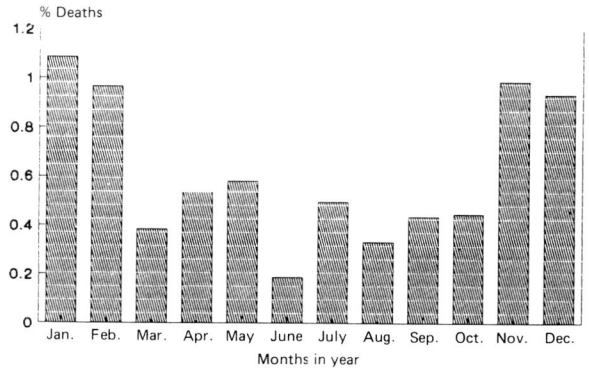

Fig. 28.2. Fatal pulmonary embolism. Seasonal variations. These variations are statistically significant.

Yearly Variations in Incidence

There is no obvious explanation for this apparently erratic, and yet in a way almost cyclic, change in the incidence of deaths resulting from the complication (Fig. 28.1). The possibilities are too numerous to contemplate or examine in detail. The questions that may be asked are more obvious than the answers offered. Some in-depth review of the subject is essential. It is only mentioned here to indicate the complexity of the problem. Is the incidence of post-operative pulmonary emboli on the decline as Fig. 28.1 would suggest? If so then what are the likely explanations?

The dramatic reduction in the incidence of the complication in 1974/1975 may in fact demonstrate the effect of Plaquenil which was introduced at that time. Its use in subsequent years has been somewhat erratic. However, the gradual reduction in the incidence was already evident before the introduction of the treatment.

Seasonal Variations in Incidence

Although mentioned before, seasonal variations in incidence have not received detailed attention to date. These variations are very obvious (Fig. 28.2) and statistically significant, and overshadow any year-to-year changes. There is a very obvious 3-monthly cycle for the incidence of fatal pulmonary emboli. Herein probably lies the answer to the *mechanics* of pulmonary embolism.

The yearly and seasonal variations in the incidence of pulmonary embolism are mentioned here only to stimulate thought and to point out possible avenues of research. Any "advances" made that do not take into account the "natural history" of the complications should be questioned.

Variations in the Incidence Between Different Patient Groups

Early mobilization of the patient following hip surgery has always been regarded as essential in the prevention of deep vein thrombosis and pulmonary embolism, but is it logical? A fatal pulmonary embolism usually occurs at the stage when the patient is fully mobile and ready for discharge. What would have been the outcome if that patient had been mobilized slowly or not at all? Would the embolism have occurred if the patient was in bed rather that on the way home? In order to shed some light on the problem a review was carried out of the author's 8 years' work. The incidence of *fatal* pulmonary emboli was compared in two groups of patients: those undergoing primary operations and those having revision surgery. The first group of patients were mobilized at 2 days and often discharged home by 2 weeks. The second group remained in bed for up to 3 weeks before mobilization. The results are shown in Table 28.2. The results seem to suggest that early mobilization may in fact do the same to the clot. Immobility it may be claimed, increases the incidence of deep vein thrombosis but appears to reduce the number of fatal pulmonary emboli, and this is contrary to the time-honoured views.

Table 28.2. The incidence of fatal pulmonary embolism (PE) in primary LFA with early mobilization and revision surgery with delayed mobilization

	Primary LFAs	Revisions
No. of cases	1043	819
No. of fatal PE	4	1
% of fatal PE	0.38	0.12

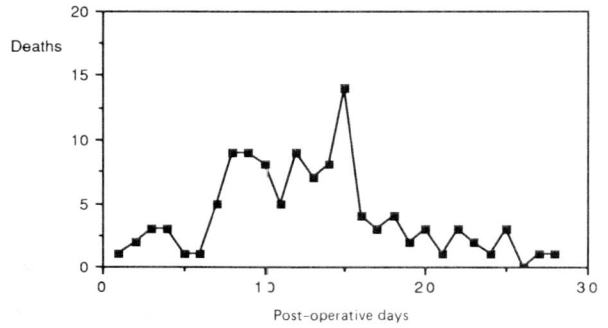

Fig. 28.3. The incidence of fatal pulmonary embolism in relation to the time of surgery. Note the gradual increase in the incidence in the first 2 weeks after surgery.

The Incidence of Fatal Pulmonary Emboli During the Post-operative Period

The incidence of fatal pulmonary emboli increases quite rapidly from the first to the fourteenth post-operative day then decreases very rapidly (Fig. 28.3). In contrast, the deaths from non-pulmonary emboli peak on the first post-operative day then decline gradually (Fig. 28.4). The two cross on the seventh day giving a third peak in the mortality figures.

Mortality Due to Causes Other than Pulmonary Embolism

It must be accepted that a fair proportion of patients undergoing total hip arthroplasty are somewhat older than average. Underlying medical conditions may therefore contribute to the morbidity and mortality associated with the operation.

Figures from a 17-year period of study during which 18 000 LFAs have been performed show quite clearly that mortality from causes other than pulmonary embolism is gradually being reduced (Fig. 28.5). Many explanations can be offered for this: possibly younger and fitter patients are being accepted for surgery; also, there may be better understanding of the post-operative complications.

A more extensive study of post-operative deaths is in progress. A vast amount of material is available extending beyond the twenty-eighth post-operative day, and the numerous parameters that may have a bearing on the results will take time to assess.

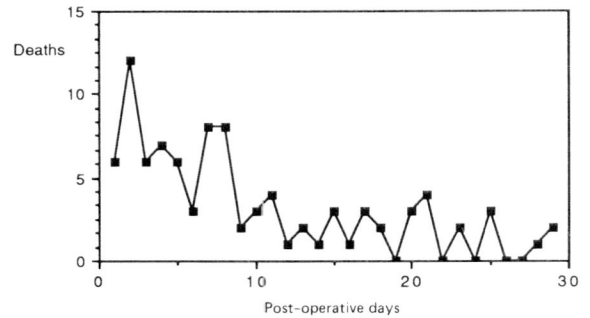

Fig. 28.4. Mortality from causes other than pulmonary embolism in relation to the time of the operation.

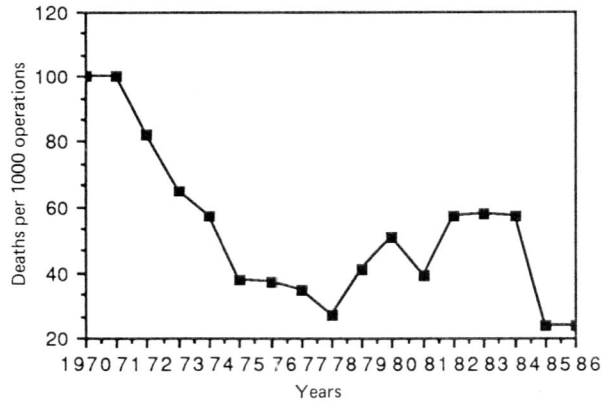

Fig. 28.5. Mortality from causes other than pulmonary embolism. Gradual decline in the incidence over the 17-year period.

Conclusions

29 Conclusions

Cemented total hip arthroplasty in general and the Charnley low-friction arthroplasty in particular have produced excellent clinical results over the past 26 years and much has been learned about these methods of treatment.

The operation marks the beginning of the treatment for a large proportion of patients. The surgeon and the system providing such care remain under obligation to provide aftercare in the form of follow-up, study of the results and further surgical interventions. Only when the materials, designs, surgical technique and the terminology are standardized can a meaningful discussion of the long-term results proceed and innovations be recommended logically.

Timely intervention will, at times, be indicated for radiographic appearances only and must be accepted before primary surgery if failures due to diminishing bone stock are to be avoided. The treatment of the arthritic hip must not be equated with soft-tissue surgery.

It is an understanding of the natural history of the arthritic hip, detailed study of results by methods other than purely clinical assessment, examination of the components ex vivo and the study of materials, patients' function and the "living/non-living" interface that are most likely to offer the best and the longest lasting results for an individual patient. If uniformly successful results cannot be achieved for all patients then at least predictability of the result for an individual patient should be aimed for.

Revision surgery can produce spectacular results, but the principles must not be forgotten in the excitement of a single clinical case. The method of treatment places ever-increasing demands on the surgeon and the system providing such care. This must be appreciated at every level and must not become a pawn of meddlesome manoeuvring.

References

Ainscow DAP, Denham RA (1984) The risk of haematogenous infection in total joint replacements. J Bone Joint Surg 66B:580–582

Allan DB, Dominguez-VA, Wroblewski BM (1990) Symptomatic socket loosening in Charnley low-friction arthroplasty. (in press)

Atkinson JR, Dowson D, Isaac GH, Wroblewski BM (1985a) Laboratory wear tests and clinical observations of the penetration of femoral heads into acetabular cups in total replacement hip joints. II. A microscopical study of the surfaces of Charnley polyethylene acetabular sockets. Wear 104:217–224

Atkinson JR, Dowson D, Isaac GH, Wroblewski BM (1985b) Laboratory wear tests and clinical observations of the penetration of femoral heads into acetabular cups in total replacement hip joints. Explanted Charnley sockets after 2–16 years in vivo and the determination of wear factors. Wear 104:225–244

Bernard AA, Brooks S (1987) The role of trochanteric wire revision after total hip replacement. J Bone Joint Surg 69B:352–354

Bisla RS, Ranawat CS, Inglis AE (1976) Total hip replacement in patients with ankylosing spondylitis with involvement of the hip. J Bohe Joint Surg 58A:233–238

Bonnin JG (1972) Editorials and annotations. Complications of arthroplasty of the hip. J Bone Joint Surg 54B:576–577

Brooker AF, Bowerman JW, Robinson RA, Riley LH (1973) Ectopic ossification following total hip replacement. J Bone Joint Surg 55A:1629–1632

Buchholz HW, Elson RA, Heinert K (1984) Antibiotic loaded acrylic cement: current concept. Clin Orthop 190:96–108

Charnley J (1960) Surgery of the hip joint. Present and future developments. Br Med J 1:821–826

Charnley J (1966) The healing of human fractures in contact with self-curing acrylic cement. Clin Orthop 47:157–163

Charnley J (1972) The long term results of low-friction arthroplasty of the hip performed as a primary intervention. J Bone Joint Surg 54B:61–76

Charnley J (1971) Operative technique of low-friction arthroplasty of the hip joint. Wrightington Hospital Internal Publication No. 6

Charnley J (1975) Fracture of the femoral prosthesis in total hip replacement. A clinical study. Clin Orthop 111:105–120

Charnley J (1979a) Long term results of low-friction arthroplasty of the hip. The hip. CV Mosby, St. Louis, Toronto, pp 42–49

Charnley J (1979b) Low-friction arthroplasty of the hip. Theory and practice. Springer, Berlin Heidelberg New York, p 84

Charnley J, Cupic Z (1973) The nine and ten year results of the low-friction arthroplasty of the hip. Clin Orthop 95: 9–25

Charnley J, Halley DK (1975) Rate of wear in total hip replacement. Clin Orthop 112:170–179

Charnley J, Ferreira A De SD (1964) Transplantation of the greater trochanter in arthroplasty of the hip. J Bone Joint Surg 46B:191–197

Charnley J, Kamanger A, Longfield MD (1969) The optimum size of prosthetic heads in relation to the wear of plastic sockets in total replacement of the hip. Med Biol Eng 7:31–39

Clegg J (1977) The results of the pseudarthrosis after removal of an infected total hip prosthesis. J Bone Joint Surg 59B:298–301

Coventry MB (1985) Late dislocations in patients with Charnley total hip arthroplasty. J Bone Joint Surg 67A:832–841

d'Aubigne RM, Postel M (1954) Functional results of hip arthroplasty with acrylic prosthesis. J Bone Joint Surg 36A:451–475

Debeyre J, Duliveux P (1954) Les arthroplasties de la hanche: étude critique a propos de 200 cas operes. Paris Editions Medicales Flammarion

DeLee J, Ferrari A, Charnley J (1976) Ectopic bone formation following low-friction arthroplasty of the hip. Clin Orthop 121:53–59

del Sel HJ, Charnley J (1979) Total hip replacement following infection in the opposite hip. Clin Orthop 141:138–142

del Sel HJ, Brittain G, Wroblewski BM (1981) Blood loss and operation time in the Charnley low-friction arthroplasty. Acta Orthop Scand 52:197–200

Dominguez VA, Allan DB, Wroblewski BM (1990) Heterotopic ossification after psoas tenotomy in Charnley low-friction arthroplasty (in press)

Dominguez VA, Allan DB, Wroblewski BM (1990) Predictability of success of one stage revision of infected cemented total hip arthroplasty (in press)

Dorr LD, Takei GK (1981) Review of total hip arthroplasties in patients 45 years or younger. (Read at the meeting of the American Academy of Orthopedic Surgeons. Las Vegas, Nevada, 2 March 1981)

Dupont JA, Charnley J (1972) Low-friction arthroplasty of the hip for the failures of previous surgery. J Bone Joint Surg 54B:77–87

Echeverri A, Shelley P, Wroblewski BM (1988) Long term result of hip arthroplasty for failure of previous surgery. J Bone Joint Surg 70B:49–51

Eftekhar NS (1984) Infection in joint replacement. Prevention and management. CV Mosby, St. Louis, Toronto

Etienne A, Cupic Z, Charnley J (1978) Post-operative dislocation after Charnley low-friction arthroplasty. Clin Orthop 132:19–23

Fahmy NRM, Wroblewski BM (1982) Reccurence of ectopic ossification after excision in Charnley low-friction arthroplasty. Acta Orthop Scand 53:799–802

Finerman GAM (1977) The role of diphosphonate in heterotopic ossification after total hip arthroplasty. J Bone Joint Surg 59B:501

Fowler JL, Gie GA, Lee AJC, Ling RSM (1988) Experience with the Exeter total hip replacement since 1970. Orthop Clin North Am 19:477–489

Fraser GA, Wroblewski BM (1981) Revision of the Charnley low-friction arthroplasty for recurrent or irreducible dislocation. J Bone Joint Surg 63B:552–555

Griffith MJ, Seidenstein MK, Williams D, Charnley J (1978) Socket wear in Charnley low-friction arthroplasty of the hip. Clin Orthop 137:37–47

Gruen TA, McNeice GM, Amstutz HC (1979) "Modes of failure" of cemented stem-type femoral components. A radiographic analysis of loosening. Clin Orthop 141:17–27

Hamblen DL, Harris WH, Rottger J (1971) Myositis ossificans as a complication of hip arthroplasty. J Bone Joint Surg 53B:764

Harris WH, White RE (1982) Socket fixation using a metal-backed acetabular component for total hip replacement. J Bone Joint Surg 64A:745–748

Hodgkinson JP, Shelley P, Wroblewski BM (1989a) Reattachment of the un-united trochanter in the Charnley low-friction arthroplasty. J Bone Joint Surg 71B(3):523–525

Hodgkinson JP, Shelley P, Wroblewski BM (1989b) The correlation between the roentgenographic appearances and operative findings at the bone–cement junction of the socket in Charnley low-friction arthroplasties. Clin Orthop 228:105–109

Isaac GH, Atkinson JR, Dowson D, Wroblewski BM (1986) The role of cement in the long term performance and premature failure of Charnley low-friction arthroplasties. Eng Med 15:19–22

Jensen NF, Harris WH (1986) A system of trochanteric osteotomy and reattachment for total hip arthroplasty with a ninety-nine per cent union rate. Clin Orthop 208:174–181

Johnson R, Loudon JR (1986) Hydroxychloroquine sulphate prophylaxis for pulmonary embolism for patients with low-friction arthroplasty. Clin Orthop 211:151–153

Jones JM (1979) Revisional total hip replacement for failed Ring arthroplasty. J Bone Joint Surg 61A:1029–1034

Josefsson G, Lindberg L, Wiklander B (1981) Systemic antibiotics and gentamicin-containing bone cement in prophylaxis of post-operative infections in total hip arthroplasty. Clin Orthop 159:194–200

Khan MAA, O'Driscoll M (1977) Fractures of the femur during total hip replacement and their management. J Bone Joint Surg 59B:36–41

Khan MAA, Brakenbury PH, Reynolds ISR (1981) Dislocation following total hip replacement. J Bone Joint Surg 63B:214–218

Lazansky MG (1973) Complications revisited: the debit side of total hip replacement. Clin Orthop 95:96–103

Lidwell OM, Lowbury EJL, Whyte W, Blowers R, Stanley SJ, Lowe D (1982) Effect of ultraclean air in operating rooms on deep sepsis in the joint after total hip and knee replacement: a randomised study. Br Med J 285:10–14

Loudon JR, Charnley J Sir (1980) Subsidence of the femoral prosthesis in total hip replacement in relation to the design of the stem. J Bone Joint Surg 62B:450–453

Lynch M, Esser MP, Shelley P, Wroblewski BM (1987) Deep infection in Charnley low-friction arthroplasty. J Bone Joint Surg 69B:355–360

Menon TJ, Wroblewski BM (1983) Charnley low-friction arthroplasty in patients with psoriasis. Clin Orthop 176:127–128

Menon TJ, Thjellesen D, Wroblewski BM (1983) Charnley low-friction arthroplasty in diabetic patients. J Bone Joint Surg 65B:580–581

McLeish RD (1977) Some aspects of forces in the human lower limb. PhD Thesis. Victoria University of Manchester

Nutton RW, Checketts RG (1984) The effects of trochanteric osteotomy on abductor power. J Bone Joint Surg 66B:180–183

Olerud S, Karlstrom G (1984) Hip arthroplasty with an extended femoral stem for salvage procedures. Clin Orthop 181:64–81

Olerud S, Karlstrom G (1985) Recurrent dislocation after total hip replacement. (Treatment by fixing an additional sector to the acetabular component.) J Bone Joint Surg 67B:402–405

Pacheco V, Shelley P, Wroblewski BM (1988) Mechanical loosening of the stem in Charnley arthroplasties. J Bone Joint Surg 70B:596–599

Patterson FP, Brown CS (1972) The McKee–Farrar total hip replacement. J Bone Joint Surg 54A:257–275

Redfern T, Wroblewski BM (1990) Failure of healing of the abductor muscles following hip arthroplasty (in press)

Reigler HF, Harris CM (1976) Heterotopic bone formation after total hip arthroplasty. J Bone Joint Surg 58A:284

Ring PA (1968) Complete replacement arthroplasty of the hip by the Ring prosthesis. J Bone Joint Surg 50B:720–731

Ritter MA, Vaughan RB (1977) Ectopic ossification after total hip arthroplasty. J Bone Joint Surg 59A:345–351

Rose RM, Nusbaum HJ, Schneider H et al. (1980) On the true wear rate of ultra-high-molecular-weight polyethylene in total hip prosthesis. J Bone Joint Surg 62A:537–549

Stauffer RN (1982) Ten year follow-up study of total hip replacement. With particular reference to Roentgenographic loosening of the components. J Bone Joint Surg 64A:983–990

Taylor AR, Kamdar BA, Arden GP (1976) Ectopic ossification following total hip replacement. J Bone Joint Surg 58B:134

Taylor TKF (1966) The place of the girdlestone pseudarthrosis in the treatment of hip disorders. J Bone Joint Surg 48A:1227–1228

Van Niekerk A, Charnley J Sir (1979) Post-operative infection after Charnley low-friction arthroplasty of the hip. J Bone Joint Surg 61B:252–253

Vernon-Roberts B, Freeman MAR (1977) The tissue response to total joint replacement prostheses. In: Swanson SAV, Freeman MAR (eds) The scientific basis of joint replacement. Pitman Medical, Tunbridge Wells pp 86–129

Volz RG, Brown FW (1977) The painful migrated un-united greater trochanter in total hip replacement. J Bone Joint Surg 59A:1091–1093

Walenkamp GHIM (1983) Gentamicin PMMA beads. A clinical, pharmacokinetic and toxicological study. Drukkerij Cliteur, Amsterdam

Weber BG, Stuhmer G (1979) Improvements in total hip prosthesis implementation technique; a cement-proof seal for the lower medullary cavity and a dihedral self-stabilizing trochanteric osteotomy. Arch Orthop Trauma Surg 93:185–189

Wiesman HS, Simon SR, Edward FC, Thomas WH, Sledge CB (1978) Total hip replacement with and without osteotomy of the greater trochanter. J Bone Joint Surg 60A:203–210

Willert HHG, Semlitsch M (1976) Reaction of the articular capsule to artificial joint prosthesis. In: Williams D (ed) Biocompatibility of implant materials. Pitman Medical, Tunbridge Wells, pp 40–48

Wilson PD, Amstutz HC, Czarniecki A, Salvati EA, Mendes DG (1972) Total hip replacement with fixation by acrylic cement. J Bone Joint Surg 54A:207–236

Woo RYG, Morrey BF (1982) Dislocations after total hip arthroplasty. J Bone Joint Surg 64A:1295–1306

Wroblewski BM (1977) Leaching out from acrylic bone cement. Experimental evaluation. Clin Orthop 124:311–312

Wroblewski BM (1979) Wear of high-density polyethylene on bone and cartilage. J Bone Joint Surg 61B:498–500

Wroblewski BM (1980) Revision of infected hip arthroplasty. In: Altemeier WA (ed) 2nd World Congress – Antisepsis. HP Publishing, New York, pp 97–98

Wroblewski BM (1982a) Revision surgery in total hip arthroplasty. Surgical technique and results. Clin Orthop 170:56–61

Wroblewski BM (1982b) Fractured stem in total hip replacement. A clinical review of 120 cases. Acta Orthop Scand 53:279–284

Wroblewski BM (1983) Revision of infected hip arthroplasty. J Bone Joint Surg 65B:224–225

Wroblewski BM (1984a) Girdlestone pseudarthrosis following deep sepsis in total hip arthroplasty. In: Eftekhar NS (ed) Infection in joint replacement. Prevention and management. CV Mosby, St. Louis, Toronto, pp 345–362

Wroblewski BM (1984b) The sources of infection in revision arthroplasty.2. Franklin Scientific Publications, London, pp 44–45

Wrosblewski BM (1985a) Charnley low-friction arthroplasty in patients under the age of 40 years. In: Sevastik J, Goldie I (eds) The young patient with degenerative hip disease. Almquist & Wiksell, Stockholm, pp 197–201

Wroblewski BM (1985b) Direction and rate of socket wear in Charnley low-friction arthroplasty. J Bone Joint Surg 67B:757–761

Wroblewski BM (1986a) 15–21 year results of the Charnley low-friction arthroplasty. Clin Orthop 211:30–35

Wroblewski BM (1986b) One-stage revision of infected cemented total hip arthroplasty. Clin Orthop 211:103–107

Wroblewski BM (1987) Wear and loosening of the socket in Charnley low-friction arthroplasty. In: Draenert K, Rutt A (eds) Current status of the art: interface histomorph. Bone and Joints 4. Munich Art and Science

Wroblewski BM, Charnley J (1982) Radiographic morphology of the osteoarthritic hip. J Bone Joint Surg 64B:568–569

Wroblewski BM, del Sel HJ (1980) Urethral instrumentation and deep sepsis in total hip replacement. Clin Orthop 146:209–212

Wroblewski BM, Shelley P (1985) Reattachment of the greater trochanter after hip replacement. J Bone Joint Surg 67B:736–740

Wroblewski BM, van der Rijt AJ (1984) Intramedullary cancellous bone block to improve femoral stem fixation in Charnley low-friction arthroplasty. J Bone Joint Surg 66B:639–644

Wroblewski BM, Esser M, Srigley DW (1986) Release of gentamicin from bone–cement. Acta Orthop Scand 57:413–414

Subject Index

Abductor integrity 18
Abductor mass 181
Abductor mechanism, loss of 32
Abductor muscle-mass fascia 26
Abductors 209
Acetabular cavity, exposure and
    examination 189
Acetabular defects
  central 202–5
  superior 203
Acetabular reinforcement ring 204
Acetabular retractor 14
Acetabular rim disruption 203
Acetabulum
  anatomical 35
  anterversion 36
  exposure of 14
  high 35
  low 35
  preparation 189–90
  replacement 175
Acrylic cement 1, 87, 88, 109, 139
    (See also Antibiotic-loaded
      acrylic cement (ALAC)
  antibiotic release from 61
  comparison with ALAC 51
  leaching out from 50
  plain 58
  removal of 193–6
Adjustable Trial Prosthesis (ATP) 22
Allografts 201
Anaesthesia in relation to bleeding
    8–9
Anaesthetic assessment 168
Angle-bore socket 43
Anteversion wire marker 36
Antibiotic-loaded acrylic beads 61
Antibiotic-loaded acrylic cement
    (ALAC) 59–51, 57–8, 60
  comparison with plain acrylic
    cement 51

Antibiotics 57, 58, 60, 219
Anti-coagulants 221, 222
Antiseptics 57
Arthritic hip assessment 163–4
Arthritis 77
Arthrography 166
Aseptic loosening 4
Aspiration 166–7
ATP 24

Bed rest 58
Betadine 57
Bleeding areas 7
Bone-cement interface 71–9, 85, 107
Bone-cement junction 84, 86, 101
    removal of fibrous or pyogenic
      granulation tissue 196
Bone grafting 202
Bone stock
  loss of 201–6
  quality 4, 175

Calcar 69, 196
Cancellous bone 65
  in heterotopic ossification 147–8
  removal of 196
Capsule 209
Capsule excision 39
Catheterization 49
Cement anchoring pegs and
    extrusions, extraction of 189
Cement-bone interface. See Bone-
    cement interface
Cement extractor 174
Cement-free bony ingrowth designs
    1
Cement ingress into socket 96
Cement removal 173
Cephradine 57

Charnley acetabular cement restrictor
    189
Charnley acetabular reamers 189
Charnley east-west (E–W) retractor
    187
Charnley gouges 189
Charnley low-friction arthroplasty
    1–2, 20, 27, 29, 74, 76, 81, 83,
    84, 87, 90, 96, 109, 112, 125,
    146, 175, 227
Charnley north-south retractor 14
Charnley pin retractor 14, 187
Charnley retractor 142
Charnley stainless steel stem 44
Charnley wire holding forceps 182
Cholecystectomy forceps 184
Claw hammer method 183
Clean air enclosure 47
Cloacae in femoral shaft 53
Component examination 186–9
Component fixation, requirements
    for 65
Component loosening 63–70
  containment and pressurization of
      cement 65–6
  definition 62
  femoral side 67–70
  radiography in 65
  stem design in 67
  study and management of 62
Component malorientation 35–41
Component selection 175–7
Components 1
Compression fixation of greater
    trochanter 44
Congenital dysplasia 33, 34

Deep fascia 209
Diabetics 49
Dislocation 28, 29–46, 156, 185

by distraction 31
by impingement 30–1
early 37
early irreducible 37
following primary surgery 31–41
following revision 29, 40–1
incidence of post-operative 41
incidence of revision for 39
late 39
management 29
management and prevention of
    post-operative 43
mechanism of 30–1
non-operative methods 41–2
operative procedures 42–6
persistent 39
recurrent 39, 42
Distal cement plug removal 173–4
Distal femoral cement, demarcation
    of 113
Distraction, dislocation by 31
Drains 210–11
Dual-purpose wire cutter-pullers 182,
    183

Ectopic ossification 150, 151
Endosteal cavitation 53, 68, 113, 123,
    129, 196
Exposure problems 11–18
Exposure requirements 11–18
Extended neck prosthesis 40
Extended neck stems 44–5, 177

Fatique fracture wave 133, 134
Fatique limit 127–8
Femoral cement extraction
    distal part 195
    middle part 194–5
    proximal part 194
Femoral cement fracture 129
    at tip of stem 113
Femoral cement restrictors 195–6
Femoral components
    extraction of 193
    revision surgery 176–7
Femoral cortex, endosteal cavitation
    of 113
Femoral defects 205–6
    major deficiencies 205–6
    minor deficiencies 205
Femoral head protector 172
Femoral shaft fracture 139–43
    associated with stem loosening 139
    distal to implant 139
Femur 193–9, 209
Fixation requirements 1–2
Follow-up
    problems to be anticipated at 155–9
    requirements 1–2
Fractured stems presented for
    revision surgery 21

Gentamicin 50, 60
    clinical use of beads 61

concentration remaining in acrylic
    cement 51
    release from acrylic cement 50–1
Gigli saw 182, 183, 184
Girdlestone pseudarthrosis 217–19
Gluteus maximus 181
Greater trochanter 181, 209
    compression fixation of 44
    reattachment 198–9
    reattachment when stem has not
        been changed 199

Haematoma 7–10
    classification of 9–10
    deep 10, 41
    infected 10
    management of 7
    superficial 8–9
Head-neck ratio 44
Heterotopic ossification 145–51
    cancellous bone in 147–8
    cause of 147
    definition 145–6
    excision 148–51
    extent of 147
    incidence of 146
    planimetric study of 150
    site of 147
High-density polyethylene (HDP) 1
    restrictor 103
    socket 43, 76, 86–8, 105
    wear particles 101
Hip joint exposure 183–90
Hohman retractor 8
Hypertrophic-type arthritis 151

Impingement
    dislocation by 30–1
    in socket wear 92
Implant-bone interface 202
Implant pivoting within bone 120
Implant pivoting within cement 120
Implant responses 2
Incision 180–1
    deep fascia 181
Infection 47–61
    classification of 53–5
    deep 47
        bone-cement junction type 53
        conservative management 55
        diabetics 49
        diagnosis of 51–3
        following previous hip surgery
            49–50
        incidence of 48
        length of follow-up 48
        males with post-operative urinary
            retention, catheterization and
            prostatectomy 49
        management of 55–61
        one-stage revision 56–8
        operative management 56
        osteitis-osteomyelitis type 53
        patients at risk 49, 155–6
        patients with psoriasis 49
        prevention of 49–50

results of revisions for 58
revisions using ALAC 50
revisions using plain acrylic
    cement 50
size of sample studied 48
two-stage revision 61
late 53–5
superficial 53
Instrumentation 169–74
Intramedullary bone block 112

Kuntscher nail 16, 139, 143

Lesser trochanter, excavation of
    196–7
Lignocaine 27
Limb shortening 32–5
Limp 27–8
Local examination 165
Loosening of components. See
    Component loosening
Lotus hip 45–6

Medullary canal 109
    distal closure 198–9
    exposure of 16–18
    position of stem within 115
    stem-cement complex slip within
        119–20
    stem position within 130
Metal-backed acetabular components
    105, 107
Metal-backed socket 105
Mobilization of proximal part of
    femur 185
Modular stem system 206
Morbidity and mortality 224
Mortality from causes other than
    pulmonary embolism 224
Muscle ischaemia 145
Muscle tone loss 39

Natural history of hip condition 77–9
Neck of the stem 181–2
Neck stem
    mechanical testing 97
    reduced diameter 96–7

Ortron wire mesh 176
Osteoarthritis 48
    deep sepsis in 48

Pain distribution 163–4
Pain in failed total hip arthroplasty
    164–5
Patient assessment for revision
    surgery 163
Patient discussion in revision
    surgery 167–8
Periosteal stripping 147, 148
Positioning the patient 179–80
Post-operative management 213

pseudarthrosis 219
Post-operative urinary retention 49
Press-fit socket 105
Prostatectomy 49
Proximal femur
  absence of 41
  mobilization of 172
Proximal support, lack or loss of
  122–3
Pseudarthrosis 217–19
  clinical results 219
  examples of 218
  indications for 217–19
  operative procedure 219
  post-operative management 219
Psoriasis 49
Pulmonary embolism 221–4
  fatal 224
  incidence variations 223–4
  mortality due to causes other
    than 224
  prediction 221
  prevention 221–2
  reviews of trends 222–4
  treatment 222

Radiography
  in component loosening 65
  correlation with long-term clinical
    results 74–5
  correlation with operative findings
    73
  in diagnosis of deep infection 52–3
  revision surgery 169
  socket wear 89–90
  stem-fixation failure 117
  stem fracture 129–31
  stem loosening 112
Radiolucent cement 166
Research Fellow in Revision Surgery
  4
Revision surgery 4
  correlation between radiological
    appearances and clinical
    function 160–71
  need for 155
  outcomes of delay 160
  patient assessment for 163
  patient discussion in 167–8
  radiography 169
  technique 179–90
  timing of 155–61
Rheumatoid arthritis 48
  deep sepsis in 48

Sardine-can method 183
Scanning techniques 166
Sedation 8–9
Sinograms 166
Skin closure 210
Socket anteversion/retroversion 35–7
Socket demarcation 71–2, 77, 159
Socket demarcation and loosening
  75–9
Socket examination 187
Socket exposure 187

testing and extraction 173
Socket extraction 188–9
Socket failure 71–9
Socket fixation 65–6, 79, 189–90
Socket loosening 81–6, 89, 101, 159
  basic mechanism of 81
  correlation between clinical,
    radiological and operative
    findings 83–6
  long-term 77
  study and management of 81
  testing for 188
  time lag between primary and
    revision surgery 81–3
Socket migration 72, 87, 90, 101
  and socket wear 74
Socket penetration 87
Socket rim, stabilizer attachment to
  44
Socket wear 39, 76–7, 87–97
  and socket migration 74
  angular movements in relation to
    96
  correlation between real and
    radiographic measurements 91
  direction of impingement with 79
  direction of wear 92
  explanted sockets 91–6
  impingement in 92
  mechanical and histological changes
    resulting from 86
  mechanical effects of 101
  radiographic measurement 89–90
Sound component fixation 58, 201
Special investigations 165
Stabilizer attachment to socket rim 44
Stainless steel 97, 127, 128
Staphylococcus 58, 60
Stem, reduced diameter neck 44
Stem-cement complex
  fracture of shaft of femur involving
    143
  pivoting of 121
  slip within medullary canal 119–20
  tilt of 120
Stem-cement separation 113
Stem corrosion 127
Stem design 109, 135
  in component loosening 67
Stem extraction 186–7
Stem fixation 109
  early radiographic signs of failure
    129–30
  failure patterns 117–21
  radiological appearances of failure
    of 117
  sequelae of failure 122
  within medullary canal 37
Stem fracture 125–38, 156
  bending of proximal fragment prior
    to 133–4
  clinical implications 137
  comparison of cases from two
    sources 131
  curved banana stem 135
  experimental confirmation of
    mechanism 137
  extractor kit 174

flat-back 127, 131
following revision surgery 135–8
fracture lip 134–5
level of fracture 135
mechanism 137
mechanism in total hip
  arthroplasty 131–5
mechanism of failure 136
obliquity of 131–2
patients' function 127
patients' weight and time to
  fracture 127–8
radiographic appearances 129–31
recent developments 138
salient features of 125
stages of 132
surgical technique 129
time to failure 127
time to revision 127
uncemented metal-to-metal
  arthroplasty 138
Stem insertion 198–9
Stem loosening 109–23, 158–9
  associated with femoral shaft
    fracture 139
  effect of previous operation 115
  Pacheco study 112–15
  problem of limited exposure 116
  radiography 112
  testing for 186
  time interval from primary to
    revision surgery 116–17
Stem position 186
  within medullary canal 115, 130
Stem removal 172
Stem selection and trial reduction
  197–8
Stem slip within cement mantle 119
Stem tilt 120
Straight leg raising 165
Subcutaneous fat 210
Subluxation, episodes of 39
Supero-lateral cavitation 76
Support and reinforcement rings 204
Surgical technique 1, 2, 179–90
  landmarks in 181–2
  layer-by-layer approach 209
  preparation 179
  pseudarthrosis 219
  socket demarcation and loosening
    75–6
  stem fracture 129

Tear drop 14, 20, 32–4
Teflon 87, 88, 217
  sockets 86, 87
  wear particles 99–101
Tight hip reduction 37
Tissue reaction to high-density
  polyethylene wear particles
  99–107
Tissue turgor loss 40
Total body exhaust suits 47
Total hip arthroplasty, failure of 164
Total hip components 209
Transverse reaming 32
Trochanteric bursa 183

Trochanteric bursitis 26
Trochanteric non-union 27, 28, 32,
      191–92
   double cross-over wire and
      compression spring fixation
      191
   examples of revision with 192
   with trochanteric migration 186
   without trochanteric migration 185
Trochanteric osteotomy 19–28, 30,

      37, 172, 181, 183
   as method of exposure 22–4
   blood loss and operating time 24–6
   controversy surrounding 22
   problems related to 24–8
Trochanteric pain 26, 27
Trochanteric reattachment 21
Trochanteric wires, removal of 172,
      182–3

Uncemented metal-to-metal
      arthroplasty, stem fracture 138

Vastus group of muscles 209

Wear debris 72
Wound closure 209–11